SMOKING AND HEALTH

A Comprehensive Bibliography

BIOMEDICAL INFORMATION GUIDES

Compiled by Alberta D. Berton
Medical Documentation Service, Philadelphia, Pennsylvania

Volume 1 ASBESTOSIS: A Comprehensive Bibliography

Volume 2 NUCLEAR MEDICINE: A Comprehensive Bibliography

Volume 3 SMOKING AND HEALTH: A Comprehensive Bibliography

Published in conjunction with Medical Documentation Service

SMOKING AND HEALTH

A Comprehensive Bibliography

Compiled by

ALBERTA D. BERTON

Assisted by

K. BERNICE ODOM

Medical Documentation Service
Philadelphia, Pennsylvania

Springer Science+Business Media, LLC

Library of Congress Cataloging in Publication Data

Berton, Alberta D 1916-
Smoking and health.

(Biomedical information guides; v. 3)
"Published in conjunction with the Medical Documentation Service... Philadelphia."
1. Tobacco–Toxicology–Bibliography. 2. Tobacco–Physiological effect–Bibliography. 3. Smoking–Bibliography. I. College of Physicians of Philadelphia. Library. Medical Documentation Service. II. Title. III. Series.
Z7882.B47 [RA1242.T6] 016.6138'5 80-25736

ISBN 978-1-4684-8865-4 ISBN 978-1-4684-8863-0 (eBook)
DOI 10.1007/978-1-4684-8863-0

Originally published by IFI/Plenum Data Company in 1980

INTRODUCTION

The objective of this series is to provide medical researchers and libraries with single sources to scattered research results in selected disciplinary and interdisciplinary fields. The topics for these books have been chosen for their timeliness to current research requirements. The literature searches to compile these books have been as extensive as possible for the years covered for each book. We plan to offer updated supplements to various volumes as the research in these fields accumulates and based on users' continued interest in the subject matter.

This major contribution to the medical literature has been made possible through the efforts of the Medical Documentation Service staff and the dedicated work of Mrs. K. Bernice Odom, who set the standards for bibliographic reporting and who spent long hours in copy-editing.

ALBERTA D. BERTON

Director
Medical Documentation Service
College of Physicians of Philadelphia

Aaberg, G. and Kopp, U.

Haemodynamic effects of the quarternary ammonium compound QX 572 in anaesthetized cats. II. Studies on the mechanism for the cardiac chronotropic effects.

Acta Pharmacol. Toxicol. (Kbh.) 44(2): 95-98, Feb. 1979.

Abanobi, S. E., et al.

Persistence of DNA damage during development of liver angiosarcoma in rats fed dimethylnitrosamine.

Cancer Res. 39(5):1592-1596, May 1979.

Abbatucci, J.-S.

Prevention en cancerologie: Responsabilities et methodes - perspectives en France. (Fr.)

Concours Med. 101(25):4229-4240, June 23, 1979.

Abdel, M. T., et al.

Urinary catecholamines in habitual smokers and non-smokers.

Acta Physiol. Acad. Sci. Hung. 52(4): 429-433, 1978.

Abdulla, M. and Svensson, S.

Nutrition of Old Age: Chromium and nickel.

Scand. J. Gastroenterol. 14(Suppl. 52): 176-180, 1979.

Abe, Y.

Measurement of estrogen receptor in relation to the prediction of hormone dependency in 7,12-dimethylbenz (a)-anthracene-induced rat breast cancer and in human breast cancer. (Jpn.)

Fukuoka Acta Med. 69(9):400-413, Sept. 1978.

Abelin, Th.

'Rauchen im Uebermass'. 'La fumee du tabac en dose exageree.' (Editorial) (Ger., Fr.)

Soz. Praventivmed. 22(4):153-154, July-Aug. 1977.

Abelin, Th., et al.

Das Fortschungsprogramm des Instituts fuer Sozial-und Praeventivmedizin der Universitaet Bern. (Ger.)

Soz. Praeventivmed. 24(4):236-239, Aug. 1979.

Abood, L. G., et al.

Electrophysiological, behavioral, and chemical evidence for a noncholinergic, stereospecific site for nicotine in rat brain.

J. Neurosci. Res. 3(5-6):327-333, 1978.

Abood, L. G., et al.

Evidence for a noncholinergic site for nicotine's action in brain: Psychopharmacological, electrophysiological and receptor binding studies.

Arch. Int. Pharmacodyn. Ther. 237(2):213-229, Feb. 1979.

Abramowicz, M. (Editor)

Aids for patients who want to stop smoking.

Med. Lett. Drugs. Ther. 20(24):107-108, Dec. 1, 1978.

Abramowicz, M. (Editor), et al.

Update: Drugs in breast milk.

Med. Lett. Drugs Ther. 21(5):21-24, Mar. 9, 1979.

Abramowicz, M., (Editor)

Toxic reactions to plant products sold in health food stores.

Med. Lett. Drugs Ther. 21(7):29-32, Apr. 6, 1979.

Abramson, E. E. and Seguest, R. C.

Predicting success in a smoking control program.

Int. J. Addict. 13(6):1009-1012, 1978.

Abramson, J. H., et al.

A case-control study of Hodgkin's disease in Israel.

JNCI 61(2):307-314, Aug. 1978.

Aceto, M. D., et al.

Optically pure (plus)-nicotine from (plus/minus)-nicotine and biological comparison with (minus)-nicotine.

J. Med. Chem. 22(2):174-177, Feb. 1979.

Adachi, K.-I. and Ishii, Y.

Vocalization response to close-arterial injection of bradykinin and other algesic agents in guinea pigs and its application to quantitative assessment of analgesic agents.

J. Pharmacol. Exp. Ther. 209(1):117-124, Apr. 1979.

Adams, W. G.

Survey of tobacco and alcohol use among undergraduates.

Med. J. Aust. 2(3):160, Aug. 11, 1979.

Adamsson, E., et al.

Pulmonary and gastrointestinal exposure to cadmium oxide dust in a battery factor.

Environ. Health Perspect. 28:219-222, Feb. 1979.

Adelstein, A. M.

Current vital statistics: Methods and interpretation.

Br. Med. J. 2(6143):983-987, Oct. 7, 1978.

Adesso, V. J. and Glad, W. R.

A behavioral test of a smoking typology.

Addict. Behav. 3(1):35-38, 1978.

Adir, J., et al.

Effect of ethanol pretreatment on the pharmacokinetics of nicotine in rats.

J. Pharmacol. Exp. Ther. 212(2):274-279, Feb. 1980.

Afanasiev, I. V. and Ivanovsky, V. B.

Smoking and tuberculosis. (Russ.)

Probl. Tuberk. (4):45-48, 1979.

Agrelo, C. E. and Schoental, R.

Synthesis of DNA in human fibroblasts treated with T-2 toxin and HT-2 toxin (the trichothecene metabolites of Fusarium species) and the effects of hydroxyurea.

Toxicol. Lett. 5(2):155-160, Feb. 1980.

Ahmed, Z. and Abuhay, M.

The prevalence of cigarette-smoking among secondary school children in Gondar City, Ethiopia.

Ethiop. Med. J. 17(2):41-46, Apr. 1979.

Aho, W. R.

Smoking, dieting, and exercise: Age differences in attitudes and behavior relevant to selected health belief model variables.

RI Med. J. 62(3):85-92, Mar. 1979.

Ahokas, J. T., et al.

The in vitro metabolism and covalent binding of benzo[a]pyrene to DNA catalysed by trout liver microsomes.

Chem. Biol. Interact. 25(1):103-111, Apr. 1979.

Aitio, A. and Parkki, M.

Effect of phthalate esters on drug metabolizing enzyme activities in rat liver.

Arch. Int. Pharmacodyn. Ther. 235(2):187-195, Oct. 1978.

Aitio, M. L. and Aitio, A.

Induction of disopyramide N-dealkylation by phenobarbital and disopyramide in rat liver.

Arch. Int. Pharmacodyn. Ther. 239(1):16-23, May 1979.

Akasu, T., et al.

Roles of electrogenic Naplus pump and Kplus conductance in the slow inhibitory postsynaptic potential of bullfrog sympathetic ganglion cells.

Life Sci. 23(24):2405-2410, Dec. 11, 1978.

Akiyama, H.

Surgery for carcinoma of the esophagus.

Curr. Probl. Surg. 17(2):55-120, Feb. 1980.

Akkermann, S., et al.

Ein Katalog von Risikofaktoren und seine Verwendungsmoeglichkeiten bei der Prophylaxe von Fruehgeburten. (Ger.)

Dtsch. Gesundheitswes. 33(9):413-417, 1978.

Al-Nuaimi, N., et al.

Purification of the cytoplasmic oestrogen receptor from mammary tumours induced in rats with dimethylbenzanthracene.

J. Endocrinol. 81(1):119-130, Apr. 1979.

Al-Saleem, T., et al.

Smoking behaviour among medical students in the University of Baghdad.

J. Fac. Med. Baghdad 20(1):4-9, Apr. 1978.

Alaily, A. B. and Carrol, K. B.

Pulmonary ventilation in pregnancy.

Br. J. Obstet. Gynaecol. 85(7):518-524, July 1978.

Alarie, Y. C. and Anderson, R. C.

Toxicologic and acute lethal hazard evaluation of thermal decomposition products of synthetic and natural polymers.

Toxicol. Appl. Pharmacol. 51(2): 341-362, Nov. 1979.

Albert, R. E., et al.

Identification of occupational settings with very high risks of lung cancer. (Letter to the Editor and Reply.)

JNCI 63(6):1289-1290, Dec. 1979.

Albertson, P.

Therapeutic potential for marijuana and its derivatives.

Med. Trib. 20(12):16-21, Mar. 28, 1979.

Alderman, M. H.

Communities with unusually short life-spans: The effects of life-style modification.

Bull. NY Acad. Med. 55(3):357-366, Mar. 1979.

Alexander, Jr., J. C., et al.

Proceedings of the International Conference on the Clinical Uses of Carcinoembryonic Antigen: CEA levels in patients with carcinoma of the esophagus.

Cancer 42(3, Suppl.):1492-1497, Sept. 1978.

Aliperta, A., et al.

Aspect histopathologique de l'inflammation bronchique chez des fumeurs exposes a l'action d'autres facteurs nocifs d'origine exogene. (Fr.)

Bronchopneumologie 28(3):205-213, May-June 1978.

Althouse, R., et al.

An evaluation of chemicals and industrial processes associated with cancer in humans based on human and animal data: IARC monographs volumes 1 to 20.

Cancer Res. 40(1):1-12, Jan. 1980.

Altland, P. D., et al.

Effects of nicotine and carbon monoxide on tissue and systemic changes in rats.

Environ. Res. 19(1):202-212, June 1979.

Altose, M. D.

The physiological basis of pulmonary function testing.

Clin. Symp. 31(2):3-39 1979.

Alvares, A. P.

Interactions between environmental chemicals and drug biotransformation in man.

Clin. Pharmacokinet. 3(6):452-477, Nov.-Dec. 1978.

Alvares, A. P., et al.

Drug Disposition in Man: Regulation of drug metabolism in man by environmental factors.

Drug Metab. Rev. 9(2):185-205, 1979.

Alvares, A. P., et al.

Intraindividual variation in drug disposition.

Clin. Pharmacol. Ther. 26(4):407-419, Oct. 1979.

Amery, A., et al.

Aging and the cardiovascular system.

Acta Cardiol. (Brux.) 33(6):443-467, 1978.

Ames, B. N.

Identifying environmental chemicals causing mutations and cancer.

Science 204(4393):587-593, May 11, 1979.

Amicarella, G., et al.

Studio clinico-statistico delle neoplasie polmonari primitive nei soggetti di eta inferiore ai 40 anni. (Ital.)

Policlinico (Sez. Med.) 85(6):403-410, Nov.-Dec. 1978.

Ammann, R., et al.

Extrapankreatische und Pankreas-karzinome bei chronischer Pankreatitis. (Abstr.) (Ger.)

Z. Gastroenterol. 17(9):576-577, Sept. 1979.

Amure, B. O.

Nicotine and the decay of the McCollough effect.

Vision Res. 18(10):1449-1451, 1978.

Anderes, C., et al.

Postoperative spontaneous breathing with CPAP to normalize late post-operative oxygenation.

Intensive Care Med. 5(1):15-21, Mar. 1979.

Anderson, A. J., et al.

Workshop on Carbon Monoxide and Cardiovascular Disease: Occlusive coronary artery disease and parental history of myocardial infarction.

Prev. Med. 8(3):419-428, May 1979.

Anderson, D. and Styles, J. A.

Appendix II: The bacterial mutation test.

Br. J. Cancer 37(6):924-930, June 1978.

Anderson, D. E.

Newer aspects of therapy for obstructive pulmonary disease.

Rocky Mt. Med. J. 76(2):72-78, Mar.-Apr. 1979.

Anderson, G. D.

Nutrition in pregnancy - 1978.

South. Med. J. 72(10):1304-1314, Oct. 1979.

Anderson, H. R.

Chronic lung disease in the Papua New Guinea Highlands.

Thorax 34(5):647-653, Oct. 1979.

Anderson, L. M., et al.

Lung tumorigenesis in mice after chronic exposure in early life to a low dose of demethylnitrosamine.

JNCI 62(6):1553-1555, June 1979.

Andrews, A. W., et al.

The relationship between mutagenicity and carcinogenicity of some nitrosamines.

Mutat. Res. 51(3):319-326, Sept. 1978.

Angelo, M. M.

Hypertension: A review.

J. Kuwait Med. Assoc. 13(1):39-50, Mar. 1979.

Anichkov, S. V. and Losev, N. A.

The relationship of structure and pharmacological action of some cholinolytics.

Gen. Pharmacol. 11(1):31-32, 1980.

Anonymous.

Memory loss can serve to spook heavy cigaret smokers.

Oncol. Times 2(2):6, Feb. 1980.

Anonymous.

Savukkeiden terva, haekae ja nikotiini. (Finn.)

Suom. Laeaekaeril. 33(7):482, Mar. 1, 1978.

Anonymous.

Breathing other people's smoke.

Br. Med. J. 2(6135):453-454, Aug. 12, 1978.

Anonymous.

Any Questions? Can nicotine be found in the blood of non-smokers after using the cigarette-making machine to make, say 40 cigarettes, as this would include firmly pressing down two ounces (56.7g) of moist tobacco with the pulp of the fingers?

Br. Med. J. 2(6134):420, Aug. 5, 1978.

Anonymous.

Il fumo di sigaretta causa di menopausa precoce?

Minerva Ginecol. 30(6):VII June 1978.

Anonymous.

Public Education about Cancer: Adult use of tobacco - 1975.

UICC Tech. Rep. Ser. 26:8-27, 1977.

Anonymous.

WHO attacks member states soft on smokers.

Asian Med. J. 21(8):60, Aug. 1978.

Anonymous.

Public Education about Cancer: 1976 Gallup survey results on smoking habits in Norway.

UICC Tech. Rep. Ser. 26:6-7, 1977.

Anonymous.

Vitamin C und Zigarettenkonsum. (Ger.)

Med. Monatsschr. Pharm. 2(1):22-23, Jan. 1979.

Anonymous.

Symposium sur les Maladies Thrombo-Emboliques. Travaux Scientifiques: I. Discussion: Les thrombo-embolies arterielles. (Fr.)

Union Med. Can. 107(2):198-203, Feb. 1978.

Anonymous.

Smoking and intrauterine growth.

Lancet 1(8115):536-537, Mar. 10, 1979.

Anonymous.

Functions of the Septo-Hippocampal System: General discussion I.

Ciba Found. Symp. 58:127-143, 1978.

Anonymous.

Obstetrics should become social science to reduce stillbirths: MD.

Can. Fam. Physician 24:958, Oct. 1978.

Anonymous.

Physicians work to eliminate smoking.

J. Med. Assoc. Ga. 68(3):193, Mar. 1979.

Anonymous.

Highlights of the surgeon general's report on smoking and health.

MMWR 28(1):1-11, Jan. 12, 1979.

Anonymous.

Study compares bacterial adherence of pharyngeal cells in smokers and nonsmokers.

Am. Fam. Physician 19(3):206, Mar. 1979.

Anonymous.

Silent prevention.

Lancet 1(8118):705-706, Mar. 31, 1979.

Anonymous.

Mind and cancer.

Lancet 1(8118):706-707, Mar. 31, 1979.

Anonymous.

Priority for action.

Br. Med. J. 1(6175):1377-1378, May 26, 1979.

Anonymous.

News from the biomedical press.

Biomedicine 30(1):17-18, Feb. 1979.

Anonymous.

Controlling The Smoking Epidemic.

WHO Tech. Rep. Ser. 636:1-87, July 1979.

Anonymous.

Clinical implications of Surgeon General's Report on Smoking and Health.

J. Natl. Med. Assoc. 71(7): 713-715, July 1979.

Anonymous.

Clinical implications of Surgeon General's Report on Smoking and Health.

FDA Drug Bull. 9(1):4-6, Feb.-Mar. 1979.

Anonymous.

Survey of health professionals: Smoking and health, 1975. Summary report from U.S. Dept. H.E.W.

UICC Tech. Rep. Ser. 31:81-87, 1978.

Anonymous.

Cigarette smoking as a risk factor in men with a prior history of myocardial infarction.

J. Chronic Dis. 32(6):415-425, 1979.

Anonymous.

Empfehlungen des Senates der Schweizerischen Akademie der Medizinischen Wissenschaften betreffend den Missbrauch von Tabak und Alkohol. (Ger.)

Bull. Schweiz. Akad. Med. Wiss. 35(1-3):261-264, Mar. 1979.

Anonymous.

Roekvaneundersoekning i Storstockholm. (Swed.)

Lakartidningen 76(26-27):2500, June 27, 1979.

Anonymous.

Photochemical oxidants.

Environ. Health Criteria No. 7 1979.

Anonymous.

Tobacco smoking in the world.

WHO Chron. 33(3):94-97, Mar. 1979.

Anonymous.

Treatment of cigarette dependence.

WHO Chron. 33(3):98-100, Mar. 1979.

Anonymous.

Drug effects can go up in smoke.

FDA Consum 13(2):17-18, Mar. 1979.

Anonymous.

Medical charities and prevention.

Br. Med. J. 2(6205):1610, Dec. 22-29, 1979.

Anonymous.

Five regulatory agencies find 'together-ness' is better.

PMA Newsl. 21(21):4-5, May 28, 1979.

Anonymous.

Carbon monoxide exposure in air-craft fuelers - New York City.

MMWR 28(22):254-255, June 8, 1979.

Anonymous.

Treatment of early diabetes.

Adv. Exp. Med. Biol. 119:419-425, 1979.

Anonymous.

A randomized, controlled trial of aspirin in persons recovered from myocardial infarction.

JAMA 243(7):661-669, Feb. 15, 1980.

Anthoine, D.

Le cancer bronchique des mineurs de fer de Lorraine. (A propos de 270 nouveaux cas observes de 1964 a 1977.) (Fr.)

Ann. Med. Nancy 18(105):461-469, Apr. 15, 1979.

Antuono, P., et al.

Perspectives in Psychopharmaco-therapy: Psychopharmacological prospectives in the treament of dementia.

Prog. Neuropsychopharmacol. 3(1-3): 75-80, 1979.

Apple, D., et al.

The syndrome of inappropiate anti-diuretic hormone secretion in multiple sclerosis.

Arch. Intern. Med. 138(11):1713-1714, Nov. 1978.

Arai, M., et al.

Long-term experiment of maximal non-carcinogenic dose of dimethylnitrosamine for carcinogenesis in rats.

Gan 70(4):549-558, Aug. 1979.

Arai, T.

Annual Meeting Symposium on Smoking and Cardiopulmonary Function: Effects of smoking on pulmonary circulation in anesthetized dogs. (Jpn.)

Jpn. J. Thorac. Dis. 15(9):595-602, Sept. 1977.

Arai, T.

Studies on early detection of obstructive impairments, expecially concerning with the significance and normal values of flow-volume curve (Vmax). (Jpn.)

J. Jpn. Soc. Intern. Med. 67(4):379-388, Apr. 1978.

Aranha, G. V., et al.

Primary tumors of the small intestine.

Am. Surg. 45(8):495-502, Aug. 1979.

Archer, V. E., et al.

Sulfur dioxide exposure in a smelter: III. Acute effects and sputum cytology.

JOM 21(5):359-364, May 1979.

Arffmann, E. and Hjoerne, N.

Influence of surface lipids on skin carcinogenesis in rats.

Acta Pathol. Microbiol. Scand. [A] 87(3): 143-149, May 1979.

Argus, M. F., et al.

Apparent absence of requirement of hydrocarbon metabolism for induction and repression of mixed-function oxidases.

Chem. Biol. Interact. 29(2):247-253, Feb. 1980.

Argus, M. F., et al.

Induction of dimethylnitrosamine-demethylase by polar solvents.

Proc. Soc. Exp. Biol. Med. 163(1):52-55, Jan. 1980.

Argyris, T. S.

Minireview: Ribosome accumulation and the regulation of epidermal hyperplastic growth.

Life Sci. 24(13):1137-1148, Mar. 26, 1979.

Armstrong, B. K., et al.

Mortality in gold and coal miners in Western Australia with special reference to lung cancer.

Br. J. Ind. Med. 36(3):199-205, Aug. 1979.

Armuth, V. and Berenblum, I.

Mechanism of ovarian carcinogenesis: Effect of 7,12-dimethylbenz[a]anthracene administration on intrasplenic ovarian grafts in unilaterally ovariectomized C3HeB/Fe mice.

JNCI 63(4):1047-1050, Oct. 1979.

Arnold, A. M. and Williams, C. J.

Small-cell lung cancer: A curable disease?

Br. J. Dis. Chest 73(4):327-348, Oct. 1979.

Aroesty, J. M., et al.

Medically refractory unstable angina pectoris. II. Hemodynamic and angiographic effects of intraaortic balloon counterpulsation.

Am. J. Cardiol. 43(5):883-888, May 1979.

Aronow, W. S.

Effect of non-nicotine cigarettes and carbon monoxide on angina.

Circulation 61(2):262-265, Feb. 1980.

Aronow, W. S.

Workshop on Carbon Monoxide and Cardiovascular Disease: Effect of carbon monoxide on cardiovascular disease.

Prev. Med. 8(3):271-278, May 1979.

Aronow, W. S., et al.

Carbon monoxide and ventricular fibrillation threshold in normal dogs.

Arch. Environ. Health 34(3):184-186, May-June 1979.

Arqueros, L., et al.

Nicotine-induced release of catecholamines from rat hippocampus and striatum.

Biochem. Pharmacol. 27(23):2667-2674, 1978.

Artvinll, M. and Baris, Y. I.

Mallgnant mesotheliomas in a small village in the Anatolian region of Turkey: An epidemiologic study.

JNCI 63(1):17-22, July 1979.

Asano, M., et al.

Annual Meeting Symposium on Smoking and Cardiopulmonary Function: Cardiac responses to cigarette smoking in healthy young male adults. (Jpn.)

Jpn. J. Thorac. Dis. 15(9):603-610, Sept. 1977.

Ashby, J.

Appendix 1: Structural analysis as a means of predicting carcinogenic potetial.

Br. J. Cancer 37(6):904-923, June 1978.

Ashby, J., et al.

Potentially carcinogenic analogues of the carcinogen hexamethylphosphoramide: Evaluation in vitro.

Br. J. Cancer 38(3):418-427, Sept. 1978.

Ashman, L. K. and Kotlarski, I.

Effect of salmonella enteritidis 11RX infection on two-stage skin carcinogenesis in mice.

Aust. J. Exp. Biol. Med. Sci. 56(Part 6): 695-701, Dec. 1978.

Ashton, H., et al.

Self-titration by cigarette smokers.

Br. Med. J. 2(6186):357-360, Aug. 11, 1979.

Ashton, W. D.

Cigarette smoking and associated disease.

J. R. Coll. Gen. Pract. 29(201):229-233, Apr. 1979.

Ashton, W. D.

Cigarette smoking and associated disease.

J. R. Coll. Gen. Pract. 29(201): 229-233, Apr. 1979.

Ashurst, S. W. and Cohen, G. M.

A benzo[a]pyrene-7,8-dihyrodiol-9,10-epoxide is the major metabolite involved in the binding of benzo[a]pyrene to DNA in isolated viable rat hepatocytes.

Chem. Biol. Interact. 29(1):117-127, Jan. 1980.

Ashurst, S. W., et al.

Importance of conjugation reactions in determining the qualitative nature of polycyclic aromatic hydrocarbon-DNA interactions.

Med. Biol. 57(5):313-320, Oct. 1979.

Ashutosh, K. and Keighley, J. F.

Passive expiration as a test of lung function.

Thorax 33(6):740-746, Dec. 1978.

Ashwell, M., et al.

Social class, smoking, and obesity.

Br. Med. J. 2(6150):1466-1467, Nov. 25, 1978.

Asselin, J. and Labrie, F.

Effects of estradiol and prolactin on steriod receptor levels in 7,12-dimethylbenz(a)anthracene-induced mammary tumors and uterus in the rat.

J. Steroid Biochem. 9(11):1079-1082, Nov. 1978.

Astrup, P.

Eraeiden tupakansavun komponenttien vaikutus sydaemeen ja verisuoniin. (Finn.)

Duodecim 93(8):543-554, 1977.

Astrup, P. and Kjeldsen, K.

Workshop on Carbon Monoxide and Cardiovascular Disease: Model studies linking carbon monoxide and/or nicotine to arteriosclerosis and cardiovascular disease.

Prev. Med. 8(3):295-302, May 1979.

Asuni, T.

The International Challenge of Drug Abuse: The drug abuse scene in Nigeria.

Natl. Inst. Drug Abuse Res. Monogr. Ser. 19:15-25, 1978.

Aubry, F., et al.

Air pollution and health in three urban communities.

Arch. Environ. Health 34(5):360-368, Sept-Oct. 1979.

Audigier, J. C. and Lambert, R.

Epidemiologie des cancers du pancreas. (Fr.)

Ann. Gastroenterol. Hepatol. 15(3): 159-162, 1979.

Auerbach, O.

Acceptance of the Trudeau Medal for 1979.

Am. Rev. Respir. Dis. 120(3):710-711, Sept. 1979.

Auerbach, O., et al.

Changes in bronchial epithelium in relation to cigarette smoking, 1955-1960 vs. 1970-1977.

N. Engl. J. Med. 300(8):381-386, Feb. 22, 1979.

Auerbach, O., et al.

Scar cancer of the lung: Increase over a 21 year period.

Cancer 43(2):636-642, Feb. 1979.

Aune, T. and Dybing, E.

Mutagenic activation of 2,4-diamino-anisole and 2-aminofluorene in vitro by liver and kidney fractions from aromatic hydrocarbon responsive and nonresponsive mice.

Biochem. Pharmacol. 28(18):2791-2797, Sept. 15, 1979.

Austin, G. E. and Moyer, G. H.

Hepatic RNA synthesis in rats treated with ethylene thiourea.

Res. Commun. Chem. Pathol. Pharmacol. 23(3):639-642, Mar. 1979.

Autrup, H.

Separation of water-soluble metabolities of benzo[a]pyrene formed by cultured human colon.

Biochem. Pharmacol. 28(11): 1727-1730, June 1, 1979.

Autrup, H., et al.

Uptake of benzo(a)pyrene-ferric oxide particulates by human pulmonary macrophages and release of benzo(a)pyrene and its metabolites.

Proc. Soc. Exp. Biol. Med. 161(3): 280-284, July 1979.

Axell, T., et al.

Snusning och munhaalecancer - en retrospektiv studie. (Swed.)

Lakartidningen 75(22):2224-2226, May 31, 1978.

Axelson, O., et al.

Lung cancer and residency- A case-referent study on the possible impact of exposure to radon and its daughters in dwellings.

Scand. J. Work Environ. Health 5(1): 10-15, Mar. 1979.

Aylsworth, C. F., et al.

Role of adrenals and estrogen in regression of mammary tumors during postpartum lactation in the rat.

Cancer Res. 39(7, Part 1):2436-2439, July 1979.

Ayres, S. M., et al.

Workshop on Carbon Monoxide and Cardiovascular Disease: The prevalence of carboxyhemoglobinemia in New Yorkers and its effects on the coronary and systemic circulation.

Prev. Med. 8(3):323-332, May 1979.

Bababunmi, E. A.

Toxins and carcinogens in the environment: An observation in the tropics.

J. Toxicol. Environ. Health 4(5-6):691-699, Sept.-Nov. 1978.

Bachmann, K., et al.

Smoking and warfarin disposition.

Clin. Pharmacol. Ther. 25(3):309-315, Mar. 1979.

Bacq, Z. M.

Quelques faits anciens et nouveaux sur l'accoutumance au tabac. (Fr.)

Rev. Med. Liege 33(20):701-705, Oct. 15, 1978.

Bacq, Z. M.

Quelques faits anciens et nouveaux sur l'accoutumance au tabac. (Fr.)

Louv. Med. 97(8):433-439, Oct. 1978.

Baden, E.

Tabac et cancers de la region oropharyngee et des bronches: Donnees actuelles. (Fr.)

Rev. Med. Toulouse 14(8):549-560, Oct. 1978.

Badre, R., et al.

Pollution atmospherique par la fumee de tabac. (Fr.)

Ann. Pharm. Fr. 36(9-10):443 452, 1978.

Bagg, L. R. and Hughes, D. T. D.

Serial pulmonary function tests in progressive systemic sclerosis.

Thorax 34(2):224-228, Apr. 1979.

Bagnato, A., et al.

Fattori professionali di rischio respiratorio e fumo di tabacco. Indagine su tre popolazioni operaie. (Ital.)

Friuli Med. 33(3):203-212, May-June 1978.

Bagnato, A., et al.

Pollution du milieu et tabagisme: Recherches effectuees sur trois populations de travailleurs exposes aux differents risques pulmonaires. (Fr.)

Bronchopneumologie 28(4):272-277, July-Aug. 1978.

Bagrov, Ya. Yu. and Manusova, N. B.

The inhibitory action of acetylcholine on the pituitrin-stimulated osmotic water flow through the frog urinary bladder wall. (Russ.)

Biull. Eksp. Biol. Med. 86(9):321-324, Sept. 1978.

Bahna, L., et al.

Carcinogenicity and polarographic behavior of dibenz[a,h]anthracene dibenz[a,h]acridine and dibenz[a,h] phenazine.

Neoplasma 25(6):641-645, 1978.

Bailar, III, J. C.

The case for cancer prevention.

JNCI 62(4):727-731, Apr. 1979.

Bain, C., et al.

Stopping smoking and coronary heart-disease. (Letter to the Editor.)

Lancet 2(8089):581, Sept. 9, 1978.

Baird, W. M., et al.

Formation of glucuronic acid conjugates of 7,12-dimethylbenz(a)anthracene phenols in 7,12-dimethylbenz(a) anthracene-treated hamster embryo cell cultures.

Cancer Res. 38(10):3432-3437, Oct. 1978.

Baird, W. M., et al.

Analysis of metabolism of carcinogenic polycyclic hydrocarbons by position-sensing proportional counting of thin-layer chromatograms.

Anal. Biochem. 99(1):165-169, Oct. 15, 1979.

Baker, M. D., et al.

Smoking habits of blacks in industry.

S. Afr. Med. J. 54(2):67-69, July 8, 1978.

Baker, M. D., et al.

Lung function insisal ropemakers.

Br. J. Ind. Med. 36(3):216-219, Aug. 1979.

Baker, R. R., et al.

Screening for bronchogenic carcinoma: The surgical experience.

J. Thorac. Cardiovasc. Surg. 78(6): 876-882, Dec. 1979.

Bakhle, Y. S., et al.

Effects of cigarette smoke on the metabolism of vasoactive hormones in rat isolated lungs.

Br. J. Pharmacol. 65(3):495-499, Mar. 1979.

Bakka, A.

Medikamentinduserte lungesjukdommar. (Norw.)

Tidsskr. Nor. Laegeforen. 98(12): 630-634; 637, Apr. 30, 1978.

Balfour, D. J. K. and Reid, A.

Effects of betamethasone on the stimulation of corticosterone secretion in rats.

Arch. Int. Pharmacodyn. Ther. 237(1): 67-74, Jan. 1979.

Ball, J. K.

Leukemogenesis by an endogenous virus isolated from the CFW mouse. II. Early effects of virus on thymus gland and bone marrow cell populations.

JNCI 62(6):1517-1522, June 1979.

Ball, J. K. and McCarter, J. A.

Biological characterization of a leukemogenic virus isolated from the CFW mouse.

Cancer Res. 39(8):3080-3088, Aug. 1979.

Ball, K.

Carbon monoxide yield of cigarrettes. (Letter to the Editor.)

Br. Med. J. 280(6211):400, Feb. 9, 1980.

Ball, K.

Carbon monoxide yield of cigarettes. (Letter to the Editor.)

Br. Med. J. 2(6192):731, Sept. 22, 1979.

Ball, K. and Stevenson, A.

Hospital action on smoking.

Br. Med. J. 2(6193):777-778, Sept. 29, 1979.

Ball, L. M., et al.

Benzo(a)pyrene oxidation, conjugation and disposition in the isolated perfused rabbit lung: Role of the glutathione s--transferases. transferases.

Med. Biol. 57(5):298-305, Oct. 1979.

Balster, R. L. and Chait, L. D.

Phencyclidine (PCP) Abuse: An Appraisal. The behavioral effects of phencyclidine in animals.

NIDA Res. Monogr. Ser. No. 21:53-65, Aug. 1978.

Barad, C. B.

Smoking on the job: The controversy heats up.

Occup. Health Saf. 48(1):21-24, Jan.-Feb. 1979.

Baranova, L. N. and Alexandrov, V. A.

Peculiarities of transplacental penetration of 7,12-dimethylbenz(a)anthracene and of its distribution in the organs of the rat fetus. (Russ.)

Biull. Eksp. Biol. Med. 86(9):477-479, Oct. 1978.

Barbason, H., et al.

Effects of discontinuation of chronic feeding of diethylnitrosamine on the development of hepatomas in adult rats.

Br. J. Cancer 40(2):260-267, Aug. 1979.

Barboriak, J. J., et al.

High density lipoprotein cholesterol and coronary artery occulsion.

Metabolism 28(7):735-738, July 1979.

Barboriak, J. J., et al.

Interrelationship between coronary artery occlusion, high-density lipoprotein cholesterol, and alcohol intake.

J. Lab. Clin. Med. 94(2):348-353, Aug. 1979.

Bardell, D.

Infectivity titers of adenovirus type 5 suspensions after exposure to cigarette smoke.

Appl. Environ. Microbiol. 36(5):774-775, Nov. 1978.

Baric, L.

Gesundheitserziehung im Rahmen der primaeren Sozialisation. (Ger.)

Med. Klin. 74(44):1648-1652, Nov. 2, 1979.

Barlow, J. W., et al.

Potentiation of steroid binding to proteins by 7,12-dimethylbenz(alpha)-anthracene.

J. Steroid. Biochem. 9(11):1027-1032, Nov. 1978.

Barnard, R. J. and Webster, J. S.

Carbon monoxide: A hazard to fire fighters.

Arch. Environ. Health 34(4):255-257, July/Aug. 1979.

Barnes, W. S. and Klekowski, Jr., E. J.

Testing the environment for dispersed mutagens: Use of plant bioconcentrators coupled with microbial mutagen assays.

Environ. Health Perspect. 27:61-67, Dec. 1978.

Barnes, W. S., et al.

Theoretical prediction of carcinogenicity: Quasi-quantification by quasi-valence. A reply to V. Veljkovic and D. I. Lalovic.

Experientia 35(4):565-567, Apr. 15, 1979.

Barrett-Connor, E., et al.

Heart disease risk factors and hormone use in postmenopausal woman.

JAMA 241(20):2167-2169, May 18, 1979.

Barrett, J. C., et al.

Correlation of in vitro growth properties and tumorigenicity of Syrian hamster cell lines.

Cancer Res. 39(5):1504-1510, May 1979.

Bartfeld, D. and Fuchs, S.

Active acetylcholine receptor fragment obtained by tryptic digestion of acetylcholine receptor from Torpedo californica.

Biochem. Biophys. Res. Commun. 89(2):512-519, July 27, 1979.

Bartho, L. and Szolcsanyi, J.

The site of action of capsaicin on the guinea-pig isolated ileum.

Naunyn Schmiedebergs Arch. Pharmacol. 305(1):75-81, Oct. 31, 1978.

Bartholomew, J. C., et al.

Modulation of the cell cycle of cultured mouse liver cells by benzo(a)pyrene and its derivatives.

Cancer Res. 39(7, Part 1):2538-2543, July 1979.

Bartlett, C. L. R.

International Symposium on Legionnaires' Disease: Sporadic cases of Legionnaires' disease in Great Britain.

Ann. Intern. Med. 90(4):592-595, Apr. 1979.

Bartlett, V., et al.

Evidence for two adenine derivative receptors in rat ileum which are not involved in the nonadrenergic, noncholinegric response.

Can. J. Physiol. Pharmacol. 57(10):1130-1137, Oct. 1979.

Bartolome Pineda, A.

Prevencion cardiovascular. Factores de riesgo. Estudio estadistico.

Med. Segur. Trab. (Madr.) 26(104): 11-39, Oct.-Dec. 1978.

Barton, E. S. and Barton, J. L.

A case report on the use of DRO in the treatment of smoking.

Addict. Behav. 3(1):1-4, 1978.

Basler, A., et al.

Effects of caffeine on sister-chromatid exchanges (SCE) in vivo.

Mutat. Res. 59(2):209-214, Feb. 1979.

Basrur, P. K. and Haraad, T.

Alterations in the nasal mucosa of Syrian golden hamsters exposed to cigarette smoke.

Prog. Exp. Tumor Res. 24:283-301, 1979.

Bassler, T. J.

The Marathon: Physiological, Medical, Epidemiological, and Psychological Studies. Marathon running and immunity to atherosclerosis.

Ann. NY Acad. Sci. 301:579-592, 1977.

Bastian, P.

Coronary heart disease in tribal Aborigines - The West Kimberley survey.

Aust. NZ J. Med. 9(3):284-292, June 1979.

Bateman, J. R. M., et al.

Regional lung clearance of excessive bronchial secretions during chest physiotherapy in patients with stable chronic airways obstruction.

Lancet 1(8111):294-297, Feb. 10, 1979.

Bateman, J. R. M., et al.

The retention of lung secretions during the night in normal subjects.

Clin. Sci. Mol. Med. 55(6):523-527, Dec. 1978.

Bates, R. C.

The hidden alcoholic: A history that reveals the early clues.

Diagnosis :22-27, Mar.-Apr. 1979.

Batt, A. M., et al.

Glucuronidation of 3-hydroxybenzo(a) pyrene in liver microsomes.

Med. Biol. 57(5):281-286, Oct. 1979.

Batt, R. A. L. and Topping, D. L.

Acute effects of nicotine on plasma free fatty acid concentrations and on the response to cold stress, in lean and obese (genotype ob/ob) mice.

Int. J. Obes. 3(1):7-13, 1979.

Battistich, V. A. and Huffman, S.

Psychoactive drug use in a midwestern high school: Extent of current use and future trends.

Int. J. Addict. 13(6):975-980, 1978.

Batzinger, R. P., et al.

Antimutagenic effects of 2(3)-tert-butyl-4-hydroxyanisole and of antimicrobial agents.

Cancer Res. 38(12):4478-4485, Dec. 1978.

Batzinger, R. P., et al.

Antimutagenic effects of 2(3)-tert-butyl-4-hydroxyanisole and of antimicrobial agents.

Cancer Res. 38(12):4478-4485, Dec. 1978.

Baulieu, E.-E.

Cell membrane, a target for steroid hormones.

Mol. Cell. Endocrinol. 12(3): 247-254, Dec. 1978.

Baulieu, E.-E., et al.

SteroiD induced meiotic division in Xenopus laevis oocytes: Surface and calcium.

Nature 275(5681):593-598, Oct. 19, 1978.

Beaglehole, B., et al.

High density lipoprotein cholesterol and other serum lipids in New Zealand Maoris.

NZ Med. J. 90(642):139-142, Aug. 22, 1979.

Beaglehole, R., et al.

A controled smoking intervention programme in secondary schools.

N.Z. Med. J. 87(610):278-280, Apr. 26, 1978.

Beaumont, J. L.

Arterielle paroxystique induite par la fumee de tabac. (Fr.)

J. Med. Chir. Prat. 149(10):391-394, May 1978.

Beaumont, V., et al.

Hormones contraceptives, risque vasculaire et precipitabilite anormale des gamma-globulines seriques. (Fr.)

Sem. Hop. Paris 55(11-12):585-591, Mar. 18-25, 1979.

Becci, P. J., et al.

The respiratory epithelium. VI. Histogenesis of lung tumors produced by benzo[a]pyrene-ferric oxide in the hamster.

JNCI 61(2):607-618, Aug. 1978.

Becci, P. J., et al.

The respiratory epithelium. IV. Histogenesis of epidermoid metaplasia and carcinoma in situ in the hamster.

JNCI 61(2):577-586, Aug. 1978.

Becci, P. J., et al.

Inhibitory effect of 13-cis-retinoic acid on urinary bladder carcinogenesis induced in C57BL/6 mice by N-butyl-N-(4-hydroxybutyl)-nitrosamine.

Cancer Res. 38(12):4463-4466, Dec. 1978.

Becci, P. J., et al.

A quantitive dosing schedule for the induction of transitional cell carcinomas in female F344 rats with the use of N-butyl-N-(4-hydroxybutyl)nitrosamine.

JNCI 62(1):187-191, Jan. 1979.

Becci, P. J., et al.

Inhibitory effect of 13-cis-retinoic acid on urinary bladder carcinogenesis induced in C57BL/6 mice by N-butyl-N-(4-hydroxybutyl)-nitrosamine.

Cancer Res. 38(12):4463-4466, Dec. 1978.

Becci, P. J., et al.

Effect of delay in administration of 13-cis-retinoic acid on the inhibition of urinary bladder carcinogenesis in the rat.

Cancer Res. 39(8):3141-3144, Aug. 1979.

Becker, C. G. and Dubin, T.

Tobacco allergy and cardiovascular disease.

Cardiovasc. Med. 3(8):851-854, Aug. 1978.

Becker, C. G., et al.

Induction of IgE antibodies to antigen isolated from tobacco leaves and from cigarette smoke condensate.

Am. J. Pathol. 96(1):249-255, July 1979.

Becker, F. F. and Sell, S.

Differences in serum alpha-fetoprotein concentrations during the carcinogenic sequences resulting from exposure to diethylnitrosamine or acetylaminofluorene.

Cancer Res. 39(5):1437-1442, May 1979.

Becker, L. C. and Haak, Jr., E. D.

Augmentation of myocardial ischemia by low level carbon monoxide exposure in dogs.

Arch. Environ. Health 34(4):274-279, July/Aug. 1979.

Becklake, M. R.

Enviromental exposure to asbestos: A factor in the rising rate of cancer in the industrialized world?

Chest 76(3):245-247, Sept. 1979.

Begemann, F., et al.

Tagung der Deutschen Gesellchaft feur Verdauungs und Stoffwechsel-krankheiten: Zigarettenrauchen stiegert den intragastralen Lysolecithingehalt. (Abstr.) (Ger.)

Z. Gastroenterol. [Verh] 14:13, 1978.

Beglinger, Ch., et al.

Beeinflussung des Rauchverhaltens durch Fernmethoden. (Ger.)

Soz. Preventivmed. 22(4):182-183, July-Aug. 1977.

Behar, J., et al.

Characterization of feline gastroduodenal junction by neural and hormonal stimulation.

Am. J. Physiol. 236(1):E45-E51, Jan. 1979.

Behar, J., et al.

Effect of glucagon, secretin, and vasoactive intestinal polypeptide on the feline lower esophageal sphincter: Mechanism of action.

Gastroenterology 77(5):1000-1007, Nov. 1979.

Belesin, D. B. and Samardzic, R.

The pharmacology of aggressive behavioural phenomena elicited by muscarine injected into the cerebral ventricles of conscious cats.

Psychopharmacology 60(2):155-158, Jan. 31, 1979.

Beleslin, D. B. and Samardzic, R.

Comparative stuly of aggressive behaviour after injection of cholinomimetics, anticholinesterases, nicotinic, and muscarinic ganglionic stimulants into the cerbral ventricles of conscious cats: Failure of nicotine drugs to evoke aggression.

Psychophamacology 60(2):147-153, Jan. 31, 1979.

Belin, L., et al.

New Approaches to the Management of Allergic Diseases: Immunological and clinical responses to humidifier fever antigens.

Monogr. Allergy 14:146-149, 1979.

Bell, B. A. and Symon, L.

Smoking and subarachnoid haemorrhage.

Br. Med. J. 1(6163):577-578, Mar. 3, 1979.

Bell, D. S. and Champion, R. A.

Deviancy, delinquency and drug use.

Br. J. Psychiatry 134:269-276, Mar. 1979.

Belman, S., et al.

Effect of phorbol myristate acetate on cyclic nucleotide levels in mouse epidermis.

Cancer Res. 38(9):2978-2982, Sept. 1978.

Belnap, L. P., et al.

Immunogenicity of chemically induced murine colon cancers.

Cancer Res. 39(4):1174-1179, Apr. 1979.

Belyaev, I. I.

Some problems of prophylaxis of carcinogenic effect of N-nitrosoamines. (Russ.)

Vestn. Akad. Med. Nauk. SSSR No. 8: 30-36, 1978.

Bem, A. and Trzeciak, B.

Zaburzenia zmyslu smaku u nalogowych palaczy tytoniu. (Pol.)

Pol. Tyg. Lek. 33(36):1413-1414, Sept. 4, 1978.

Ben-Barak, J. and Dudai, Y.

Cholinergic binding sites in rat hippocampal formation: Properties and ontogenesis.

Brain Res. 166(2):245-257, Apr. 27, 1979.

Ben-Sira, Z. and Padeh, B.

"Instrumental coping" and "affective defense": An additional perspective in health promoting behavior.

Soc. Sci. Med. 12(3A):163-168, May 1978.

Benatar, S. R.

Smoking and chronic respiratory symptoms in 11-15 year-old children.

S. Afr. Med. J. 56(8):301-304, Oct. 25, 1979.

Benatar, S. R.

Current concepts in asthma therapy.

S. Afr. Med. J. 56(16):627-630, Oct. 13, 1979.

Bend, J. R., et al.

Aquatic Pollutants and Biologic Effects with Emphasis on Neoplasia: In vitro metabolism of xenobiotics in some marine animals.

Ann. NY Acad. Sci. 298:505-521, Sept. 29, 1977.

Bensaid, J.

Idiopathic hypertrophic subaortic stenosis and associated coronary artery disease: Clinical, hemodynamic, and therapeutic features from a review of 57 cases of the literature.

Angiology 30(9):585-593, Sept. 1979.

Benson, A. M., et al.

Elevation of hepatic glutathione S-transferase activities and protection against mutagenic metabolites of benzo(a)pyrene by dietary antioxidants.

Cancer Res. 38(12):4486-4495, Dec. 1978.

Benson, A. M., et al.

Elevation of hepatic glutathione S-transferase activities and protection against mutagenic metabolites of benzo(a)pyrene by dietary antioxidants.

Cancer Res. 38(12):4486-4495, Dec. 1978.

Benson, A. M., et al.

Elevation of extrahepatic glutathione S-transferase and epoxide hydratase activities by 2(3)-tert-butyl-4-hydroxyanisole.

Cancer Res. 39(8):2971-2977, Aug. 1979.

Benwell, M. E. M. and
Balfour, D. J. K.

Effects of nicotine administration and its withdrawal on plasma corticosterone and brain 5-hydroxyindoles.

Psychopharmacology 63(1):7-11, May 8, 1979.

Berend, N., et al.

Correlation between the function and structure of the lung in smokers.

Am. Rev. Respir. Dis. 119(5):695-705, May 1979.

Berg, K., et al.

Effect of smoking on serum levels of HDL apoproteins.

Atherosclerosis 34(3):339-343, Nov. 1979.

Berger, L. R.

Factors influencing breast feeding.

J. Contin. Educ. Pediatr. 20(9):13-29, Sept. 1978.

In human lactation arthraquinone derivatives (cascara, casanthranol) and dioctyl sodium sulfosuccinate should not be used while bulk-forming, saline and stool-softening types do not affect infant feeding.

Berger, L. R.

Factors influencing breast feeding.

J. Contin. Educ. Fam. Med. 26(4): 17-30, Apr. 1979.

Cascara, casauthranol and dioctyl sodium should not be used by breast-feeding mothers.

Berglund, G., et al.

Modell foer omhaendertagande av patienter med hoegt blodtryck. (Swed.)

Lakartidningen 75(46):4253-4256, Nov. 15, 1978.

Bergofsky, E. H.

Respiratory failure in disorders of the thoracic cage.

Am. Rev. Respir. Dis. 119(4):643-669, Apr. 1979.

Bergstrand, R., et al.

Myocardial infarction among men below age 40.

Br. Heart J. 40(7):783-788, July 1978.

Bergstrand, R., et al.

Sekundaar prevention efter hjaertinfarkt. (Swed.)

Lakartidningen 75(20):2038-2044, May 17, 1978.

Bergstrom, P.

Riskfaktorer, prevention och terapi. (Swed.)

Sven. Farm. Tidskr. 82(8):397-407, Aug. 1978.

Berkman, L. F. and Syme, S. L.

Social networds, host resistance, and mortality: A nine-year follow-up study of Alameda county resisdents.

Am. J. Epidemiol. 109(2):186-204, Feb. 1979.

Berkman, Y. M.

Aspiration and inhalation pneumonias.

Semin. Roentgenol. 15(1):73-84, Jan. 1980.

Berman, J. J., et al.

Intestinal tumors induced by a single intraperitoneal injection of methyl-(acetoxymethyl)nitrosamine in three strains of rats.

Cancer Res. 39(5):1462-1466, May 1979.

Berman, J. J., et al.

Dependence of tumor spectrum on route of administration in Sprague-Dawley rats as a result of single or multiple injections of methyl(acetoxymethyl)nitrosamine.

JNCI 63(1):93-100, July 1979.

Berman, L. B. and Kuehn, S. H.

Biochemical screening for lung cancer. (Letters to the Editor.)

Chest 75(3):408, Mar. 1979.

Bernard, J. P.

Epidemiologie des cancers primitifs broncho-pulmonaires. (Fr.)

Cah. Med. 5(7):433-436, Nov. 5, 1979.

Bernard, J., et al.

Bronchoalveolar lavage.

Thorax 35(1):1-8, Jan. 1980.

Bernfeld, P., et al.

Cigarette smoke inhalation studies in inbred Syrian golden hamsters.

JNCI 63(3):675-689, Sept. 1979.

Bernfeld, P., et al.

Cigarette smoking-induced cancer of the larynx in hamsters (CINCH): A method to assay the carcinogenicity of cigarette smoke.

Prog. Exp. Tumor Res. 24:315-319, 1979.

Bernow, R. and Wilhelmsen, L.

Minskande roekning bland Sveriges laekare 1969-1977. (Swed.)

Lakartidningen 75(48):4490-4492, Nov. 29, 1978.

Berry, G., et al.

Asbestosis: A study of dose-response relationships in an asbestos textile factory.

Br. J. Ind. Med. 36(2):98-112, May 1979.

Bertram, B., et al.

Carcinogenicity of di(N-nitroso)-perhydropyrimidine (DNPP) after intraperitoneal application to rats.

Cancer Lett. 6(1):57-60, Jan. 1979.

Best, J. A.

Stopping smoking by finding alternatives.

Contin. Educ. Fam. Physician 9(1):36-45, July 1978.

Best, J. A. and Hakstian, A. R.

A situation-specific model for smoking behavior.

Addict. Behav. 3(2):79-92, 1978.

Best, J. A., et al.

Comparison of satiation and rapid smoking in self-managed smoking cessation.

Addict. Behav. 3(2):71-78, 1978.

Bewley, B. R., et al.

Teacher's smoking.

J. Epidemiol. Commun. Health 33(3): 219-222, Sept. 1979.

Beyer-Boon, M. E. and Rubio, C. A.

Kinetics of cell replication of the uterine cervix: II. Parabasal cell production in atypical epithelium.

Oncology 37(1):27-29, 1980.

Beyhl, F., et al.

The Induction of Drug Metabolism. Regulation of Protein Synthesis: Discussion.

Symp. Med. Hoechst 14:113-129, 1979.

Bhargava, V. K., et al.

Effect of cholinergic drugs on the brainstem auditory evoked reponses (far-field) in rats.

Neuroscience 3(9):821-826, 1978.

Bhargava, V. K., et al.

Effects of cholinergic drugs on auditory evoked responses (CER) of rat cortex.

Neuropharmacology 17(12):1009-1013, Dec. 1978.

Bhuyan, B. K.

Kinetics of cell kill by hyperthermia.

Cancer Res. 39(6, Part 2):2277-2284, June 1979.

Bialik, O., et al.

British Region Abstracts: Indexing of air pollution based on photodynamic activity of organic pollutants. (Abstr.)

Biometrics 34(4):726, Dec. 1978.

Bibby, M. C., et al.

Autoradiography of deposition of tobacco smoke particulate matter in isolated perfused rat lung.

Eur. J. Drug Metab. Pharmacokinet. 3(3):141-145, July-Sept. 1978.

Bickers, D. R. and Kappas, A.

Human skin aryl hydrocarbon hydroxylase: Induction by coal tar.

J. Clin. Invest. 62(5):1061-1068, Nov. 1978.

Biener, K.

Neue Sonderstudien zum Tabakkonsum der Bevoelkerung. (Ger.)

Praxis 67(40):1467-1470, Oct. 3, 1978.

Biener, K.

Einflussfaktoren fuer das Rauchen der Jugend. (Ger.)

Bull. Schweiz. Akad. Med. Wiss. 35(1-3):111-117, Mar. 1979.

Biener, K. and Ritter, R.

Sport und Lebensverlaengerung. (Ger.)

Munch. Med. Wochenschr. 120(35): 1119-1122, Sept. 1, 1978.

Bierenbaum, M. L., et al.

Effect of cigarette smoking upon in vivo platelet function in man.

Thromb. Res. 12(6):1051-1057, June 1978.

Bignon, J. and Bernaudin, J. F.

Les cellules pulmonaires et leurs fonctions. (Fr.)

Med. Hyg. 36(1301):3080-3089, Sept. 27, 1978.

Bilgi, C., et al.

Pulmonary manifestations in patients with malignant melanoma during BCG immunotherapy: A preliminary report.

Chest 75(6):685-687, June 1979.

Bingham, S., et al.

Dietary fibre and regional large-bowel cancer mortality in Britain.

Br. J. Cancer 40(3):456-463, Sept. 1979.

Binns, R. and Wilton, L. V.

Inhalation toxicity studies on cigarette smoke (VIII). 6-Week comparative experiments using modified flue-cured cigarettes: General toxicology.

Toxicology 11(3):207-218, Nov. 1978.

Birch, C. D.

Desaminooksytocin-induceret foedsel og neonatal hyperbilirubinaemi: En prospektiv undersoegelse. (Dan.)

Ugeskr. Laeger 140(21):1234-1235, May 22, 1978.

Birnbaum, L. S. and Baird, M. B.

Induction of hepatic mixed function oxidases in senescent rodents.

Exp. Gerontol. 13(5):299-303, 1978.

Bismuth, H. and Malt, R. A.

Current concepts in cancer: Carcinoma of the bilary tract.

N. Engl. J. Med. 301(13):704-706, Sept. 27, 1979.

Bissel, M. J., et al.

Culture systems for studying malignancy.

Cancer Res. 39(10):4293-4295, Oct. 1979.

Biswas, N. M., et al.

Adrenogonadal interactions in nicotine-induced alteration of steroidogenesis in male rat.

Andrologia 11(3):227-233, May-June 1979.

Bjartveit, K., et al.

The Cardiovascular Disease Study in Norwegian Counties: Background and organization.

Acta Med. Scand. Suppl. 634:1-70, 1979.

Bjerke, R. D., et al.

Small airways in progressive systemic sclerosis (PSS).

Am. J. Med. 66(2):201-209, Feb. 1979.

Bjordal, M., et al.

Bly- og karbonmonoksydnivaa i blod hos anleggsarbeidere i Bergen. (Norw. Engl. Summ.)

Tidsskr. Nor Laegeforen. 98(17-18):886-887;912, June 20, 1978.

Black, Jr., O.

Histofluorescence of 3-methylcholanthrene metabolites in the rat pancreas.

Gastroenterology 75(3):438-444, Sept. 1978.

Blake, C. A.

Paradoxical effects of drugs acting on the central nervous system on the preovulatory release of pituitary luteinizing hormone in pro-oestrous rats.

J. Endocrinol. 79(3):319-326, Dec. 1978.

Blazsek, I., et al.

Binding of benzo(a)pyrene into lung and thymocyte nuclear fractions.

Res. Commun. Chem. Pathol. Pharmacol. 23(3):611-626, Mar. 1979.

Bloch, R. J.

Dispersal and reformation of acetylcholine receptor clusters of cultured rat myotubes treated with inhibitors of energy metabolism.

J. Cell. Biol. 82(3):626-643, Sept. 1979.

Block, J. R. and Goodman, N.

Illicit drug use and consumption of alcohol, tobacco, and over-the-counter medicine among adolescents.

Int. J. Addict. 13(6):933-946, 1978.

Blog, F. B. and Szabo, G.

The effects of UVB and 7, 12 dimethylbenz(a)anthracene (DMBA) on epidural melanocytes of the tail in C57BL mice.

J. Invest. Dermatol. 73(6):538-544, Dec. 1979.

Blohmke, M.

Neue Aspekte in der Vorsorgemedizin. (Ger.)

Fortschr. Med. 96(43):2179-2180, Nov. 16, 1978.

Blot, W. J. and Fraumeni, Jr., J. F.

Studies of respiratory cancer in high risk communities.

JOM 21(4):276-278, Apr. 1979.

Blot, W. J., et al.

Lung cancer after employment in shipyards during World War II.

N. Engl. J. Med. 299(12):620-624, Sept. 21, 1978.

Bloxham, C. A., et al.

Malignant hypertension and cigarette smoking.

Br. Med. J. 1(6163):581-583, Mar. 3, 1979.

Bluemchen, G., et al.

Langezeitbeobachtung bei 27 Patienten mit nichtoperierten linksventrikulaeren Aneurysmen. (Ger.)

Z. Kardiol. 67(11):736-748, Nov. 1978.

Blum, A.

Medicine vs. Madison avenue: Fighting smoke with smoke.

JAMA 243(8):739-740, Feb. 22/29. 1980.

Bock, K. W.

Increase of liver microsomal benzo (a)pyrene monooxygenase activity by subsequent glucuronidation.

Naunyn Schmiedebergs Arch. Pharmacol. 304(1):77-79,Aug. 1978.

Bock, K. W. and Lilienblum, W.

Activation and induction of rat liver microsomal UDP-glucuronyltransferase with 3-hydroxybenzo(a)pyrene and N-hydroxy-2-naphthylamine as substrates.

Biochem. Pharmacol. 28(5):695-700, Mar. 1, 1979.

Bockman, D. E., et al.

Metabolism of benzo(a)pyrene by multinucleated giant cells.

J. Reticuloendothel. Soc. 25(1):39-47, Jan. 1979.

Boddy, K.

Fetal breathing: Its physiologic and clinical implications.

Hosp. Pract. 14(2):89-96, Feb. 1979.

Bodendorfer, T. W., et al.

Obtaining drug exposure histories during pregnancy.

Am. J. Obstet. Gynecol. 135(4):490-494, Oct. 15, 1979.

Bodwin, J. S. and Cho-Chung, Y. S.

Dibutyryl cyclic-AMP mimics the effect of ovariectomy on a dehydrogenase in hormone-dependent mammary tumors.

Eur. J. Cancer 15(4):443-449, Apr. 1979.

Bodwin, J. S., et al.

Inverse relation between estrogen receptors and cyclic adenosine 3':5'-monophospahte-binding proteins in hormone-dependent mammary tumor regression due to dibutyryl cyclic adenosine 3':5'-monophosphate treatment or ovaruectomy.

Cancer Res. 38(10):3410-3413, Oct. 1978.

Boelens, R. and Wever, R

Electron-transfer processes in carboxy-cytochromec oxidase after photodissociation of cytochrome A3 2-plus.CO.

Biochim. Biophys. Acta 547(2):296-310, Aug. 14, 1979.

Boer, P., et al.

Measurement of cardiac output by impedance cardiography under various conditions.

Am. J. Phsyiol. 237(4):H491-H496, Oct. 1979.

Boillat, M.-A., et al.

Fluorose industrielle: Etude Multi-disciplinaire de 43 Ouvriers de L'industrie de L'-luminium. (Fr.)

Schweiz. Med. Wochenschr. (Suppl. 8): 1-28, 1979.

Boisson, J., et al.

La barriere muqueuse gastrique: Essai de synthese des acquisitions recentes. (Fr.)

Ann. Gastroenterol. Hepatol. 14(5):331-344, Oct.-Nov. 1978.

Boksay, I. J. E., et al.

Synthesis and pharmacological activity of befuraline (N-benzo[b]furan-2-ylcarbonyl-N'-benzylpiperazine), a New antidepressant compound.

Arzneim. Forsch. 29(2):193-204, 1979.

Boland, J. and De Landsheere, C.

Epidemiologie et histoire naturelle de l'insuffisance coronarienne. (Fr.)

Rev. Med. Leige 34(Suppl 1):5-13, June 1979.

Bonardi, O.

Fumo e carcinoma laringeo. (Ital.)

Minerva Chir. 33(6):IX, Mar. 31, 1978.

Bond, J. A., et al.

Metabolism of benzo[a]pyrene and 7,12-dimethylbenz[a]anthracene in chicken aortas: Monooxygenation, bioactivation to mutagens, and covalent binding to DNA in vitro.

Toxicol. Appl. Pharmacol. 52(2):323-335, Feb. 1980.

Bondi, K. R.

Current submarine carbon monoxide and estimated carboxyhemoglobin levels and interpretation of their possible effects on mental performance and health risk.

Nav. Submar. Med. Res. Lab. Rep. No. 883:1-13, Nov. 27, 1978.

Bone, R. C., et al.

Medical Grand Rounds: University of Arkansas for Medical Sciences. Tobacco and the lung.

J. Arkansas Med. Soc. 75(12):458-463, May 1979.

Bonnevie, O., et al.

Double-blind randomised clinical trial of a pepsin-inhibitory pentapeptide (pepstatin) in the treatment of duodenal ulcer.

Gut 20(7):624-628, July 1979.

Bonnevie, P., et al.

Aendring af danskernes rygevaner 1958-1976. (Letters to the Editor.) (Dan.)

Ugeskr. Laeger 140(47):2964-2965, Nov. 20, 1978.

Boobis, A. R., et al.

Carcinogenic benzo(a)pyrene metabolites bound to DNA: Metabolic formation by human cultured lymphocytes and by human liver microsomes.

Pharmacology 17(5):241-248, 1978.

Boobis, A. R., et al.

Effects of microsomal enzyme inducers in vivo and inhibitors in vitro on the covalent binding of benzo[a]pyrene metabolites to DNA catalyzed by liver microsomes from genetically responsive and nonresponsive mice.

Biochem. Pharmacol. 28(1):111-121, 1979.

Boobis, A. R., et al.

Genetic differences in the binding of benzo[a]pyrene metabolites to DNA in the mouse.

Cancer Detect. Prev. 2(1):83-111, 1979.

Boobis, A. R., et al.

Monooxygenase activity of human liver in microsomal fractions of needle biopsy specimens.

Br. J. Clin. Pharmacol. 9(1):11-19, Jan. 1980.

Borenfreund, E., et al.

Intermediate-sized filaments in cultured rat liver tumor cells with Mallory body-like cytoplasm abnormalities.

JNCI 64(2):323-333, Feb. 1980.

Borenfreund, E., et al.

Carcinogen-induced abnormalities in rat liver cells and their modification by chemical agents.

Cancer Res. 39(3):800-807, Mar. 1979.

Borgers, D. and Junge, B.

Workshop on Carbon Monoxide and Cardiovascular Disease: Thiocyanate as an indicator of tobacco smoking.

Prev. Med. 8(3):351-357, May 1979.

Borlee, I. and Lechat, M. F.

Resultats d'une enquete sur les malformations congenitales dans le Hainaut. (Fr.)

Arch. Belg. Med. Soc. 36(2):77-99, Feb. 1978.

Bornstein, W. A., et al.

Comparison of nuclear and microsomal epoxide hydrase from rat liver.

Arch. Biochem. Biophys. 197(2):436-446, Oct. 15, 1979.

Borrie, J.

Lung cancer.

NZ Med. J. 89(635):354-357, May 9, 1979.

Borrie, J. and Hilless, A. D.

Peripheral early stage lung cancer: Superiority of six-monthly over random chest films.

NZ Med. J. 89(628):56-58, Jan. 24, 1979.

Botvin, G. J., et al.

Preventing the onset of cigarette smoking through life skills training.

Prev. Med. 9(1):135–143, Jan. 1980.

Bouhuys, A., et al.

Do present levels of air pollution outdoors affect respiratory health?

Nature 276(5687):466–471, Nov. 30, 1978.

Bouhuys, A., et al.

Pulmonary function in young smokers: Male-female differences. (Letter to the Editor.)

Am. Rev. Respir. Dis. 119(3):515–516, Mar. 1979.

Bouhuys, A., et al.

Priorities in prevention of chronic lung diseases.

Lung 156(2):129–148, May 18, 1979.

Bouhuys, A., et al.

Epidemiology of enviromental lung disease.

Yale J. Biol. Med. 52(2):191–210, July 1979.

Boulton, T. J. C. and Rowley, M. P.

Nutritional studies during early childhood incidental observations of temperment, habits, and experiences of ill-health.

Aust. Paediatr. J. 15(2):87–90, June 1979.

Bour, H.

Prevention et traitement de l'atherosclerose. (Fr.)

Rev. Prat. 29(7):657-673, Feb. 1, 1979.

Bousser, M.-G.

Le role du medecin traitant dans la prevention des accidents vasculaires cerebraux. (Fr.)

Rev. Med. 20(18):929-933, Apr. 30, 1979.

Bouveng, R., et al.

Effects of LS 1727, a nitrosocarbamate of 19-nortestosterone, on dimethylbenz (a)anthracene-induced mammary tumors in the rat.

Eur. J. Cancer 15(4):407-414, Apr. 1979.

Bowden, G. T. and Yuspa, S. H.

Repair of daughter strand gaps in nascent DNA from mouse epidermal cell treated with dihydrodiol epoxide derivatives of benzo[a]pyrene.

Biochim. Biophys. Acta 565(1):67-83, Nov. 22, 1979.

Bowley, N. B., et al.

The chest X-ray in pulmonary capillary haemorrhage: Correlation with cabon monoxide uptake.

Clin. Radiol. 30(4):413-417, July 1979.

Boyd, G.

The Current Role of Oral Theophylline Derivatives in Respiratory Medicine: The problem of the bronchitic patient.

J. Int. Med. Res. 7(Suppl. 1):36-39, 1979.

Boykin, J., et al.

Role of plasma vasopressin in impaired water excretion of glucocorticoid deficiency.

J. Clin. Invest. 62(4):738-744, Oct. 1978.

Boyland, E.

The history and future of chemical carcinogenesis.

Br. Med. Bull. 36(1):5-10, Jan. 1980.

Bracken, M. B. and Holford, T. R.

Induced abortion and congenital malformations in offspring of subsequent preganancies.

Am. J. Epidemiol. 109(4):425-432, Apr. 1979.

Bracken, M. B., et al.

Role of oral contraception in congential malformations of offspring.

Int. J. Epidemiol. 7(4):309-317, Dec. 1978.

Bradby, G. V. H., et al.

Serum high-density lipoproteins in peripheral vascular disease.

Lancet 2(8103):1271-1274, Dec. 16, 1978.

Bradby, G. V. H., et al.

Serum high-density lipoproteins in peripheral vascular disease.

Lancet 2(8103):1271-1274, Dec. 16, 1978.

Brady, M. E., et al.

Animal model and pharmacokinetic interpretation of nicotine poisoning in man.

Int. J. Clin. Pharmacol. Biopharm. 17(1):12-17, Jan. 1979.

Braeuer, R. and Otto, C.

Die Kupierung pektanfinoeser Schmerzen mit inhaliertem isosorbiddinitrat: Auswertung einer Gragebogenaktion. (Ger.)

Praxis 68(4):117-123, Jan. 23, 1979.

Brailey, Jr., A. G.

The promotion of health through health insurance.

N. Engl. J. Med. 302(1):51-52, Jan. 3, 1980.

Brain, J. D. and Valberg, P. A.

Deposition of aerosol in the respiratory tract.

Am. Rev. Respir. Dis. 120(6):1325-1373, Dec. 1979.

Brambilla, G., et al.

DNA repair synthesis in primary cultures of kidneys from BALB/c and C3H mice treated with dimethylnitrosamine.

Cancer Lett. 5(3):153-159, Sept. 1978.

Brandaenge, S. and Lindblom, L.

The enzyme "aldehyde oxidase" is an iminium oxidase. Reaction with nicotine delta1' (5')iminium ion.

Biochem. Biophys. Res. Commun. 91(3):991-996, Dec. 14, 1979.

Brandeburg, J.

Inhalation injury: Carbon monoxide poisoning.

Am. J. Nurs. 80(1):98-100, Jan. 1980.

Brandsborg, O., et al.

The effect of exercise, smoking and propranolol on serum gastrin in patients with duodenal ulcer and in vagotomized subjects.

Scand. J. Clin. Lab. Invest. 38(5): 441-446, Sept. 1978.

Brant, N. K. and Stevenson, T. D.

Ohio Cancer Information Service.

Ohio State Med. J. 75(7):440-441, July 1979.

Brass, A.

American letter: Where there's smoke.

Br. J. Hosp. Med. 21(3):316, Mar. 1979.

Braun, S. R. and Tsiatis, A.

Pulmonary abnormalities in art glassblowers.

JOM 21(7):487-489, July 1979.

Braun, S. R., et al.

Farmer's lung disease: Long-term clinical and physiologic outcome.

Am. Rev. Respir. Dis. 119(2):185-191, Feb. 1979.

Brecher, E. M.

Smoking: For most, a sentence to nicotine addiction.

Med. World News 20(5):61-68;72-73, Mar. 5, 1979.

Breckenridge, A. M., et al.

The Induction of Drug Metabolism. Biochemical Characterization and Toxicological Effects of Drug Metabolism. Discussion.

Symp. Med. Hoechst 14:327-340, 1979.

Breddin, K., et al.

Transactions of the Annual Meeting of the International Committee on Thrombosis and Haemostasis. Secondary prevention of myocardial infarction. Comparison of acetylsalicylic acid, phenprocoumon and placebo: A multicenter two-year prospective study.

Thromb. Haemost. 40(1):225-236, Feb. 28, 1979.

Breithaupt, H. and Walter, P.

Behandlung der Angina pectoris (I). (Ger.)

Med. Welt 30(2):39-46, Jan. 12, 1979.

Bremond, G., et al.

A propos de deux cas de coincidence d'un epithelioma spino-cellulaire larynge et d'un epithelioma papillaire thyroidien. (Fr.)

J. Fr. Otolrhinolaryngol. 27(8):547-551, Oct. 1978.

Bresnick, E., et al.

Benzo[a]pyrene metabolism in neonatal rat liver nuclei.

Chem. Biol. Interact. 24(1):111-115, Jan. 1979.

Bridges, J. W. and Fry, J. R.

The Induction of Drug Metabolism: The Effects of pretreatment with various inducing agents on extrahepatic induction.

Symp. Med. Hoechst 14:453-469, 1979.

Bridges, J. W. and Fry, J. R.

The Induction of Drug Metabolism. Chairman's introductory statement: The use of isolated liver cell preparations for studying the induction of mixed function oxidase.

Symp. Med. Hoechst 14:343-354, 1979.

Bridges, R. A., et al.

Cigarette smoking - Does it carry a genetic risk?

Mutat. Res. 65(1):71-81, Mar. 1979.

Brin, M. and Roe, D.

Drug-diet interactions.

J. Fla. Med. Assoc. 66(4):424-428, Apr. 1979.

Osteomalacia may be due to abuse of certain laxatives including mineral oil and phenolphthalein.

Broder, I., et al.

Comparison of respiratory variables in grain elevator workers and civic outside workers of Thunder Bay, Canada.

Am. Rev. Respir. Dis. 119(2):193-203, Feb. 1979.

Brodie, A. M. H., et al.

Proceedings of the International Congress on Hormonal Steroids: Aromatase inhibitors and their use in controlling oestrogen-dependent processes.

J. Steroid Biochem. 11(1A):107-112, July 1979.

Brodie, A. M. H. and Lomgcope, C.

Inhibition of peripheral aromatization by aromatase inhibitors, 4-hydroxy-and 4-acetoxy-androstene-3,17-dione.

Endocrinology 106(1):19-21, Jan. 1980.

Broll, M., et al.

Etude pharmacologique d'un antiparkinsonien potentiel: La diprobutine.(Fr.)

J. Pharmacol. (Paris) 9(2):121-131, Apr.-June 1978.

Brookes, P.

The binding to mouse skin DNA of benzo[a]pyrene, its 7,8-diol and 7,8-diol-9,10-epoxides in relation to the tumourigenicity of these compounds.

Cancer Lett. 6(4-5):285-289, Apr. 1979.

Brown, E. R., et al.

Aquatic Pollutants and Biologic Effects with Emphasis on Neoplasia: Chemical pollutants in relation to diseases in fish.

Ann. NY Acad. Sci. 298:535-546, Sept. 29, 1977.

Brown, H. S., et al.

Formation of DNA adducts in 10T1/2 mouse embryo fibroblasts incubated with benzo(a)pyrene or dihydrodiol oxide derivatives.

Cancer Res. 39(5):1673-1677, May 1979.

Brown, J. S.

A coronary screening programme in general practice.

J. R. Coll. Gen. Pract. 28(197):735-742, Dec. 1978.

Brown, M. M.

Literature survey of bacterial, fungal, and Drosophila assay systems used in the evaluation of selected chemical compounds for mutagenic activity.

JNCI 62(4):841-871, Apr. 1979.

Brown, T. R., et al.

Effect of the Tfm locus on the hepatic ethylmorphine N-demethylase system in mice.

Endocrinology 103(4):1374-1382, Oct. 1978.

Brown, W. T.

Human mutations affecting aging - A review.

Mech. Ageing Dev. 9(3-4):325-336, Feb. 1979.

Bruce, R. A., et al.

Noninvasive screening criteria for enhanced 4-year survival after aorto-coronary bypass surgery.

Circulation 60(3):638-646, Sept. 1979.

Brunnemann, K. D. and Hoffmann, D.

Environmental Aspects of N-Nitroso Compounds: Chemical studies on tobacco smoke LIX. Analysis of volatile nitrosamines in tobacco smoke and polluted indoor environments.

IARC Sci. Publ. No. 19:343-356, 1978.

Bruppacher, R., et al.

Entwicklung von Risikofaktoren fuer kardiovaskulaere Krankheiten im Laufe der Adoleszenz: Erste Resultate des Follow-up der Adoleszenten-studie Basel-Stadt. (Ger.)

Soz. Praeventivmed. 24(4):234-235, Aug. 1979.

Brusick, D. J.

Alterations of germ cells leading to mutagenesis and their detection.

Environ. Health Perspect. 24:105-112, June 1978.

Buchanan-Davidson, D. J.

Cancer epidemiology: Part IV.

Wis. Med. J. 77(9):18, Sept. 1978.

Buchkremer, G.

Raucherbehandlung. (Ger.)

Fortschr. Neurol. Psychiatr. 46(11):613-624, nov. 1978.

Buechler, J. R.

Cigarette smoking in family practice.

J. Indiana State Med. Assoc. 72(5):360-361, May 1979.

Buecker, M., et al.

Mutagenicity of phenanthrene and phenanthrene K-region derivatives.

Mutat. Res. 66(4):337-348, Apr. 1979.

Buening, M. K., et al.

Tumorigenicity of the optical enantiomers of the diastereomeric benzo[a]pyrene 7,8-diol-9,10-epoxides in newborn mice: Exceptional activity of (plus)-7beta,8alpha-dihydroxy-9alpha, 10alpha-epoxy-7,8,9,10-tetrahydrobenzo[a]pyrene.

Proc. Natl. Acad. Sci. USA 75(11):5358-5361, Nov. 1978.

Buening, M. K., et al.

Tumorigenicity of the dihydrodiols of dibenzo(a,h)anthracene on mouse skin and in newborn mice.

Cancer Res. 39(4):1310-1314, Apr. 1979.

Buening, M. K., et al.

Tumorigenic activity of benzo(e) pyrene derivatives on mouse skin and in newborn mice.

Cancer Res. 40(2):203-206, Feb. 1980.

Buerki, H. R.

Pharmacological Methods in Toxicology: Extrapyramidal side-effects.

Pharmacol. Ther. 5(1-3, Suppl.):325-534, 1979.

Buffler, P. A., et al.

Mortality experience of workers in a vinyl chloride monomer production plant.

JOM 21(3):195-203, Mar. 1979.

Buhl, J. M., et al.

Smokers vs. nonsmokers: Understanding their differences.

Health Educ. 8(1):11-12, Jan.-Feb. 1977.

Buhr, J. and Schuetz, J.

Diabetes mellitus und koronare Herzerkrankung - gemeinsame Probleme bei der Langzeitbetreuung. (Ger.)

Z. Gesamte Inn. Med. 34(2):82-86, Jan. 15, 1979.

Buist, A. S.

The relative contributions of nature and nurture in chronic obstructive pulmonary disease.

West. J. Med. 131(2):114-121, Aug. 1979.

Buist, A. S., et al.

Relationship between the single-breath N2, test and age, sex, and smoking habit in three North American cities.

Am. Rev. Respir. Dis. 120(2): 305-318, Aug. 1978.

Buist, A. S., et al.

The effect of smoking cessation on pulmonary function: A 30-month follow-up of two smoking cessation clinics.

Am. Rev. Respir. Dis. 120(4):953-957, Oct. 1979.

Buist, A. S., et al.

Pulmonary function in heterozygotes for alpha,-antitrypsin deficiency: A case control study.

Am. Rev. Respir. Dis. 120(4):759-766, Oct. 1979.

Buist, S. and Nagy, J.

Proceedings of the Aspen Lung Conference. A longitudinal study of smokers and nonsmokers: 5-6 Year follow-up using spirometry and the single breath N2 test.

Chest 77(2 Suppl.):259, Feb. 1980.

Bulay, O. and Mirvish, S. S.

Carcinogenesis in rat esophagus by intraperitoneal injection of different doses of methyl-n-amylnitrosamine.

Cancer Res. 39(9):3644-3646, Sept. 1979.

Bulay, O., et al.

Carcinogenicity test of six nitrosamides and a nitrosocyanamide administered orally to rats.

JNCI 62(6):1523-1528, June 1979.

Burch, P. R. J.

Coronary disease: Risk factors, age and time.

Am. Heart J. 97(4):415-419, Apr. 1979.

Burdon, J. G. W. and Cade, J. F.

"Barbiturate burns" caused by glutethimide.

Med. J. Aust. 1(3):101-102, Feb. 10, 1979.

Burger, R., et al.

Rationelle Therapie uunter Beruecksichtigung von Uebergewicht, Rauchen, Alkolholmissbranch und chronischer Selbstmedikation als Krankheitsfaktoren. (Ger.)

Therapiewoche 28(45):8687-8690, Nov. 8, 1978.

Burgess, R. E., et al.

Brain metastases in small cell carcinoma of the lung.

JAMA 242(19):2084-2086, Nov. 9, 1979.

Burke, D. H.

Cobaltous chloride-induced hypothermia in mice I: Effect of pretreatment with anticholinergic drugs.

J. Pharm. Sci. 67(6):799-801, June 1978.

Burke, M. J., et al.

Trigeminal neuropathy as the presenting symptom of systemic sclerosis.

Postgrad. Med. J. 55(644):423-425, June 1979.

Burleson, G. R., et al.

Ozonation of mutagenic and carinogenic polyaromatic amines and polyaromatic hydrocarbons in water.

Cancer Res. 39(6, Part 1):2149-2154, June 1979.

Burman, L. G.

DNA-skadande agens vaar tids stoersta hot mot folkhaelsan? (Swed.)

Lakartidningen 76(19):1823-1825, May 9, 1979.

Burnet, F. M.

Cancer: Somatic-genetic considerations.

Adv. Cancer Res. 28:1-29, 1978.

Burnett, A. K.

Thyroid hormone in 7,12-dimethylbenz(a)anthracene-induced leukemia in rats.

Cancer Res. 39(10):4252-4255, Oct. 1979.

Burr, J. M., et al.

Miami Multiple Risk Factor Intervention Trial (MRFIT). An experiment in coronary heart disease prevention in high risk med age 35-57: Preliminary report.

J. Fla. Med. Assoc. 66(4):482-488, Apr. 1979.

Burrows, B.

Proceedings of the Aspen Lung Conference: Course and prognosis of patients with chronic airways obstruction.

Chest 77(2 Suppl.):250-251, Feb. 1980.

Busch, F. W., et al.

Mutagenic activity of marihuana smoke condensates.

Cancer Lett. 6(6):319-324, May 1979.

Busch, S., et al.

Kongress der Deutschen Gesellschaft fuer Lungekrankheiten und Tuberlose: Fruehergassung bronchialer Erkrankungen bei jugendlichen Rauchern. (Ger.)

Prax. Klin. Pneumol. 33(Spec. Issue 1):651-654, Apr. 1979.

Buynitzky, S. J., et al.

Effect of viral infection on drug metabolism and pesticide disposition in ducks.

Toxicol. Appl. Pharmacol. 46(2):267-278, Nov. 1978.

Bylock, A., et al.

Surface ultrastructure of human arteries with special reference to the effects of smoking.

Acta Pathol. Microbiol. Scand. [A] 87(3): 201-209, May 1979.

Byng, G. S., et al.

Biosynthesis of phenazine pigments in mutant and wild-type cultures of Pseudomonas aeruginosa.

J. Bacteriol. 138(3):846-852, June 1979.

Cadwell, E. J., et al.

Serum alpha-1-antitrypsin deficiency in Maine young people.

J. Maine Med. Assoc. 69(9):252-256, Sept. 1978.

Cady, B.

Smokers should pay the medical costs of smoking.

Resident Staff Physician 25(4):44, Apr. 1979.

Cain, H. D., et al.

Preoperative pulmonary function and complications after cardiovascular surgery.

Chest 76(2):130-135, Aug. 1979.

Calabrese, E. J.

Should the concept of the recommended dietary allowance be altered to incorporate interactive effects of ubiquitous pollutants?

Med. Hypotheses 5(12):1273-1285, Dec. 1979.

Calaresu, F. R., et al.

Electrophysiological characteristics of renorenal reflexes in the cat.

J. Physiol. (Lond.) 283:141-154, 1978.

Calleman, C. J., et al.

Monitoring and risk assessment by means of alkyl groups in hemoglobin in persons occupationally exposed to ethylene oxide.

J. Environ. Pathol. Toxicol. 2(2):427-442, Nov.-Dec. 1978.

Calsini, L., et al.

Effet de la fumee de cigarette sur les properties elastiques du poumon du rat. (Fr.)

Bronchopneumologie 28(4):278-282, July-Aug. 1978.

Calvert, J. P. and Richards, C. J.

Fetal breathing movements and fetal distress.

Br. J. Obstet. Gynaecol. 86(8):607-611, Aug. 1979.

Cam, G. R., et al.

The action of nicotine on the pituitary-adrenal cortical axis.

Arch. Int. Pharmacodyn. Ther. 237(1): 49-66, Jan. 1979.

Camarasa, G. and Alomar, A.

Menthol dermatitis from cigarettes.

Contact Dermatitis 4(3):169-170, June 1978.

Cameron, E., et al.

Ascorbic acid and cancer: A review.

Cancer Res. 39(3):663-681, Mar. 1979.

Camner, P., et al.

Elimination of test particles from the human tracheobronchial tract by voluntary coughing.

Scand. J. Respir. Dis. 60(2):56-62, Apr. 1979.

Campbell, E. J., et al.

Receptor-mediated binding and internalization of leukocyte elastase by alveolar macrophages in vitro.

J. Clin. Invest. 64(3):824-833, Sept. 1979.

Campbell, M. D., et al.

The lack of an effect of cholinergic agonists on anterior pituitary prolactin production in vitro.

Experientia 34(11):1522-1523, Nov. 15, 1978.

Campbell, M. J., et al.

Sequential immunological studies in an asbestos-exposed population: Factors affecting lymphocyte function.

Clin. Exp. Immunol. 39(1):176-182, Jan. 1980.

Campbell, R. L., et al.

Rat liver microsome-mediated N-demethylation and mutagenicity of azoxymethane.

Cancer Res. 38(12):4585-4590, Dec. 1978.

Campbell, R. L., et al.

Rat liver microsome-mediated N-demethylation and mutagenicity of azoxymethane.

Cancer Res. 38(12):4585-4590, Dec. 1978.

Campbell, T. C., et al.

Dietary lipotropes, hepatic microsomal mixed-function oxidase activities, and in vivo covalent binding of aflatoxin B1 in rats.

Cancer Res. 38(12):4569-4573, Dec. 1978.

Cantrell, E. T., et al.

Secondary metabolism of benzo(a) pyrene in human cells.

Proc. West. Pharmacol. Soc. 22:273-276, 1979.

Capdevila, J., et al.

The existence of a benzo(a)pyrene-3, 6-quinone reductase in rat liver microsomal fractions.

Biochem. Biophys. Res. Commun. 83(4):1291-1298, Aug. 29, 1978.

Capel, I. D., et al.

The effect of anti-cancer drugs on the plasma disposition of antipyrine and the biliary excretion of phenolphthalein in the rat.

Biochem. Pharmacol. 27(10):1413-1416, May 15, 1978.

Card, J. P. and Mitchell, J. A.

The effects of nicotine on implantation in the rat.

Biol. Reprod. 20(3):532-539, Apr. 1979.

Carlens, E.

Jagar vi fel bov i cigaretten? (Swed.)

Lakartidningen 75(40):3531-3533, Oct. 4, 1978.

Carlson, L. A., et al.

Risk factors for myocardial infarction inthe Stockholm prospective study: A 14-year old follow-up focusing on the role of plasma triglycerides and cholesterol.

Acta Med. Scand. 206(5):351-360, 1979.

Carluccio, L., et al.

Serial CEA levels in colorectal carcinoma on adjuvant immuno (chemo) therapy.

J. Surg. Oncol. 10(6):511-517, 1978.

Carp, H. and Janoff, A.

Possible mechanisms of emphysema in smokers: In vitro suppression of serum elastase-inhibitory capacity by fresh cigarette smoke and its prevention by antioxidants.

Am. Rev. Respir. Dis. 118(3):617-621, Sept. 1978.

Carter, P. K.

Carinoid tumors at MMC - 1955-1978: Part-1 bronchial.

J. Maine Med. Assoc. 70(10):402-405, Oct. 1979.

Carter, S. K.

Introduction - What has happened in the last five years.

Prog. Cancer Res. Ther. 11:1-12, 1979.

Carver, J. H., et al.

Estimating maximum limits to mutagenic potency from cytotoxic potency.

Nature 279(5709):154-156, May 10, 1979.

Castellano, C.

Effects of mescaline and psilocin on asquistion, consolidation, and performance of light-dark discrimination in two inbred strains of mice.

Psychopharmacology 59(2):129-137, Oct. 31, 1978.

Castello, D., et al.

Indagine sulle relazioni intercorrenti fra fumo di sigaretta nell'ambiente e patologia respiratoria pediatrica: Primi resultati. (Ital.)

Minerva Pediatr. 30(19):1489-1496, Oct. 15, 1978.

Castonguay, A. and Van Vunakis, H.

Radioimmunoassay of N'-nitrosonornicotine.

Anal. Biochem. 95(2):387-396, June 1979.

Castro, A., et al.

Automated radioimmunoassay of nicotine.

Clin. Chim. Acta 95(3):473-481, Aug. 1, 1979.

Casula, D., et al.

Changes in respiratory symptoms in the pulmonary function in a 3-year follow-up study of dust exposed workers.

Bronchopneumologie 28(6):463-478, Nov.-Dec. 1978.

Caulfield, M. J., et al.

Ozonation of mutagenic and carinogenic alkylating agents, pesticides, aflatoxin B1, and benzidine in water.

Cancer Res. 39(6, Part 1):2155-2159, June 1979.

Cerniglia, C. E. and Gibson, D. T.

Oxidation of benzo[a]pyrene by the filamentous fungus Cunninghamella elegans.

J. Biol. Chem. 254(23):12174-12180, Dec. 10, 1979.

Cerutti, H.

Der Krebs als geographisches Problem. (Ger.)

Ther. Ggw. 118(4):485-509, Apr. 1979.

Cha, Y.-N.

Inducibility of the hepatic drug-metabolizing capacity of mice infected with Schistosoma mansoni.

Am. J. Trop. Med. Hyg. 27(6):1181-1187, Nov. 1978.

Cha, Y.-N. and Bueding, E.

Effect of 2(3)-tert-butyl-4-hydroxy anisole administration on the activities of several hepatic microsomal and cytoplasmic enzymes in mice.

Biochem. Pharmacol. 28(12): 1917-1921, June 15, 1979.

Cha, Y.-N., et al.

Enhancement of liver microsome epoxide hydratase activity in rodents by treatment with 2(3)-tert-butyl-4-hydroxyanisole.

Cancer Res. 38(12):4496-4498, Dec. 1978.

Cha, Y.-N., et al.

Enhancement of liver microsome epoxide hydratase activity in rodents by treatment with 2(3)-tert-butyl-4-hydroxyanisole.

Cancer Res. 38(12):4496-4498, Dec. 1978.

Chahl, L. A. and Cross, R. B.

The nature of the pressor response to carotid artery occlusion in the hexamethonium-treated rat.

Clin. Exp. Pharmacol. Physiol. 5(5):495-502, Sept.-Oct. 1978.

Chakravorty, R. C., et al.

Necrotizing sialometaplasia of palate.

Br. J. Surg. 66(4):283-284, Apr. 1979.

Chalmers, D. M., et al.

Sex-related differences in the haematological effects of excessive alcohol consumption.

J. Clin. Pathol. 33(1):3-7, Jan. 1980.

Chalmers, D. M., et al.

Mean cell volume in a working population: The effect of age, smoking alcohol and oral contraception.

Br. J. Haematol. 43(4):631-636, Dec. 1979.

Chalon, J., et al.

Tracheobronchial cytologic changes in malignant melanoma.

Arch. Pathol. Lab. Med. 102(12):631-634, Dec. 1978.

Chalon, J., et al.

Humidity and the anesthetized patient.

Anesthesiology 50(3):195-198, Mar. 1979.

Chamberlain, G.

Background to perinatal health.

Lancet 2(8151):1061-1063, Nov. 17, 1979.

Chamberlain, W. J., et al.

Analysis of a tumor-inhibiting fraction of tobacco smoke condensate.

J. Anal. Toxicol. 2(5):138-140, July-Aug. 1978.

Chan-Yeung, M., et al.

Respiratory abnormalities among grain elevator workers.

Chest 75(4):461-467, Apr. 1979.

Chan, W. C., et al.

Bronchial cancer in Hong Kong 1976-1977.

Br. J. Cancer 39(2):182-192, Feb. 1979.

Chang, C.-C., et al.

Effects of harman and norharman on spontaneous and ultraviolet light-induced mutagenesis in cultured Chinese hamster cells.

Cancer Res. 38(12):4527-4533, Dec. 1978.

Chang, G. T., et al.

Inactivation of SV40 replication by derivatives of benzo[a]pyrene.

Biochem. Biophys. Res. Commun. 88(2): 688-695, May 28, 1979.

Chang, R. L., et al.

Carcinogenicity of 2-hydroxybenzo(a)-pyrene and 6-hydroxybenzo(a)pyrene in newborn mice.

Cancer Res. 39(7, Part 1):2660-2664, July 1979.

Chang, R. L., et al.

Differences in mutagenicity and cytotoxiciy of (plus)- and (minus)-benzo[a] pyrene 4,5-oxide: A synergistic interaction of enantiomers.

Proc. Natl. Acad. Sci. USA 76(9): 4280-4284, Sept. 1979.

Chang, S.-K., et al.

Accelerating effect of ascorbic acid on n-nitrosamine formation and nitrosation by oxyhyponitrite.

Cancer Res. 39(10):3871-3874, Oct. 1979.

Chapman, P. H., et al.

Activity of aryl hydrocarbon hydroxylase in psoriatic skin.

Lancet 1(8111):297-298, Feb. 10, 1979.

Chappell, F.

Smoking health hazards reduced after quitting: Smoking halt can be tough.

Phila. Med. 75(6):253, June 1979.

Chaput, J.-C., et al.

Relations entre le volume globulaire moyen, les consommations alcooliques et tabagiques et l'existence de maladies alcoooliques du foie chez des malades hospitalises. (Fr.)

Gastroenterol. Clin. Biol. 3(3):221-226, Mar. 1979.

Charan, N. B., et al.

Pulmonary injuries associated with acute sulfur dioxide inhalation.

Am. Rev. Respir. Dis. 119(4):555-560, Apr. 1979.

Charpin, D., et al.

Bronchodilator effects of antiasthmatic cigarette smoke (Datura stramonium).

Thorax 34(2):259-261, Apr. 1979.

Chase, M. W.

Irreverent recollections from Cooke and Coca 1928-1978.

J. Allergy Clin. Immunol. 64(5): 306-320, Nov. 1979.

Chau, I. Y. and Archer, M. C.

Inhibition of rat hepatic dimethylnitrosamine demethylase by cyclic and acyclic nitrosamines and secondary amines.

Experientia 34(11):1505-1506, Nov. 15, 1978.

Chau, I. Y., et al.

Kinetic studies on the hepatic microsomal metabolism of dimethylnitrosamine, diethylnitrosamine, and methylethylnitrosamine in the rat.

JNCI 61(2):517-521, Aug. 1978.

Chen, C. B.

Assay for microsomal alpha-hydroxylation of N'-nitrosonornicotine and determination of the deuterium isotope effect for alpha-hydroxylation.

Cancer Res. 39(12):5057-5062, Dec. 1979.

Chenery, R. J. and McLean, A. E. M.

Stimulation of aryl hydrocarbon hydroxylase activity in cultured cells by human and animal sera: A new approach to human drug metabolism.

Biochem. Pharmacol. 29(3):271-276, Feb. 1, 1980.

Cheng, J.-T. and Araki, H.

Inhibitory mechanisms of dexamethasone on contractions induced by drugs and by transmural stimulations in isolated guinea pig ileum.

Jpn. J. Pharmacol. 28(5):755-762, Oct. 1978.

Chernow, B. and Castell, D. O.

Diet and heartburn.

JAMA 241(21):2307-2308, May 25, 1979.

Chernow, B., et al.

Pulmonary aspiration as a consequence of gastroesophageal reflux: A diagnostic approach.

Digest. Dis. Sci. 24(11):839-844, Nov. 1979.

Cherrier, F., et al.

Profil epidemiologique des sujets porteurs d'un infarctus avec coronarographie normale. (Fr.)

Arch. Mal. Coeur 72(1):26-31, Jan. 1979.

Chester, E. H. and Schwartz, H. J.

Study session on occupational asthma.

J. Allergy Clin. Immunol. 64(6, Part 2): 665-666, Dec. 1979.

Chevrier, A., et al.

Isolation and characterization of a mesenchyme associated antigen from dimethylbenzanthracene induced rat fibrosarcoma.

Biomedicine 30(4):219-223, Oct. 1979.

Chicou, F. J.

La lutte antitabagique en France. (Fr.)

Med. Hyg. 36(1301):3058-3062, Sept. 27, 1978.

Chien, P. T. and Thomas, M. H.

Evaluation of a degradation method for nitrosamine wastes.

J. Environ. Pathol. Toxicol. 2(2):513-516, Nov.-Dec. 1978.

Chilvers, C., et al.

Alcohol and oesophgeal cancer: An assessment of the evidence from routinely collected data.

J. Epidemiol. Commun. Health 33(2): 127-133, June 1979.

Cho-Chung, Y. S., et al.

Nuclear protein phosphorylation and hormone-dependent mammary tumor regression following dibutyryl cyclic adenosine 3':5'-monophosphate treatment or ovariectomy.

Cancer Res. 38(10):3405-3409, Oct. 1978.

Cho-Chung, Y. S. and Doud, F. J.

Antagonistic action between cyclic AMP and estrogen in phosphorylation of mammary tumor nuclear proteins.

Cancer Lett. 5(4):219-224, Oct. 1978.

Cho, D. K., et al.

Effects of smoking on lung volume and intrapulmonary gas mixing. (Korean)

Korean J. Intern. Med. 20(12):1098-1102, Dec. 1977.

Chodynicki, S. and Tupalska, M.

Wplyw palenia tytoniu i innych czynnikow drazniacych na blone sluzowa krtani i tchawicy. (Pol.)

Wiad. Lek. 32(5):299-304, Mar. 1, 1979.

Chole, R. A. and Domb, G. H.

Differential diagnosis of superficial ulcerations of the oral mucosa.

Otolaryngol. Head Neck Surg. 87(6):734-740, Nov.-Dec. 1979.

Choo, L. K. and Mitchelson, F.

Antagonism of cholinomimetics by troxypyrrolidinium in guinea-pig atria and longitudinal ileal muscle: Comparison with hemicholinium-3.

Eur. J. Pharmacol. 52(3-4):313-322, Dec. 1, 1978.

Chopra, J. S. and Prabhakar, S.

Clinical features and risk factors in stroke in young.

Acta Neurol. Scand. 60(5):289-300, 1979.

Chopra, P., et al.

Kupffer cell sarcoma in rats after exposure to small doses of dimethylnitrosamine and N-2-acetylaminofluorene during hepatic regeneration.

JNCI 62(4):1089-1095, Apr. 1979.

Chopra, S. K., et al.

Lung clearance of soluble radioaerosols of different molecular weights in systemic sclerosis.

Thorax 34(1):63-67, Feb. 1979.

Chouroulinkov, I., et al.

Biological activities of dihydrodiols derived from two polycyclic hydrocarbons in rodent test systems.

Br. J. Cancer 39(4):376-382, Apr. 1979.

Chovil, A. C.

Occupational lung cancer and smoking: A review in the light of current theories of carcinogenesis.

Can. Med. Assoc. J. 121(5):548-555, Sept. 8, 1979.

Chretien, J.

Le role du tabac dans les perturbations des defenses immunitaires pulmonaires. (Fr.)

Nouv. Presse Med. 8(25):2131-2134, June 7, 1979.

Chretien, J.

Quelques reflexions sur la prevention du tabagisme. (Fr.)

Med. Hyg. 37(1330):1472-1474, Apr. 25, 1979.

Christ, D.

Effects of nicotine and hexamethonium on discharge in the stellate ganglion.

Eur. J. Pharmacol. 54(3):243-249, Mar. 1, 1979.

Christen, A. G. and Cooper, K. H.

Stategic withdrawal from cigarette smoking.

CA 29(2):96-107, Mar.-Apr. 1979.

Christensen, A.

Kost, levevaner og sundhed. (Dan.)

Ugeskr. Laeger 140(37):2250-2252, Sept. 1978.

Christensen, J. M. and Angelo, H.

A rapid direct determination of cadmium in blood by anodic stripping voltammetry.

Scand. J. Clin. Lab. Invest. 38(7):655-658, Nov. 1978.

Christianson, M. L. and Chiscon, J. O.

Use of haploid plants as bioassays for mutagens.

Environ. Health Perspect. 27:77-83, Dec. 1978.

Christianson, R. E.

Gross differences observed in the placentas of smokers and nonsmokers.

Am. J. Epidemiol. 110(2):178-187, Aug. 1979.

Chu, J. T. and Jurs, P. C.

Computer assisted structure-activity studies of chemical carcinogeUy pn N-nitroso compound data set.

J. Med. Chem. 22(7):792-797, July 1979.

Churg, A. M. and Warnock, M. L.

Analysis of the cores of ferruginous (asbestos) bodies from the general population: III. Patients with environmental exposure.

Lab. Invest. 40(5):622-626, May 1979.

Churg, A. M. and Warnock, M. L.

Numbers of asbestos bodies in urban patients with lung cancer and gastrointestinal cancer and in matched controls.

Chest 76(2):143-149, Aug. 1979.

Clague, H. W. and Hall, D. R.

Effect of posture on lung volume: Airway closure and gas exchange in hemidiaphragmatic paralysis.

Thorax 34(4):523-526, Aug. 1979.

Clapp, N. K., et al.

Selective sex-related modification of diethylnitrosamine-induced carcinogenesis in BALB/c mice by concomitant administration of butylated hydroxytoluene.

JNCI 61(1):177-182, July 1978.

Clark, R. R.

Reactions to other people's cigarette smoking.

Int. J. Addict. 13(8):1237-1244, 1978.

Clarke, G., et al.

Effects of cholinoceptor antagonists on the suckling-induced and experimentally evoked release of oxytocin.

Br. J. Pharmacol. 63(3):519-527, July 1978.

Classen, W. and Baettig, K.

Wirkung von Nikotin und amphetamine auf die Regulation des Koerpergewichts. (Ger.)

Soz. Praventivmed. 22(4):197-198, July-Aug. 1977.

Claus, D. and Kornhuber, H. H.

Vor allem das inhalierende Zigarettenrauchen reduzieren. (Ger.)

MMW 121(48):1583-1584, Nov. 30, 1979.

Clayton, J. K., et al.

Effect of cigarette smoking on subsequent postoperative thromboembolic disease in gynaecological patients.

Br. Med. J. 2(6134):402, Aug. 5, 1978.

Clemmesen, J.

Luftvejssygdomme blandt skoleboern i Fredericia. (Letter to the Editor.) (Dan.)

Ugeskr. Laeger 140(7):380-381, Feb. 13, 1978.

Clemmesen, J. and Hjalgrim-Jensen, S.

Is isonicotinic acid hydrazide (INH) carcinogenic to man? A 24-year follow up of 3371 tuberculosis cases.

Ecotoxicol. Environ. Safety 3(4):439-450, Dec. 1979.

Clemmesen, J., et al.

Epidemiologi, bronchitis og lungekraeft. (Letters to the Editor.) (Dan.)

Ugeskr. Laeger 140(18):1067-1068, May 1, 1978.

Cleveland, P. H., et al.

Tumour-associated antigens of chemically-induced murine tumors: The emergence of MuLV and fetal antigens after serial passage in culture.

Int. J. Cancer 23(3):380-391, Mar. 15, 1979.

Clinton, S. K., et al.

Dietary protein, aryl hydrocarbon hydroxylase and chemical carcinogenesis in rats.

J. Nutr. 109(1):55-62, Jan. 1979.

Clive, D., et al.

Validation and characterization of the L5178Y/TKplus/minus mouse lymphoma mutagen assay system.

Mutat. Res. 59(1):61-108, Jan. 1979.

Clothier, C.

Symposium. Awkward Medicolegal Problems in Asbestos-Induced Disease: Problems in law.

J. R. Soc. Med. 71(12):922-925, Dec. 1978.

Coburn, R. F.

Workshop on Carbon Monoxide and Cardiovascular Disease: Mechanisms of carbon monoxide toxicity.

Prev. Med. 8(3):310-322, May 1979.

Coco, R., et al.

L'incidenza di alcuni fattori di rischio in una casistica ospedaliera di primi infarti miocardici acuti. (Ital.)

Boll. Soc. Ital. Cardiol. 22(2):205-212, 1977.

Coffman, J. D.

Intermittent claudication and rest pain: Physiologic concepts and therapeutic approaches.

Prog. Cardiovasc. Dis. 22(1):53-72, July/Aug. 1979.

Cohen, A. B.

Potential adverse effects of lung macrophages and neutrophils.

Fed. Proc. 38(12):2644-2647, Nov. 1979.

Cohen, A. B.

Opportunities for the development of specific therapeutic agents to treat emphysema.

Am. Rev. Respir. Dis. 120(4): 723-727, Oct. 1979.

Cohen, B. H.

Is pulmonary dysfunction the common denominator for the multiple effects of cigarette smoking?

Lancet 2(8089):1024-1027, Nov. 11, 1978.

Cohen, B. H., et al.

Proceedings of the Aspen Lung Conference: Multiple factors in airways obstruction.

Chest 77(2 Suppl.):257-159, Feb. 1980.

Cohen, B. M.

Respiratory responses to one year or daily use of a cosmetic hair spray.

Lung 155(4):309-320, Dec. 15, 1978.

Cohen, B. S., et al.

Distribution of polonium-210 in the human lung.

Radiat. Res. 79(1):162-168, July 1979.

Cohen, C. I. an Cohen, E. J.

Health education: Panacea, pernicious or pointless?

N. Engl. J. Med. 299(13):718-720, Sept. 28, 1978.

Cohen, C. R., et al.

Calcification of the basal ganglia as visualized by computed tomography.

Radiology 134(1):97-99, Jan. 1980.

Cohen, D., et al.

Smoking impairs long-term dust clearance from the lung.

Science 204(4392):514-516, May 4, 1979.

Cohen, F. L.

A survey of smoking in institutions that educate health professionals.

Public Health Rep. 94(6):544-552, Nov.-Dec. 1979.

Cohen, G. M., et al.

Comparative metabolism of benzo(a)pyrene in organ and cell cultures derived from rat tracheas.

Cancer Res. 39(6, Part 1):1980-1984, June 1979.

Cohen, G. M., et al.

Anticarcinogenic effects of 2,3,7,8-tetrachlorodibenzo-p-dioxin on benzo (a)pyrene and 7,12-dimethlybenz(a) anthracene tumor initiation and its relationship to DNA binding.

Cancer Res. 39(10):4027-4033, Oct. 1979.

Cohen, G. M., et al.

Metabolism and macromolecular binding of carcinogenic and noncarcinogenic metabolites of benzo(a)pyrene by hamster embryo cells.

Cancer Res. 40(2):207-211, Feb. 1980.

Cohen, I. K., et al.

Collagen synthesis in capsules surrounding dimethylbenzanthracene-induced rat breast tumors and the effect of pretreatment with beta-aminopropiontrile.

Cancer Res. 39(8):2923-2927, Aug. 1979.

Cohen, S.

The volitional disorders.

Clin. Toxicol. 13(5):633-639, 1978.

Cohen, W. R. and Friedman, E. A.

Etiology and management of premature labor.

Curr. Probl. Obstet. Gynacol. 1(9): 1-42, May 1978.

Cohn, V. H.

Cigarette smoking and the response to drugs.

Am. Pharm. NS18(10):32-36, Sept. 1978.

Coles, S. J., et al.

Hypersecretion of mucus glycoproteins in rat airways induced by tobacco smoke.

Am. J Pathol. 94(3):459-472, Mar. 1979.

Collan, Y., et al.

Laeaekaerien kuolleisuus vuosina 1953-1972: II. Mieslaeaekaerien kuolemansyyt. (Finn.)

Soum. Laaeaekaeril. 33(35):2797-2799, Dec. 10, 1978.

Collimedaglia, P., et al.

Il cancro bronchiale: Studio retrospettivo su 1000 casi. (Ital.)

Friuli Med. 32(3):147-158, May-June 1977.

Collins, Jr., F. L. and Epstein, L. H.

Temporal analysis of cigarette smoking.

Addict. Behav. 3(2):93-97, 1978.

Collins, R. L., et al.

Cardiopulmonary manifestations of systemic lupus erythematosus.

J. Rheumatol. 5(3):299-306, Fall 1978.

Colonna, J., et al.

L'importance de l'intoxication tabagique en pheumologie. (Fr.)

Med. Hyg. 36(1311):4050-4053, Dec. 6, 1978.

Colpaert, F. C.

Discriminative stimulus properties of narcotic analgesic drugs.

Pharmacol. Biochem. Behav. 9(6):863-887, Dec. 1978.

Commens, C. A. and Greaves, M. W.

Tests to establish the diagnosis in cholinergic urticaria.

Br. J. Dermatol. 98(1):47-51, Jan. 1978.

Concina, E., et al.

Sensibilita delle curve flusso volume nel dimostrare la compromissione funzionale delle piccole vie aeree in soggetti fumatoriasintomatici. (Ital.)

Arch. Monaldi 33(3):143-156, May June 1979.

Conley, J. J. and Baker, D. C.

Catastrophic necrosis of the neck.

Otolaryngol. Head Neck Surg. 87(5): 610-613, Sept.-Oct. 1979.

Conn, H. F. (Editor)

Angina pectoris. Method of Mudge, G. H.

Curr. Ther. 1979, p. 168-173.

Conn, H. F. (Editor)

Degenerative arterial disease. Method of Towne, J. B.

Curr. Ther. 1979, p. 230-234.

Conn, H. F. (Editor)

Chronic bronchitis and emphysema. Method of Kelsen, S. G., et al.

Curr. Ther. 1979, p. 114-118.

Conn, H. F. (Editor)

Chronic bronchitis and bronchiectasis. Method of Barbee, R. A.

Curr. Ther. 1979, p. 120-123.

Conn, H. F. (Editor)

Peptic ulcer. Method of Griffiths, W. J. and Welsh, J. D.

Curr. Ther. 1979, p. 378-381.

Conn, H. F. (Editor)

Disorders of the mouth (benign). Method of Bloom, M. G.

Curr. Ther. 1979, p. 613-628.

Conn, H. F. (Editor.)

Diabetes mellitus syndrome in the adult. Method of Shipp, J. C.

Curr. Ther. 1979, p.400-404.

Conn, H. F. (Editor)

Disorders of the mouth (malignant). Method of Lanier, Jr., V. C.

Curr. Ther. 1979, p. 628-630.

Conn, H. F. (Editor)

Acute miscellaneous poisoning. Method of Arena, J. M.

Curr. Ther. 1979, p. 888-908.

Conn, H. F. (Editor)

Contraception. Method of Connell, E. B.

Curr. Ther. 1979, p. 837-849.

Conn, H. F. (Editor)

Scleroderma: (Progressive systemic sclerosis). Method of Fries, J. F.

Curr. Ther. 1979, p. 658-661.

Conney, A. H., et al.

The Induction of Drug Metabolism: Role of environment and diet in the regulation of human drug metabolism.

Symp. Med. Hoechst 14:583-605, 1979.

Conney, A. H., et al.

The Induction of Drug Metabolism. Prenatal Development of Drug Metabolism. Discussion.

Symp. Med. Hoechst 14:545-548, 1979.

Constantinidis, K., et al.

Pulmonary function in coal workers with Caplan's syndrome and non-rheumatoid complicated pneumoconiosis.

Thorax 33(6):764-768, Dec. 1978.

Conte-Devolx, B., et al.

Dosages plasmatiques radioimmunologiques de la 8-arginine vasopressine: Reponse a la stimulation par la nicotine. (Fr.)

Ann. Endocrinol. (Paris) 38(1):61-72, Jan.-Feb. 1977.

Cook-Mozaffari, P. J., et al.

Oesophageal cancer studies in the Caspian littoral of Iran: Results of a case-control study.

Br. J. Cancer 39(3):293-309, Mar. 1979.

Cooke, N. T.

Male pattern alopecia and coronary artery disease in men.

Br. J. Dermatol. 101(4):455-458, Oct. 1979.

Coombs, M. M., et al.

Identification of the proximate and ultimate forms of the carcinogen 15, 16-dihydro-11-methylcyclopenta a phenanthren-17-one.

Cancer Res. 39(10):4160-4165, Oct. 1979.

Coon, M. J.

Oxygen activation in the metabolism of lipids, drugs and carcinogens.

Nutr. Rev. 36(11):319-328, Nov. 1978.

Coon, M. J. et al.

The Induction of Drug Metabolism. The Drug Metabolizing Enzyme System: Discussion.

Symp. Med. Hoechst 14:243-250, 1979.

Coon, M. J., et al.

The Induction of Drug Metabolism: Chemical characterization of the enzymes involved in drug metabolism.

Symp. Med. Hoechst 14:201-211, 1979.

Cooreman, J., et al.

L'adolescent et le tabagisme: Responsabilite des parents et des professeurs. Resultats d'une campagne de sensibilisation. (Fr.)

J. Med. Strasb. 9(9):483-488, Oct. 1978.

Corberand, J., et al.

Effect of tobacco smoking on the functions of polymorphonuclear leukocytes.

Infect. Immun. 23(3):577-581, Mar. 1979.

Corbin, R. P., et al.

A four-year follow-up study of lung mechanics in smokers.

Am. Rev. Respir. Dis. 120(2): 293-304, Aug. 1978.

Cordasco, E. M. and Van Ordstrand, H. S.

Newer environmental aspects of lung cancer-medical-legal aspects.

Med. Trial Tech. Q. 25(3):332-338, Winter 1979.

Corkery, J. C., et al.

Kids who really shouldn't smoke. (Letter to the Editor.)

N. Engl. J. Med. 300(22):1279, May 31, 1979.

Cornet, A., et al.

A propos des formes radiosensibles du cancer de l'oesophage. (Fr.)

Bull. Acad. Natl. Med. (Paris) 162(7): 629-633, Oct. 3-24, 1978.

Corrin, B. and Soliman, S. S.

Cholesterol in the lungs of heavy cigarette smokers.

Thorax 33(5):565-568, Oct. 1978.

Costall, B., et al.

Hyperactivity induced by injection of dopamine into the accumbens nucleus: Actions and interactions of neuroleptic cholinomimetic and cholinolytic agents.

Neuropharmacology 18(8-9):661-665, Aug.-Sept. 1979.

Costlow, M. E., et al.

Prolactin receptors in primary cultures of carcinogen-induced rat-mammary tumors.

Mol. Cell. Endocrinol. 14(1):81-97, Apr. 1979.

Cotruvo, J. A., et al.

Aquatic Pollutants and Biologic Effects with Emphasis on Neoplasia: Investigation of mutagenic effects of products of ozonation reactions in water.

Ann. NY Acad. Sci. 298:124-140, Sept. 29, 1977.

Coulam, C. B., et al.

Pituitary adenoma and oral contraceptives: A case-control study.

Fertil. Steril. 31(1):25-28, Jan. 1979.

Covelli, V., et al.

Life-span and spontaneous tumours in mice with high and low antibody responses (Biozzi mice).

Br. J. Cancer 38(3):472-475, Sept. 1978.

Cowles, S. R.

Medical effects of combined industrial exposures.

JOM 21(6):413-416, June 1979.

Cox, R.

DNA methylase inhibition in vitro by N-Methyl-N-nitro-N-nitrosoguanidine.

Cancer Res. 40(1):61-63, Jan. 1980.

Cox, R. and Irving, C. C.

O6-methylguanine accumulates in DNA of mammary glands after administration of N-methyl-N-nitrosourea to rats.

Cancer Lett. 6(4-5):273-278, Apr. 1979.

Crandall, D. C. and Leopold, I. H.

Symposium on Drugs: The influence of systemic drugs on tear constituents.

Ophthalmology 86(1):115-125, Jan. 1979.

Criqui, M. H., et al.

The effect of non-response on risk ratios in a cardiovascular disease study.

J. Chronic Dis. 32(9-10):633-638, 1979.

Crisp, A. J. and Sherry, K. M.

Fatal carbon monoxide poisoning - A new circumstance. (Letter to the Editor.)

Br. Med. J. 2(6202):1438, Dec. 1, 1979.

Crittenden, I. H.

"Risk factors" in coronary heart disease - A childhood concern.

J. Sch. Health 49(4):210-212, Apr. 1979.

Crittin, J., et al.

Left main coronary artery stenosis in young patients.

Chest 76(5):508-513, Nov. 1979.

Crivelli, M., et al.

Verarbeitung von frei verfassten Anamnesen durch den Computer. (Ger.)

Schweiz. Med. Wochenschr. 108(27): 1026 1031, July 8, 1978.

Cruise, J. S., et al.

An evaluation of a smoking withdrawal clinic.

J. Med. Assoc. Ga. 68(9):819-822, Sept. 1979.

Cryer, P. E. and Kissane, J. M. (Editors)

Clinicopathologic Conference: Erythrocytosis.

Am. J. Med. 65(6):1007-1014, Dec. 1978.

Cubilla, A. L. and Fitzgerald, P. J.

Pancreas cancer (non-endocrine): A review - Part I.

Clin. Bull. 8(3):91-99, 1978.

Cubilla, A. L. and Fitzgerald, P. J.

Pancreas cancer (non-endocrine): A review - Part II.

Clin. Bull. 8(4):143-155, 1978.

Cucu, Fl.

Carbon monoxide and its implications in atherosclerosis etiopathogeny.

Rev. Roum. Med. [Med. Interne] 16(3):229-242, July-Sept. 1978.

Culliton, B. J. and Waterfall, W. K.

Nitrites - To ban or not to ban?

Br. Med. J. 2(6152):1613-1614, Dec. 9, 1979.

Cunningham, A. S.

Morbidity in breast-fed and artificially fed infants. II.

J. Pediatr. 95(5, Part1):685-689, Nov. 1979.

Cuthbert, J. W.

Attitudes to occupational health hazards within the EEC.

J. R. Soc. Med. 72(4):287-292, Apr. 1979.

Cviklinski, E., et al.

La bronchite chronique: Quelques reflexions sur le bilan d'une annee d'hospitalisation dans un Service de pneumologie. (Fr.)

Med. Hyg. 36(1311):4042-4046, Dec. 6, 1978.

D'Ambrosio, S. M., et al.

DNA repair in syrian hamster embryo cells treated with 7,12-dimethylbenz[a] anthracene and its weakly carcinogenic 5-fluoro analog.

Cancer Lett. 6(4-5):255-261, Apr. 1979.

D'Souza, S. W., et al.

Effect of smoking during pregnancy upon the haematological values of cord blood.

Br. J. Obstet. Gynaecol. 85(7):495-499, July 1978.

Da Silva, A., et al.

Asymptomatic hyperglycemia and Coronary Heart Disease. The Basle longitudinal study: Report on the relation of initial glucose level to baseline ECG abnormalities, peripheral artery disease, and subsequent mortality.

J. Chronic Dis. 32(11/12):797-803, 1979.

Dagle, G. E., et al.

Pulmonary carcinogenesis in rats given implants of cigarette smoke condensate in beeswax pellets.

JNCI 61(3):905-910, Sept. 1978.

Dalbey, W. E., et al.

Chronic inhalation of cigarette smoke by F344 rats.

JNCI 64(2):383-390, Feb. 1980.

Dales, L. G., et al.

A case-control study of relationships of diet and other traits to colorectal cancer in American blacks.

Am. J. Epidemiol. 109(2):132-144, Feb. 1979.

Dales, L. G., et al.

Evaluating periodic multiphasic health checkups: A controlled trial.

J. Chronic. Dis. 32(5):385-404, May 1979.

Dalhamn, T. and Pira, U.

Isoelectric analysis of respiratory mucus from normal rats and rats exposed to tobacco smoking.

Am. Rev. Respir. Dis. 119(5):779-783, May 1979.

Dallner, G., et al.

The Induction of Drug Metabolism. Morphological and Chemical Changes of the Cell: Discussion.

Symp. Med. Hoechst 14:177-184, 1979.

Dally, S., et al.

Blood cadmium level and hypertension in humans.

Clin. Toxicol. 13(3):403-408, 1978.

Danaher, B. G., et al.

A smoking cessation program for pregnant women: An exploratory study.

Am. J. Public Health 68(9):896-898, Sept. 1978.

Danhof, M.

De bepaling van het farmaconmetaboliserend vermogen bij de mens. (Dut.)

Pharm. Weekbl. 114(6):129-149, Feb. 9, 1979.

Daniel, F. B., et al.

Comparative metabolism and DNA binding of 7,12-dimethylbenz[a]anthracene and its weakly carcinogenic 5-fluoro analog.

Cancer Lett. 6(4-5):263-272, Apr. 1979.

Daniels, L. M., et al.

Hypertension control on an urban university campus.

J. Am. Coll. Health Assoc. 27(5):234-238, Apr. 1979.

Dansette, P. M., et al.

Continuous fluorometric assay of epoxide hydrase activity.

Anal. Biochem. 97(2):340-345, Sept. 1, 1979.

Dantzker, D. R. and Bower, J. S.

Mechanisms of gas exchange abnormality in patients with chronic obliterative pulmonary vascular disease.

J. Clin. Invest. 64(4):1050-1055, Oct. 1979.

Danz, M., et al.

N,N-diethyl-4-aminoazobenzene (DEAB): Acute actions with respect to possible carcinogenicity as well as the role of solvents. Morphological and pharmacological investigations.

Exp. Pathol. (Jena) 16(1-6):245-253, 1978.

Danz, R. M., et al.

A possible short-term prediction of potential carcinogenicity of chemical compounds in vivo by means of a promoting activity test (PAT).

Exp. Pathol. (Jena) 16(1-6):109-120, 1978.

Darby, T. D., et al.

An evaluation of a polyurethane for use as a medical grade plastic.

Toxicol. Appl. Pharmacol. 46(2):449-453, Nov. 1978.

Dauber, J. H., et al.

Bronchoalveolar cell populations in acute sarcoidosis: Observations in smoking and nonsmoking patient.

J. Lab. Clin. Med. 94(6):862-871, Dec. 1979.

Daune, M.

Mechanisms of DNA Repair: Changement de conformation du DNA modifie par des agents chimiques. (Fr.)

Biochimie 60(10):1097-1110, 1978.

Dave, K. C., et al.

Characterization of ultraviolet light-induced relaxation of the isolated duodenum of the rat.

Br. J. Pharmacol. 66(2):197-201, June 1979.

Davidoff, G. N., et al.

Elevations in serum copper, erythrocytic copper, and ceruloplasmin concentrations in smokers.

Am. J. Clin. Pathol. 70(5):790-792, Nov. 1978.

Davidson, K. A., et al.

Qualitative alterations in plasma esterases in BALB/c mice following the administration of diethylnitrosamine.

Chem. Biol. Interact. 21(1):19-27, Apr. 1978.

Davies, D. and Darke, C. S.

Sulfametopyrazine prophylaxis in chronic bronchitis.

Br. J. Dis. Chest 72(3):231-234, July 1978.

Davies, J. M., et al.

Smoking and doctors' mortality. (Letters to the Editor.)

Br. Med. J. 280(6211):400, Feb. 9, 1980.

Davies, J. M., et al.

Effects of stopping smoking for 48 hours on oxygen availability from the blood: A study on pregnant women.

Br. Med. J. 2(6186):355-356, Aug. 11, 1979.

Davies, P., et al.

Stereology of lavaged populations of aveolar macrophages: Effects of in vivo exposure to tobacco smoke.

Exp. Mol. Pathol. 29(2):170-182, Oct. 1978.

Davies, P., et al.

Effects of experimental marijuana and tobacco smoke inhalation on alveolar macrophages: A comparative stereologic study.

Lab. Invest. 41(3):220-223, Sept. 1979.

Davies, R. E.

Interaction of light and chemicals in carcinogenesis.

Natl. Cancer Inst. Monogr. 50:45-50, Dec. 1978.

Davis, G. S., et al.

Aspen Lung Conference: Immunology of the Lung. Functional and physiologic correlates of human alveolar macrophage cell shape and surface morphology.

Chest 75(2, Suppl.):280-282, Feb. 1979.

Davis, J. W. and Davis, R. F.

Acute effect of tobacco cigarette smoking on the platelet aggregate ratio.

Am. J. Med. Sci. 278(2):139-143, Sept.-Oct. 1979.

Davis, N.

Carbon monoxide poisoning. (Letter to the Editor.)

Br. Med. J. 2(6204):1584, Dec. 15, 1979.

Dax, E. M., et al.

Individual neurophysin concentrations in the pituitary and circulation of humans.

Clin. Endocrinol. 10(3):253-263, Mar. 1979.

Dayal, P. K., et al.

Prevalence of oral cancer and precancerous lesions in 'pan'/'supari' chewers.

Indian J. Public Health 22(3):234-245, July-Sept. 1978.

Daynes, R. A., et al.

Skin cancer development in mice exposed chronically to immunosuppressive agents.

JNCI 62(4):1075-1081, Apr. 1979.

De Backer, G., et al.

Intermittent claudication-epidemiology and natural history.

Acta Cardiol. (Brux.) 34(3):115-124, 1979.

de Ferreyra, E. C., et al.

Therapeutic effectiveness of cystamine and cysteine to reduce liver cell necrosis induced by several hepatotoxins.

Toxicol. Appl. Pharmacol. 48(2):221-228, Apr. 1979.

De Geest, H., et al.

Secondary Prevention of Ischaemic Heart Disease: A Long-term Controlled Lidoflazine Study.

Acta Cardiol. (Brux.) Suppl. 24: 1-116, 1979.

de Gennes, J. L., et al.

Accidents cardio-vasculaires ischemiques au cours d'un traitement par progestatifs seuls: A propos de 3 observations. (Fr.)

Ann. Endocrinol. (Paris) 40(1):47-48, Jan.-Feb. 1979.

De Matteis, F.

Loss of microsomal components in drug-induced liver damage, in cholestasis and after administration of chemicals which stimulate heme catabolism.

Pharmacol. Ther. [A] 2(4):693-725, 1978.

de Menezes, A. P. and da Silva, P. P.

Fat droplet formation in rat lactating mammary gland and mammary carcinomas viewed by freeze-fracture.

Lab. Invest. 40(5):545-553, May 1979.

de Munter, H. K., et al.

Studies on lung tumours. IV. Correlation between [3H]thymidine labelling of lung and liver cells and tumour formation in GRS/A and C3Hf/A male mice following administration of dimethylnitrosamine.

Chem. Biol. Interact. 24(3):299-316, Mar. 1979.

De Raat, W. K.

Comparison of the induction by cigarette smoke condensates of sister-chromatid exchanges in Chinese hamster cells and of mutations in Salmonella typhimurium.

Mutat. Res. 66(3):253-259, Mar. 1979.

Dean, G.

The effects of air-pollution and smoking on health in England, South Africa and Ireland: A personal odyssey.

Ir. J. Med. 72(7):284-289, July 27, 1979.

DeBacker, G., et al.

Ventricular premature contractions: A randomized non-drug intrevention trial in normal men.

Circulation 59(4):762-769, Apr. 1979.

Decoufle, P.

Cancer risks associated with employment in the leather and leather products industry.

Arch. Environ. Health 34(1):33-37, Jan.-Feb. 1979.

DeGood, D. E. and Valle, R. S.

Self-reported alcohol and nicotine use and the ability to control occipital EEG in a biofeedback situation.

Addict. Behav. 3(1):13-18, 1978.

Deivanayagam, C. N.

Bronchogenic carcinoma.

Antiseptic 75(12):780-784, Dec. 1978.

Del Bono, N., et al.

Functional and clinical evaluation of feprazone-bromhexine association in bronchopulmonary diseases.

Panminerva Med. 20(2):117-122, Apr.-June 1978.

Delanoy, R. L., et al.

Behavioral responses to intracerebroventricularly administered neurohypophyseal peptides in mice.

Horm. Behav. 11(3):348-362, Dec. 1978.

Delashaw, Jr., J. B.

Cholinergic mechanisms and cataplexy in dogs.

Exp. Neurol. 66(3):745-757, Dec. 1979.

Demarest, G. B., et al.

Impaired alveolar macrophage chemotaxis in patients with acute smoke inhalation.

Am. Rev. Respir. Dis. 119(2):279-286, Feb. 1979.

Demirhan, A.

Tutunun evrimsel gelisimi ve folklorik tiptaki yeri. (Turk.)

Istanbul Univ. Istanbul Tip Fak. Mecm. 40(4):985-994, 1977.

Denhey, C. and Laflamme, L.-E. K.

Le programme de sante du centre de jour pour personnes agees: Rapport de la premiere annee. (Fr.)

Union Med. Can. 108(2):139-145, Feb. 1979.

Dent, J. G., et al.

Constitutive and induced hepatic microsomal cytochrome P-450 monooxygenase activities in male Fischer-344 and CD rats. A comparative study.

Toxicol. Appl. Pharmacol. 52(1):45-53, Jan. 1980.

Dent, P. B., et al.

Proceedings of the International Conference on the Clinical Uses of Carcinoembryonic Antigen: Measurement of carcinoembryonic antigen in patients with bronchogenic carcinoma.

Cancer 42(3, Suppl.):1484-1491, Sept. 1978.

Deutsch, J., et al.

Catalytic activity and stereoselectivity of purified forms of rabbit liver microsomal cytochrome P-450 in the oxygenation of the (minus) and (plus) enantiomers of trans-7,8-dihydroxy-7,8-dihydrobenzo-[alpha]pyrene.

Mol. Pharmacol. 16(3):1011-1018, Nov. 1979.

Dev. N. B. and Loeschcke, H. H.

Topography of the respiratory and circulatory responses to acetylcholine and nicotine on the ventral surface of the medulla oblongata.

Pfluegers Arch. 379(1):19-27, Feb. 14, 1979.

Dieter, H. H., et al.

Additional induction of microsomal cytochrome(s) P450 in mouse liver by consecutive application of cadmium chloride and phenobarbital.

Res. Commun. Chem. Pathol. Pharmacol. 24(2):377-388, May 1979.

DiGiovanni, J., et al.

Covalent binding of polycyclic aromatic hydrocarbons to adenine correlates with tumorigenesis in mouse skin.

Cancer Lett. 7(1):39-43, June 1979.

DiGiovanni, J., et al.

Effects of 7,8-benzoflavone on skin tumor-initiating activities of various 7- and 12-substituted derivatives of 7,12-dimethylbenz[a]anthracene in mice.

JNCI 61(1):135-140, July 1978.

DiGiovanni, J., et al.

Effects of pretreatment with 2,3,7,8-tetrachlorodibenzo-p-dioxin on the capacity of hepatic and extrahepatic mouse tissues to convert procarcinogens to mutagens for Salmonella typhimurium auxotrophs.

Toxicol. Appl. Pharmacol. 50(2): 229-239, Sept. 15, 1979.

Dill, J. R., et al.

Cellular immunity to a lung homogenate in asymptomatic cigarette smokers.

Clin. Allergy 8(4):321-327, July 1978.

Dillon, P. and Seasholtz, J.

Oral contraceptives and myocardial infarction.

Cardiovasc. Nurs. 15(2):5-9, Mar.-Apr. 1979.

Dipalma, J. R.

Clinical Pharmacology: Activated charcoal - A neglected antidote.

Am. Fam. Physician 20(5):155-156, Nov. 1979.

DiPaolo, J. A. and Casto, B. C.

Quantitative studies of in vitro morphological transformation of Syrian hamster cells by inorganic metal salts.

Cancer Res. 39(3):1008-1013, Mar. 1979.

DiPaolo, J. A. and Donovan, P. J.

Transformation frequency of Syrian golden hamster cells and its modulation by ultraviolet irradiation.

Natl. Cancer Inst Mongr. 50:75-80, Dec. 1978.

Dipple, A., et al.

Comparison of metabolism-mediated binding to DNA of 7-hydroxymethyl-12-methylbenz(a)anthracene and 7,12-dimethylbenz(a)anthracene.

Cancer Res. 39(4):1154-1158, Apr. 1979.

Ditter, H. and Matthias, R.

Verschluss der aorta abdominalis: Ein kasuistischer Beitrag. (Ger.)

Med. Welt 29(34):1317-1321, Aug. 25, 1978.

Divekar, M. V.

Progress in medicine (Part II).

Bombay Hosp. J. 20(2):57-73, Apr. 1978.

Dixon, R. L. and Lee, I. P.

Pharmacokinetic and adaption factors involved in testicular toxicity.

Fed. Proc. 39(1):66-72, Jan. 1980.

Dodds, W. J., et al.

Pharmacologic investigation of primary peristalsis in smooth muscle portion of opossum esophagus.

Am. J. Physiol. 237(6):E561-E566, Dec. 1979.

Dodge, Jr., R. E.

Atherosclerotic cardiovascular disease in small town office practice.

J. Fla. Med. Assoc. 66(12):1213-1214, Dec. 1979.

Dodson, R. A. and Johnson, W. E.

Effects of ethanol, arecoline, atropine and nicotine, alone and in various combinations, on rat cerebellar cyclic guanosine 3',5'monophosphate.

Neuropharmacology 18(11):871-876, Nov. 1979.

Doelle, W., et al.

Congress International, Societe Royale Belge de Gastroenterologie. The New Peptide Hormones of the Gut: The effect of cimetidine on inpatients with duodenal ulcer - A double blind trial.

Acta Gastroenterol. Belg. 41(7-8):424-426, July-Aug. 1978.

Doerjer, G., et al.

Reaction of 7,12-dimethylbenz(a)-anthracene with DNA of fetal and maternal rat tissues in vivo.

Int. J. Cancer 22(3):288-291, Sept. 15, 1978.

Dofuku, R., et al.

Trisomy of chromosome number 13 in spontaneous mammary tumors of GR, C3H, and noninbred Swiss mice.

JNCI 63(3):651-654, Sept. 1979.

Dohi, T. and Tsujimoto, A.

Possible mechanisms of sustained tremor induction by nicotine in pilocarpine treated animals.

Arch. Int. Pharmacodyn. Ther. 235(1):62-72, Sept. 1978.

Dolan, M.

Smoking: Still a burning issue.

Am. Pharm. NS18(10):27-31, Sept. 1978.

Dolan, M.

Alcoholism: The all-American addiction.

Am. Pharm. NS19(1):26-29, Jan. 1979.

Doll, R.

Prevention: Some future prespectives.

Prev. Med. 7(4):486-497, Dec. 1978.

Dollery, C. T., et al.

Drug Disposition in Man: Contribution of environmental factors to variability in human drug metabolism.

Drug Metab. Rev. 9(2):207-220, 1979.

Dominguez De Villoto, E., et al.

Invariabilidad en el tiempo de la capacidad de combinacion de la hemoglobina con el oxigeno. Estudio secuencial en siete varones fumadores. (Span.)

Rev. Clin. Esp. 153(1):53-56, Apr. 15, 1979.

Done, A. K.

The Toxic Emergency: The great equalizers? I. Insecticides.

Emergency Med. 95 107, May 15, 1979.

Dosman, J. A., et al.

Proceedings of the Aspen Lung Conference: Sensitivity of variables derived from the single breath nitrogen test in smokers.

Chest 77(2 Suppl.):286-289, Feb. 1980.

Dosman, J. A., et al.

Chronic bronchitis and exposure to cereal grain dust.

Am. Rev. Respir. Dis. 120(3):477-480, Sept. 1979.

Dosman, J. A., et al.

Chronic bronchitis and decreased forced expiratory flow rates in lifetime non-smoking grain workers.

Am. Rev. Respir. Dis. 121(1):11-16, Jan. 1980.

Douglas, G. R. and Grant, C. E.

DNA damage, cell survival and DNA repair in Chinese hamster ovary cells after in vitro metabolic activation of dimethylnitrosamine and benzo[a]pyrene.

Mutat. Res. 77(3):259-269, Mar. 1980.

Douglass, F. M. and Khavari, K. A.

The drug use index: A measure of the extent of polydrug usage.

Int. J. Addict. 13(6):981-993, 1978.

Douglass, Jr., H. O., et al.

Selectivity of the micro-leukocyte adherence inhibition assay in pancreatic cancer.

Cancer 43(3):1084-1088, Mar. 1979.

Douglass, M. L., et al.

The chemistry of nitrosamine formation, inhibition and destruction.

J. Soc. Cosmet. Chem. 29(9):581-605, Sept. 1978.

Doyle, J. T.

Workshop on Carbon Monoxide and Cardiovascular Disease: Risk factors in arteriosclerosis and cardiovascular disease with special emphasis on cigarette smoking.

Prev. Med. 8(3):264-270, May 1979.

Drevon, C. A.

Nyere synspunkter paa forholdet mellom plasma-lipoproteiner og utvikling av atherosklerose. (Norw.; Engl. Abstr.)

Tidsskr. Nor. Laegeforen. 98(13):669-673;698, May 10, 1978.

Drew, J. H.

Biliary reflux: Postoperative and idiopathic.

Med. J. Aust. 2(3):125-128, Aug. 11, 1979.

Drew, W. L., et al.

Growth of herpes simplex and cytomegalovirus in cultured human alveolar macrophages.

Am. Rev. Respir. Dis. 119(2):287-291, Feb. 1979.

Drinkwater, N. R., et al.

Covalent intercalative binding to DNA in relation to the mutagenicity of hydro carbon epoxides and N-acetoxy-2-acetylaminofluorene.

Cancer Res. 38(10):3247-3255, Oct. 1978.

Du Melle, F.

"You go ahead and smoke if you have to. I just don't like it."

Am. Lung. Assoc. Bull. 65(1):2-5, Jan.-Feb. 1979.

Duane, T. D., et al.

White centered hemorrhages: Their significance.

Ophthalmology 87(1):66-69, Jan. 1980.

Dubois, P., et al.

Entretiens de Physiopathologie Respiratoire: Facteurs fonctionnels respiratoires limitant la capacite physique chez des sujets ages. (Fr.)

Bull. Eur. Physiopathol. Respir. 15(2):385-394, 1979.

Dubrow, R., et al.

Different responses to drugs and serum of cells transformed by various means.

Cancer Res. 39(7, Part 1):2718-2726, July 1979.

Ducimetiere, P., et al.

Asymptomatic Hyperglycemia and Coronary Heart Disease. Relationship of glucose tolerance to prevalance of ECG abnormalities and to annual mortality from cardiovascular disease: Results of the Paris prospective study.

J. Chronic Dis. 32(11/12):759-766, 1979.

Ducommun, S. and Mounoud, R.-L.

Education pour la sante: Prevention du tabagisme. (Fr.)

Bull. Schweiz. Akad. Med. Wiss. 35(1 3):119-121, Mar. 1979.

Dudai, Y. and Yavin, E.

Ontogenesis of muscarinic receptors and acetylcholinesterase in differentiating rat cerebral cells in culture.

Brain Res. 155(2):368-373, Oct. 27, 1978.

Dufour, A.

Cent ans de lutte antitabagique. (Fr.)

Hist. Sci. Med. 12(2):136-142, 1978.

Dugan, Jr., W. M.

Cancer Corner.

J. Indiana State Med. Assoc. 71(9): 847;861, Sept. 1978.

Duncan, S. J. and Brooks, P.

Lack of oestradiol-DNA binding in mouse embryo cell cultures or following rat-liver microsomal metabolism.

Cancer Lett. 6(6):351-355, May 1979.

Dunnill, M. S.

Some aspects of pulmonary defence.

J. Pathol. 128(4):221-236, Aug. 1979.

Dunnill, M. S.

Aetiology of emphysema.

Bull. Eur. Physiopathol. Respir. 15(5):1015-1029, 1979.

DuPont, R. L.

The International Challenge of Drug Abuse. The international challenge of drug abuse: A perspective from the United States.

Natl. Inst. Drug Abuse Res. Monogr. Ser. 19:3-14, 1978.

Dutau, G., et al.

Societe Francaise de la Tuberculose et des Maladies Respiratoires: Inhalation passive de fumee de tabac chez l'enfant prescolaire etude clinique et biologique. (Fr.)

Rev. Fr. Mal. Respir. 6(5):549-553, Sept.-Oct. 1978.

Dutau, G., et al.

Manifestations respiratoires liees a l'inhalation passive de fumee de tabac chez l'enfant d'age pre-scolaire. (Fr.)

Poumon Coeur 35(2):63-69, Mar.-Apr. 1979.

Dutau, G., et al.

Inhalation passive de fumee de tabac chez l'enfant prescolaire: Etude clinique et biologique. (Fr.)

Bord. Med. 12(14):933-936, May 1979.

Dutu, St., et al.

Functia ventilatorie si tusea productiva cronica la o populatie in virsta de 60-85 de ani. (Contributtii la studiul dezvoltarii sindromului obstructiv in bronsita cronica. (Rum.)

Rev. Ig. [Pneumoftiziol.] 27(1):43-52, Jan.-Mar. 1978.

Dybing, E., et al.

In vitro metabolism and activation of carcinogenic aromatic amines by subcellular fractions of human liver.

Cancer Res. 39(10):4206-4211, Oct. 1979.

Dyer, A. R., et al.

Alcohol consumption and 17-year mortality in the Chicago Western Electric Company study.

Prev. Med. 9(1):78-90, Jan. 1980.

Dyer, A. R., et al.

A self-scoring five-question risk test for coronary heart disease.

Circulation 60(4):914-920, Oct. 1979.

Dyer, C., et al.

Cyanide reactivity of cytochrome c derivatives.

Biochem Biophys. Acta 579(2):253-268, Aug. 28, 1979.

Eagles, J.

Are all animal experiments necessary?

Nurs. Times 75(10):398-399, Mar. 8, 1979.

Eastman, A. and Bresnick, E.

Persistent binding of 3-methylcholanthrene to mouse lung DNA and the correlation with susceptibility to pulmonary neoplasia.

Cancer Res. 39(7, Part 1):2400-2405, July 1979.

Eastman, A. and Bresnick, E.

Metabolism and DNA binding of 3-methylcholanthrene.

Cancer Res. 39(11):4316-4321, Nov. 1979.

Ebenstein, P., et al.

Expression of endogenous xenotropic retrovirus by methylcholanthrene-induced squamous cell carcinoma of the mouse respiratory tract.

J. Exp. Med. 150(6):1567-1570, Dec. 1, 1979.

Ebert, R. V.

Cessation of cigarette smoking and pulmony disease.

JAMA 240(20):2159-2161, Nov. 10, 1978.

Edgar, R. T., et al.

Air pollution analysis used in operating an environmental control unit.

Ann. Allergy 42(3):166-173, Mar. 1979.

Edinger, J. D., et al.

Modification of smoking behaviors in a correctional institution.

J. Clin. Psychol. 34(4):991-998, Oct. 1978.

Edlich, R. F., et al.

The initial management of the burn patient.

Compr. Ther. 5(1):59-68, Jan. 1979.

Edmonds, Jr., H. L., et al.

The anticonvulsant activity of ropizine in the rat.

J. Pharmacol. Exp. Ther. 208(2):236-242, Feb. 1979.

Edwards, D. P., et al.

Estrogen and progesterone receptor proteins in breast cancer.

Biochim. Biophys. Acta 560(4):457-486, Dec. 19, 1979.

Edwards, G. S., et al.

Volatile nitrosamine contamination of laboratory animal diets. (Letter to the Editor.)

Cancer Res. 39(5):1857-1858, May 1979.

Edwards, G. S., et al.

Long-term treatment with cis-dichloro-diammineplatinum(II)-vinblastine-bleomycin: Possible association with severe coronary artery disease. (Letter to the Editor.)

Cancer Treat. Rep. 63(4):551-552, Apr. 1979.

Edwards, L. E., et al.

Pregnancy in the underweight woman. Course, outcome, and growth patterns of the infant.

Am. J. Obstet. Gynecol. 135(3):297-302, Oct. 1, 1979.

Efthymiou, M.-L.

Arteriopathie et intoxication chronique par l'oxyde de carbone. (Fr.)

Concours Med. 101(17):2829-2830, Apr. 28, 1979.

Egle, Jr., J. L. and Gochberg, B. J.

Respiratory retention and acute toxicity of furan.

Am. Ind. Hyg. Assoc. J. 40(4): 310-314, Apr. 1979.

Ehmann, U. K. and Wheeler, K. T.

Cinemicrographic determination of cell progression and division abnormalities after treatment with 1, 3 bis(2-chloroethyl)-1-nitrosourea.

Eur. J. Cancer 15(4):461-473, Apr. 1979.

Eidler, F.-J. and Slotkin, T. A.

Presynaptic and postsynaptic contributions to ontogeny of sympathetic control of heart rate in the preweanling rat.

Br. J. Pharmacol. 65(3):431-434, Mar. 1979.

Einfeldt, H., et al.

Moeglichkeiten zur aktiven Praevention von Gefaesserkrankungen: Eine Pilotstudie mit Fabrikarbeitern. (Ger.)

Munch. Med. Wochenschr. 121(11):387-388, Mar. 16, 1979.

Eisele, T. A., et al.

Effects of dietary cyclopropene fatty acids on the mixed function oxidase system of the rainbow trout (Salmo gairdneri).

J. Environ. Pathol. Toxicol. 1(6):773-778, July-Aug. 1978.

Eiser, J. R.

Discrepancy, dissonance, and the "dissonant" smoker.

Int. J. Addict. 13(8);1295-1305, 1978.

Eiser, J. R., et al.

Can television influence smoking?

Br. J. Addict. 73(2):215-219, June 1978.

Eiser, J. R., et al.

Can television influence smoking? Further evidence.

Br. J. Addict. 73(3):291-298, Sept. 1978.

Eiser, J. R., et al.

"Consonant" and "dissonant" smokers and the self-attribution of addiction.

Addict. Behav. 3(2):99-106, 1978.

Ekelman, K. B. and Milo, G. E.

Cellular uptake, transport, and macromolecular binding of benzo(a)-pyrene and 7,12-dimethylbenz(a)-anthracene by human cells in vitro.

Cancer Res. 38(9):3026-3032, Sept. 1978.

Ekstedt, R. D.

Enhancement of experimental tumors in mice by treatment with concanavalin A.

JNCI 63(4):1065-1069, Oct. 1979.

El-Desouky, M. A., et al.

Exposure to pesticides in Kuwait.

J. Kuwait Med. Assoc. 12(4):215 227, Dec. 1978.

Elcombe, C. R. and Lech, J. J.

Induction and characterization of hemoprotein(s) P-450 and monooxygenation in rainbow trout (salmo gairdneri).

Toxicol. Appl. Pharmacol. 49(3):437-450, July 1979.

Elespuru, R. K.

Deuterium isotope effects in mutagenesis by nitroso compounds.

Mutat. Res. 54(3):265-270, Dec. 1978.

Elinder, C.-G., et al.

Haelsoeffekter av kadmium. (Swed.)

Lakartidningen 75(47):4365-4368, Nov. 22, 1978.

Elliott, J.

Maternal smoking and the fetus: One fear buried but others arise.

JAMA 241(9):867-868, Mar. 2, 1979.

Elliott, J.

Are contaminants the culprit and not tobacco?

JAMA 241(15):1556, Apr. 13, 1979.

Ellis, E. N.

Helping individuals in apparent good health who might develop cancer.

UICC Tech. Rep. Ser. 31:9-17, 1978.

Ellis, H.

Review of general surgery 1978.

Postgrad. Med. J. 55(642):223-240, Apr. 1979.

Elovainio, L.

Finns are smoking less and less.

UICC Tech. Rep. Ser. 31:41-46, 1978.

Emura, M., et al.

Toxic and transforming effects of polycyclic hydrocarbons in fetal hamster lung-cell cultures. I. Benzo(a)pyrene.

Cancer Lett. 4(5):343-348, June 1978.

Engel, H.-J.

Nebenwirkungen oraler Kontrazeptiva. (Ger.)

Med. Monatsschr. Pharm. 2(7):199-204, July 1979.

Enjeti, S., et al.

Pulmonary function in young smokers: Male-female differences.

Am. Rev. Respir. Dis. 118(4):667-676, Oct. 1978.

Enstrom, J. E.

Cancer and total mortality among active Mormons.

Cancer 42(4):1943-1951, Oct. 1978.

Enstrom, J. E.

Rising lung cancer mortality among nonsmokers.

JNCI 62(4):755-760, Apr. 1979.

Entrican, J. H. and Douglas, A. S.

Circannual rhythm of arterial and venous thromboembolic disease.

Scott. Med. J. 24(4):273-278, Oct. 1979.

Epler, J. L., et al.

Energy-related pollutants in the environment: Use of short-term tests for mutagenicity in the isolation and identification of biohazards.

Environ. Health Perspect. 27:11-20, Dec. 1978.

Epstein, F. H., et al.

Praevention der Atherosklerose: Grundlagen heute. (Ger.)

Schweiz. Med. Wochenschr. 109(32):1171-1180, Aug. 25, 1979.

Epstein, J. H.

Stimulation of ultraviolet-induced carcinogenesis by 1,3-bis(2-chloroethyl)-1-nitrosourea.

Cancer Res. 39(2, Part 1):408-410, Feb. 1979.

Epstein, S. S., et al.

Carcinogenicity of a composite organic extract of urban particulate atmospheric pollutants following subcutaneous injection in infant mice.

Environ. Res. 19(1):163-176, June 1979.

Ericson, A., et al.

Cigarette smoking as an etiologic factor in cleft lip and palate.

Am. J. Obstet. Gynecol. 135(3):348-351, Oct. 1, 1979.

Erikssen, J. and Enger, S. Chr.

Smoking, lung function, physical performance and latent coronary heart disease in presumably healthy middle-aged men.

Acta Med. Scand. 203(6):509-516, 1978.

Eriksson, S.

Emfysemets biokemi, naagra nyare roen. (Swed.)

Kvartalsskrift 73(4):111-120, 1978.

Erzengin, F., et al.

Sigara ve kalb. (Turk.)

Istanbul Univ. Istanbul Tip Fak. Mecm. 40(4):747-757, 1977.

Eschwege, E., et al.

Blood cells and alcohol consumption with special reference to smoking habits.

J. Clin. Pathol. 31(7):654-658, July 1978.

Eskes, T. K. A. B.

Het foetale alcoholsyndroom. (Dut.)

Ned. Tijdschr. Geneeskd. 123(29):1276-1279, July 21, 1979.

Etherton, J. E., et al.

Quantitative comparisons of the pulmonary toxicity of tobacco and NSM smoke.

J. Pathol. 127(4):185-190, Apr. 1979.

Evans, D. J., et al.

Enzyme inhibition by tobacco smoke: A comparison of the effects of four filters.

Arch. Environ. Health 34(2): 103-106, Mar.-Apr. 1979.

Evans, D. L., et al.

Immunobiological characterizations of tumor-associated fetal antigens.

Cancer Res. 39(5, Part 1):2016-2025, June 1979.

Evans, D. L., et al.

Biochemical and physical characterizations of tumor-associated fetal antigens.

Cancer Res. 39(5, Part 1):2006-2015, June 1979.

Evans, D. R., et al.

Maternal smoking habits and congenital malformations: A population study.

Br. Med. J. 2(6183):171-173, July 21, 1979.

Evans, H. E. and Bognacki, N.

Alpha1-antitryspin deficiency and susceptibility to lung disease.

Environ. Health Perspect. 29:57-61, Apr. 1979.

Evans, O. B.

Pediatrics for the Clinician: Polyneuropathy in childhood.

Pediatrics 64(1):96-105, July 1979.

Evarts, R. P. and Mostafa, M. H.

Dimethylnitrosamine demethylase activity of rat liver microsomes after partial hepatectomy.

Biochem. Pharmacol. 27(23):2751-2753, 1978.

Evarts, R. P., et al.

The effect of hydroxylamine on the morphology of the rat mammary gland and on the induction of mammary tumors by 7,12-dimethylbenz[a] anthracene.

Exp. Mol. Pathol. 30(3):337-348, June 1979.

Eyre, P. and Deline, T. R.

Cholinergic modulation of anaphylactic dopamine release from calf lung.

Int. Arch. Allergy Appl. Immunol. 59(4):443-446, 1979.

Fabro, S.

Penetration of chemicals into the oocyte, uterine fluid, and preimplantation blastocyst.

Environ. Health Perspect. 24:25-29, June 1978.

Fagerstroem, K.-O.

Measuring degree of physical dependence to tobacco smoking with reference to individualization of treatment.

Addict. Behav. 3(3-4):235-241, 1978.

Fahl, W. E., et al.

UDP-glucuronosyl transferase and the conjugation of benzo(a)pyrene metabolites to DNA.

Biochem. Biophys. Res. Commun. 85(3): 891-899, Dec. 14, 1978.

Fairshter, R. D. and Wislon, A. F.

Relative sensitivities and specificities of tests for small airways obstruction.

Respiration 37(6):301-308, 1979.

Fajen, J. M., et al.

N-nitrosamines in the rubber and tire industry.

Science 205(4412):1262-1264, Sept. 21, 1979.

Falk, H. L.

Extrapolating carcinogenesis data from animal to humans.

Fed. Proc. 39(1):76-80, Jan. 1980.

Famaey, J. P., et al.

Inhibition of angiotensin-induced contractions of guinea-pig isolated ileum by high concentrations of non-steroidal antiinflammatory drugs and various steroids and its reversal by prostaglandin E1.

Prostaglandins 16(5):725-732, Nov. 1978.

Famaey, J.-P., et al.

The effects of antiinflammatory steroids on the response of the guinea pig isolated ileum to acetylcholine, histamine, nicotine, 5-hydroxytryptamine and electrical stimulation.

Naunyn Schmiedebergs Arch. Pharmacol 309(2):191-195, Nov. 1, 1979.

Fang, W.-F. Strobel, H. W.

Activation of carcinogens and mutagens by rat colon mucosa.

Cancer Res. 38(9):2939-2944, Sept. 1978.

Fardy, P. S., et al.

A comparison of habitual lifestyle, aerobic power and systolic time intervals in former athletes and non-athletes.

J. Sports Med. Phys. Fitness 18(3):287-299, Sept. 1978.

Farebrother, M. J. B.

Respiratory function and cardiorespiratory response to exercise in obesity.

Br. J. Dis. Chest 73(3):211-229, July 1979.

Farebrother, M. J. B., et al.

Propranolol and giving up smoking.

Br. J. Dis. Chest 74(1):95-96, Jan. 1980.

Farinaro, E., et al.

Asymptomatic Hyperglycemia and Coronary Heart Disease. The olivetti survey: Asymptomatic hyperglycemia and ECG abnormalities at baseline.

J. Chronic Dis. 32(11/12):773-777, 1979.

Farrell, G. C., et al.

Drug metabolism in liver disease: Activity of hepatic microsomal metabolizing enzymes.

Clin. Pharmacol. Ther. 26(4):483-492, Oct. 1979.

Farrell, P. M. and Hamosh, M.

Symposium on the Respiratory System: The biochemistry of fetal lung development.

Clin. Perinatol. 5(2):197-229, Sept. 1978.

Farwell, D. C., et al.

Liver ornithine decarboxylase during phenobarbital promotion of nitrosamine carcinogenesis.

Cancer Lett. 5(3):139-144, Sept. 1978.

Favez, G.

L'atteinte des voies aeriennes peripheriques. (Fr.)

Rev. Med. Suisse Romande 99(4):193-196, Apr. 1979.

Fay, H. T.

Risk factors in scrotal epithelioma.

J. R. Soc. Med. 71(10):741-747, Oct. 1978.

Fee, J. P. H., et al.

A prospective study of liver enzyme and other changes following repeat administration of halothane and enflurane.

Br. J. Anaesth. 51(12):1133-1141, Dec. 1979.

Feger, J., et al.

Pharmacological properties of acetylcholine-induced excitation of subthalamic nucleus neurones.

Br. J. Pharmacol 65(3):511-515, Mar. 1979.

Fein, A., et al.

Pathophysiology and management of the complications resulting from fire and the inhaled products of combustion: A review of the literature.

Crit. Care Med. 8(2):94-98, Feb. 1980.

Feinendegen, L. E.

Minimal transit times.

Nuklearmedizin 17(5):185-193, Oct. 1978.

Feinleib, M., et al.

A comparison of blood pressure, total cholesterol and cigarette smoking in parents in 1950 and their children in 1970.

Am. J. Epidemiol. 110(3):291-303, Sept. 1979.

Feisal, K. A. and Fuleihan, F. J. D.

Pulmonary gas exchange during exercise in young asthmatic patients.

Thorax 34(3):393-396, June 1979.

Fergusson, D. M., et al.

Smoking during pregnancy.

NZ Med. J. 89(628):41-43, Jan. 24, 1979.

Fernandez, J., et al.

Etiopatogenia de la arteriosclerosis. I. Etiologia. (Span.)

Rev. Clin. Esp. 152(2):93-98, Jan. 31, 1979.

Feron, V. J.

Effects of exposure to acetaldehyde in Syrian hamsters simultaneously treated with benzo(a)pyrene or diethylnitrosamine.

Prog. Exp. Tumor Res. 24:162-176, 1979.

Ferris, B. G.

Epidemiology Standardization Project: II. Recommended respiratory disease questionnaires for use with adults and children in epidemiological research.

Am. Rev. Respir. Dis. 118(6, Part 2):7-53, Dec. 1978.

Ferris, B. G.

Epidemiology Standardization Project: III. Recommended standardized procedures for pulmonary function testing.

Am. Rev. Respir. Dis. 118(6, Part 2):55-88, Dec. 1978.

Ferris, Jr., B. G., et al.

Effects of sulfur oxides and respirable particles on human health: Methodology and demography of populations in study.

Am. Rev. Respir. Dis. 120(4):767-779, Oct. 1979.

Feurstein, G., et al.

Lithium-induced increase in the metabolism of benzo[a]pyrene and drugs in rat liver.

Biochem. Pharmacol. 28(21):3167-3170, Nov. 1, 1979.

Feyerabend, C. and Russell, M. A. H.

Improved gas-chromatographic method and microextraction technique for the measurement of nicotine in biological fluids.

J. Pharm. Pharmacol. 31(2):73-76, Feb. 1979.

Fiala, E. S., et al.

Inhibition of the metabolism of the colon carcinogen, azoxymethane, by pyrazole.

Cancer Res. 38(12):4515-4521, Dec. 1978.

Fichardt, T. and Sandison, A. G.

Management of urinary bladder cancer.

S. Afr. Med. J. 54(18):731-740, Oct. 28, 1978.

Fiddler, W., et al.

Environmental Aspects of N-Nitroso Compounds: Observations on the use of the thermal energy analyzer as a specific detector for nitrosamines.

IARC Sci. Publ. No. 19:33-39, 1978.

Fiehring, H.

Pathophysiologie und klinische Diagnostik von chronisch ischaemischer Herzkrankheit, Herzinsuffizienz und Herzrhythmusstoerungen. (Ger.)

Pharmazie 34(8):472-476, Aug. 1979.

Fielding, J. E. and Yankauer, A.

The pregnant smoker. (Editorial.)

Am. J. Public Health 68(9):835-836, Sept. 1978.

Fielding, J. E.

Successes of prevention.

Milbank Mem. Fund. Q. 56(3):274-302, Summer 1978.

Fielding, J. E., et al.

A program for prevention in Massachusetts.

Prev. Med. 7(4):564-640, Dec. 1978.

Fielding, S. and Hoffmann, I.

Symposium on Clobazam: Pharmacology of anti-anxiety drugs with special reference to clobazam.

Br. J. Clin. Pharmacol. 7(Suppl. 1):7S-15S, 1979.

Fields, W. S., et al.

Controlled trial of aspirin in cerebral ischemia. Part II: Surgical group.

Stroke 9(4):309-319, July-Aug. 1978.

During therapy for cerebral ischemia, a male patient had skin ecchymoses thought to be due to ingestion of a laxative containing phenolphthalein.

Fine, D. H.

Environmental Aspects of N-Nitroso Compounds: An assessment of human exposure to N-nitroso compounds.

IARC Sci. Publ. No. 19:267-278, 1978.

Fischbein, A., et al.

Drywall construction and asbestos exposure.

Am. Ind. Hyg. Assoc. J. 40(5):402-407, May 1979.

Fischer, T., et al.

Luftverunreinigung durch Tabakrauch in Gaststaetten. (Ger.)

Int. Arch. Occup. Environ. Health 41(4):267-280, July 14, 1978.

Fishbein, L.

Mutagenesis. Environmental sources of chemical mutagens: II. Synthetic mutagens.

Adv. Mod. Toxicol. 5:257-348, 1978.

Fishbein, L.

Mutagenesis. Environmental sources of chemical mutagens: I. Naturally occuring mutagens.

Adv. Mod. Toxicol. 5:175-256, 1978.

Fishbein, L.

Overview of potential mutagenic problems posed by some pesticides and their trace impurities.

Environ. Health Perspect. 27:125-131, Dec. 1978.

Fisher, P. B., et al.

Phenotypic properties and tumor promoter-induced alterations in rat embryo cells transformed by adenovirus.

Cancer Res. 39(8):3051-3057, Aug. 1979.

Fishman, A. P.

How safe can cigarettes be?

N. Engl. J. Med. 300(8):428-430, Feb. 22, 1979.

Fitzpatrick, T. B. and Sober, A. J.

Workshop: The role of ultraviolet light in the etiology of human melanoma.

Natl. Cancer Inst. Monogr. 50:197-198, Dec. 1978.

Flaxman, J.

Affect-management and habit mechanisms in the modification of smoking behavior.

Addict. Behav. 4(1):39-46, 1979.

Flenley, D. C., et al.

Ventilatory response to steady-state exercise in hypoxia in humans.

J. Appl. Physiol. 46(3):438-446, Mar. 1979.

Fletcher, Ch. and Peto, R.

Historia naturalna przewlklego zwezenia drog oddechowych. (Pol.)

Przegl. Lek. 35(10):747-752, 1978.

Fletcher, G. F.

Exercise and the coronary patient.

Curr. Probl. Cardiol. 4(3):1-75, June 1979.

Florey, E. and Rathmayer, M.

Pharmacological characterization of cholinoreceptors of cardiac ganglion cells of crustaceans.

Gen. Pharmacol. 11(1):47-53, 1980.

Floyd, R. A., et al.

Singlet Oxygen and Related Species in Chemistry and Biology. Proceedings of the International Conference: Spin trapping of free radicals produced from nitrosoamine carcinogens.

Photochem. Photobiol. 28(4-5): 857-862, Oct. Nov. 1978.

Fogelholm, R.

Aivohalvauksen riskitekijaet ja ennalta ehkaeisy. (Finn.)

Suom. Laeaekaeril. 33(11):871-879, Apr. 10, 1978.

Foley, W. T.

Studies of vasospasm. II. The use of nitroglycerin cigarettes.

J. Clin. Pharmacol. 19(1):75-79, Jan. 1979.

Fontana, R. S.

Smoking and lung cancer: A review.

Bull. Schweiz. Akad. Med. Wiss. 35(1-3):25-31, Mar. 1979.

Ford, C. N., et al.

Distant metastasis of locally controlled supraglottic laryngeal carcinoma: A report of two cases.

Henry Ford Hosp. Med. J. 26(2):19-21, Summer 1978.

Fornace, Jr., A. J. and Little, J. B.

DNA-protein cross-linking by chemical carcinogens in mammalian cells.

Cancer Res. 39(3):704-710, Mar. 1979.

Forsberg, L., et al.

Impotence, smoking, and beta-blocking drugs.

Fertil. Steril. 31(5):589-591, May 1979.

Fortson, J. K. and Janfaza, P.

Endotracheal and tracheostomy tube cytology: A nonivasive technique for early detection of carcinoma of the lung and aerodigestive tract.

Ann. Otol. Rhinol. Laryngol. 88(6, Part 1):809-812, Nov.-Dec. 1979.

Foster, K. J., et al.

Prevalence of diverticular disease of the colon in patients with ischaemic heart disease.

Gut 19(11):1054-1056, Nov. 1978.

Fournier, Cl. and Gerbaux, A.

Effets physio-pathologiques du tabac sur le coeur. (Fr.)

Coeur Med. Interne 18(2):221-227, Apr.-June 1979.

Fox, A.

What can be done about smoking in the schools?

Health Educ. 9(3):4-5, May-June 1978.

Frankel, H. H.

Another cowboy selling cancer. (Letter to the Editor.)

West. J. Med. 130(3):270-271, Mar. 1979.

Franklin, M. R.

Proceedings of the International Symposium on Microsomes and Drug Oxidations: The inhibition of mixed-function oxidation reactions by amphetamines in liver and lung microsomes.

Biochem. Pharmacol. Suppl.:284-291, 1977.

Fransen, H. and Endtz, L. J.

De neurologische complicaties van chronisch alcoholisme. (Dut.)

Ned. Tijdschr. Geneeskd. 123(29):1273-1276, July 21,19798.

Fraser, G. E.

Sudden death in Auckland.

Aust. NZ J. Med. 8(5):490-499, Oct. 1978.

Fraser, H. and Bishop, S.

Smoking and deep-vein thrombosis. (Letter to the Editor.)

Br. Med. J. 2(6150):1499, Nov. 25, 1978.

Fraser, H. S., et al.

Environmental factors affecting antipyrine metabolism in London factory and office workers.

Br. J. Clin. Pharmacol. 7(3): 237-243, Mar. 1979.

Fraumeni, Jr., J. F.

Proceedings of Alcohol and Cancer Workshop: Epidemiological opportunities in alcohol-related cancer.

Cancer Res. 39(7, Part 2): 2851-2852, July 1979.

Frederiksen, L. W. and Martin, J. E.

Carbon monoxide and smoking behavior.

Addict. Behav. 4(1):21-30, 1979.

Freedman, H. J., et al.

Aryl hydrocarbon hydroxylase in a stable human b-lymphocyte cell line, RPMI-1788, cultured in the absence of mitogens.

Cancer Res. 39(11):4605-4611, Nov. 1979.

Freedman, H. J., et al.

Induction, inhibition, and biological properties of aryl hydrocarbon hydroxylase in a stable human b-lympocyte cell line,RPMI-1788.

Cancer Res. 39(11):4612-4619, Nov. 1979.

Frei, J. V., et al.

Alkylation of deoxyribonucleic acid in vivo in various organs of C57BL mice by the carcinogens N-methyl-N-nitrosourea, N-ethyl-N-nitrosourea and ethyl methanesulphonate in relation to induction of thymic lymphoma: Some applications of high-pressure liquid chromography.

Biochem. J. 174(3):1031-1044, Sept. 15, 1978.

Freour, P., et al.

Les praticiens girondins et le tabagisme: Evolution des connaissances et des attitudes de 1971 a 1976. (Fr.)

Bord. Med. 11(18):1615-1620, June 1978.

Friedberg, T., et al.

The identification, solubilization, and characterization of microsome-associated glutathione S-transferases.

J. Biol. Chem. 254(23):12028-12033, Dec. 10, 1979.

Friedel, H. and Preisler, J.

Tagungsbericht der Gesellschaft fuer Innere Medizin der DDR: Das Bronchialkarzinom. (Ger.)

Z. Gesamte Inn. Med. 34(4):25-29, Feb. 15, 1979.

Friedman, A. L. and Segar, W. E.

Antidiuretic hormone excess.

J. Pediatr. 94(4):521-526, Apr. 1979.

Friedman, G. D.

Cigarette smoking and coronary heart disease: New evidence and old reactions.

Am. Heart J. 99(3):398-399, Mar. 1980.

Friedman, G. D., et al.

Mortality in middle-aged smokers and nonsmokers.

N. Engl. J. Med. 300(5):213-217, Feb. 1, 1979.

Friedman, G. D., et al.

The Case Control Study: Consensus and Controversy. Characteristics predictive of coronary heart disease in ex-smokers before they stopped smoking: Comparison with persistant smokers and non-smokers.

J. Chron. Dis. 32(1-2):175-190, 1979.

Frolkis, V. V. and Bezrukov, K.

Aging of the Central Nervous System: CNS reactions to humoral factors.

Interdiscip. Top. Gerontol. 16:90-99, 1979.

Froment, A. and Milon, H.

Comment evisager la prevention de l'infarctus myocardique. (Fr.)

Cah. Med. 4(3):175-179, Sept. 25, 1978.

Fuentes, J. F.

Les malalties respiratories, el tabac i els metges. (Catalan)

Ann. Med. (Barc.) 64(10):1477-1478, Dec. 1978.

Fujii, S., et al.

Effect of uracil and its derivatives on antitumor activity of 5-fluorouracil and 1-(2-tetrahydrofuryl)-5-fluorouracil.

Gann 69(6):763-772, Dec. 1978.

Fujino, T., et al.

The effect of norharman on the metabolism of benzo[a]pyrene by rat-liver microsomes in vitro in relation to its enhancement of the mutagenicity of benzo[a]pyrene.

Mutat. Res. 58(2-3):151-158, Nov. 1978.

Fujita, K., et al.

Increase of urinary putrescine in 3,4-benzopyrene carcinogenesis and its inhibition by putrescine.

Cancer Res. 38(10):3509-3511, Oct. 1978.

Fuller, J. H., et al.

Asymptomatic Hyperglycemia and Coronary Heart Disease. Hyperglycaemia and coronary heart disease: The Whitehall study.

J. Chronic Dis. 32(11/12):721-728, 1979.

Fulmer, J. D., et al.

Morphologic-physiologic correlates of the severity of fibrosis and degree of cellularity in idiopathic pulmonary fibrosis.

J. Clin. Invest. 63(4):665-676, Apr. 1979.

Furst, A., et al.

Pulmonary tumor induction: Three hydrocarbons compared.

Proc. West. Pharmacol. Soc. 22:269-271, 1979.

Furukawa, K.

Mechanisms of contraction and relaxation in the response to 5-hydroxytriptamine of isolated rat ileum. (Jpn.)

Folia Pharmacol. Jpn. 74(4):525-537, May 1978.

Fysh, J. M. and Okey, A. B.

Aryl hydrocarbon (benzo[a]pyrene) hydroxylase development in rat mammary tissue.

Biochem. Pharmacol. 27(24):2968-2972, 1978.

Fysh, J. M. and Okey, A. B.

Aryl hydrocarbon (benzo[a]pyrene) hydroxylase in rat mammary tissue during pregnancy and lactation.

Can. J. Physiol. Pharmacol. 57(1):112-117, Jan. 1979.

Gad, A., et al.

Necrotizing sialometaplasia of the lip simulating squamous cell carcinoma.

Histopathology 4(1):111-121, Jan. 1980.

Gadek, J. E., et al.

Collagenase in the lower respiratory tract of patients with idiopathic pulmonary fibrosis.

N. Engl. J. Med. 301(14):737-742, Oct. 4, 1979.

Gadek, J. E., et al.

Cigarette smoking induces functional antiprotease deficiency in the lower respiratory tract of humans.

Science 206(4424):1315-1316, Dec. 14, 1979.

Gaensler, E. A. and Mark, E. J.

Pleuritic pain, recurrent pleural effusions and a pulsatile mass in a 58-year-old man.

N. Engl. J. Med. 299(21):1179-1185, Nov. 23, 1978.

Gage, M. I.

Automotive exhaust and mouse activity: Relationships between pollutant concentrations and decreases in wheel running.

Arch. Environ. Health 34(3):164-168, May-June 1979.

Gagne, C., et al.

Heterozygous familial hypercholesterolemia: Relationship between plasma lipids, lipoproteins clinical manifestations and ischaemic heart disease in men and women.

Atherosclerosis 34(1):13-24, Sept. 1979.

Gahmberg, C. G., et al.

Induction of aryl hydrocarbon hydroxylase activity and pulmonary carcinoma.

Int. J. Cancer 23(3):302-305, Mar. 15, 1979.

Galbraith, A. I., et al.

Distribution of 7-methylguanine and of replication sites in the different kinetic classes of DNA from rats treated with dimethylnitrosamine.

Nucleic Acids Res. 5(9):3357-3364, Sept. 1978.

Galbraith, A. I., et al.

Methylation of DNAase-digestible DNA and of RNA in chromatin from rats treated with dimethylnitrosamine.

Biochim. Biophys. Acta 561(2):334-344, Feb. 27, 1979.

Galloway, R. W.

Symposium. Awkward Medicolegal Problems in Asbestos-Induced Disease: Problem radiographs.

J. R. Soc. Med. 71(12):916-919, Dec. 1978.

Gambhir, S. S. and Das, P. K.

A vasoconstrictor action of eserine not related to blockade of cholinesterase.

Blood Vessels 16(1):58-60, 1979.

Gamble, J. F., et al.

An epidemiologic study of a group of talc workers.

Am. Rev. Respir. Dis. 119(5):741-753, May 1979.

Ganley, J. P. and Comstock, G. W.

Association of cats and toxoplasmosis.

Am. J. Epidemiol. 111(2):238-246, Feb. 1980.

Garfinkel, L.

Changes in the cigarette consumption of smokers in relation to changes in tar/nicotine content of cigarettes smoked.

Am. J. Public Health 69(12):1274-1276, Dec. 1979.

Garn, S. M., et al.

Dose-response effect of maternal smoking. (Letters to the Editor.)

Pediatrics 62(5):861-863, Nov. 1978.

Garn, S. M., et al.

Is there nutritional mediation of the "smoking effect" on the fetus. (Letter to the Editor.)

Am. J. Clin. Nutr. 32(6):1181-1184, June 1979.

Garraway, W. M., et al.

The declining incidence of stroke.

N. Engl. J. Med. 300(9):449-452, Mar. 1, 1979.

Garrett, R. J. B.

Collagen and non-collagen protein synthesis in developing lung exposed to tobacco smoke.

Environ. Res. 17(2):205-215, Oct. 1978.

Garrett, R. J. B. and Jackson, M. A.

Effect of acute smoke exposure on hepatic protein synthesis.

J. Pharmacol. Exp. Ther. 209(2): 215-218, May 1979.

Garrison, R. J., et al.

The association of total cholesterol, triglycerides and plasma lipoprotein cholesterol levels in first degree relatives and spouse pairs.

Am. J. Epidemiol. 110(3):313-321, Sept. 1979.

Garrow, J. S.

Weight penalties.

Br. Med. J. 2(6199):1171-1172, Nov. 10, 1979.

Gaspard, U.

Les repercussions metaboliques de la contraception orale. (Fr.)

J. Pharm. Belg. 33(5):312-324, Sept.-Oct. 1978.

Gaston, S. F. and Schumann, L. L.

Inhalation injury: Smoke inhalation.

Am. J. Nurs. 80(1):95-97, Jan. 1980.

Gautam, S. C. and Deodhar, S. D.

Presence of suppressor cells in spleens of mice bearing a weakly immunogenic syngeneic tumor.

Cancer Res. 39(8):2945-2951, Aug. 1979.

Gebauer, C.

Bedeutung kanzerogener Noxen fuer die Entstehung pulmonaler Hamartochondrome - eine aetiologische Vergleichsstudie zu Karzinomen und Sarkomen der Lungen. (Ger.)

Arch. Geschwulstforsch. 48(8):761-769, 1978.

Gebauer, C.

Zur aetiologie des primaeren Lungensarkoms in Gegenueberstellung zum Lungenkarzinom. (Ger.)

Z. Erkr. Atmungsorgane 152(1):51-60, 1979.

Geddes, D. M.

The natural history of lung cancer: A review based on rates of tumour growth.

Br. J. Dis. Chest 73(1):1-17, Jan. 1979.

Geddes, D. M., et al.

Airways obstruction in rheumatoid arthritis.

Ann. Rheum. Dis. 38(3):222-225, June 1979.

Gee, J. B. L., et al.

Proceedings of the Aspen Lung Conference: Human alveolar macrophage and obstructive lung disease.

Chest 77(2 Suppl.):271-272, Feb. 1980.

Gehlbach, S. H., et al.

Protective clothing as a means of reducing nicotine absorption in tobacco harvesters.

Arch. Environ. Health 34(2):111-114, Mar.-Apr. 1979.

Gehly, E. B., et al.

The metabolism of benzo(a)pyrene by cytochrome P-450 in transformable and nontransformable C3H mouse fibroblasts.

J. Biol. Chem. 254(12):5041-5048, June 25, 1979.

Geier, A., et al.

Estradiol binding to nuclear receptors in human breast cancer tissue (MCF-7 cell line) and in dimethylbenz(a)anthracene-induced mammary carcinoma.

J. Clin. Endocrinol. Metab. 49(1): 34-39, July 1979.

Gelb, A. F., et al.

Site of airway obstruction after acute cigarette smoking and mild smoke inhalation.

Bull. Eur. Physiopathol. Respir. 15(3):481-490, 1979.

Gelboin, H. V. and Whitlock, Jr., J. P.

The Induction of Drug Metabolism. Chairman's introductory statement: On the mechanism of mixed-function oxidase induction.

Symp. Med. Hoechst 14:67-79, 1979.

Geltman, E. M., et al.

The influence of location and extent of myocardial infarction on long-term ventricular dysrhythmia and mortality.

Circulation 60(4):805-814, Oct. 1979.

Gentleman, J. F., et al.

Smoking and its effect on mortality of the elderly.

Am. J. Med. Sci. 276(2):173-183, Sept.-Oct. 1978.

Georgiev, V. P. and Petkova, B. P.

Apomorphine stereotypies and transmitter mechanisms in the striatum. II. Interactions between GABA-ergic and cholinergic transmission.

Acta Physiol. Pharmacol. Bulg. 4(3):65-70, 1978.

Georgiev, V. P., et al.

Apomorphine sterotypies and transmitter mechanisms in the striatum. I. Changes in the apomorphine stereotypies caused by drugs acting on the GABA-ergic, ergic, dopaminergic and cholinergic transmission.

Acta Physiol. Pharmacol. Bulg. 4(3):56-64, 1978.

Georgiou, V.

Theprevention of the coronary disease. (Greek)

Iatriki 32(5):255-263, Nov. 1977.

Gerlach, D.

Post-mortem investigations of fatal cases of narcotic addiction.

Forensic Sci. Int. 15(1):31-39, Jan.-Feb. 1980.

Geroulanos, S. and Senning, A.

Indikation und Ergebnisse operativer Therapie beim Bronchuskarzinom. (Ger.)

Ther. Umsch. 35(12):1029-1036, Dec. 1978.

Gerrard, J. M. and White, J. G.

Prostaglandins and thromboxanes: "Middlemen" modulating platelet function in hemostasis and thrombosis.

Prog. Hemostasis Thromb. 4:87-125, 1978.

Gerrard, J. W.

Nonsmoking grain handlers in Saskatchewan: Airways reactivity and allergic status.

JOM 21(5):342-346, May 1979.

Gertz, I.

Blood volume and arterial blood gases in patients with chronic obstructive lung disease during acute respiratory failure.

Scand. J. Respir. Dis. 60(1):6-16, Feb. 1979.

Gessner, T., et al.

Presence of glucuronyltransferase activity in human lymphocytes.

Res. Commun. Chem. Pathol. Pharmacol. 22(1):187-197, Oct. 1978.

Ghosh, S. K., et al.

Studies on occupational health problems during agricultural operation of Indian tobacco workers: A preliminary survey report.

JOM 21(1):45-47, Jan. 1979.

Ghosh, S. K., et al.

A tumor-associated organ-specific antigen characteristic of spontaneously metastatic rat mammary carcinomas.

JNCI 62(5):1229-1233, May 1979.

Ghosh, S., et al.

Indentification of anaemia with the help of an anaemia recognition card.

Indian Pediatr. 15(9):751-753, Sept. 1978.

Gibbs, G. W. and Horowitz, I.

Lung cancer mortality in aluminum reduction plant workers.

JOM 21(5):347-353, May 1979.

Gibel, JC and Blumberg, H.-H.

Die Auswirkungen der Rauchgewohnheiten von Eltern auf das ungeborene und neugeborene Kind. (Ger.)

Z. Aerztl. Fortbild. (Jena) 73(7):341-342, Apr. 1, 1979.

Gibson, G. J., et al.

Exponential description of the static pressure-volume curve of normal and diseased lungs.

Am. Rev. Respir. Dis. 120(4):799-811, Oct. 1979.

Gibson, J., et al.

Lung function in an Australian population: 2. Spirometric performance and cigarette-smoking habits.

Med. J. Aust. 1(8):354-358, Apr. 24, 1979.

Gibson, R. E., et al.

The distribution of the muscarinic acetylcholine receptor antagonists, quinuclidinyl benzilate and quinuclidinyl benzilate methiodide (both tritiated), in rat, guinea pig, and rabbit.

J. Nucl. Med. 20(8):865-870, Aug. 1979.

Gilbert, D. G.

Paradoxical tranquilizing and emotion-reducing effects of nicotine.

Psychol. Bull. 86(4):643-661, July 1979.

Gilbert, R. M.

Coffee, tea and cigarette use. (Letter to the Editor.)

Can. Med. Assoc. J. 120(5):522-524, Mar. 3, 1979.

Gill, R. S., et al.

Multicentric metachronous primary carcinoma of the upper alimentary tract in 'Biri' smokers.

J. Laryngol. Otol. 93(5):527-531, May 1979.

Gilli, G., et al.

Ossido di carbonio: Aspetti di tipo ambientale e biologico. (Ital.)

Arch. Sci. Med. (Torino) 135(4):561-584, Oct.-Dec. 1978.

Gilmore, G. D. and Papenfuss, R. L.

Working together: Community and school health education.

Health Educ. 9(3):16-17, May-June 1978.

Giner-Sorolla, A., et al.

N6(methylnitroso)adenosine: A carcinogenic nitrosamine derived from a naturally-occurring nucleoside.

Cancer Lett. 6(2):79-82, Feb. 1979.

Gitlitz, G. F.

How many heart attack victims are not smokers? (Letter to the Editor.)

NY State J. Med. 76(3):420-422, Mar. 1979.

Giuliano, A. E., et al.

Serum-mediated immunosuppression in lung cancer.

Cancer 43(3):917-924, Mar. 1979.

Glatt, H. R., et al.

Reduction of benzo(alpha)pyrene mutagenicity by dihydrodiol dehydrogenase.

Nature 277(5694):319-320, Jan. 25, 1979.

Glatt, H. R., et al.

Mutagenicity of 43 structurally related heterocyclic compounds and its relationship to their carcinogenicity.

Mutat. Res. 66(4):307-328, Apr. 1979.

Glatt, M. M., et al.

Neurological and Mental Disturbances in the Elderly. Proceedings of a Conference: Alcoholic problems in the elderly.

Age Ageing 7(Suppl.):64-71, 1978.

Glaven, P.

Rygning eller sundhed. (Dan.)

Nord. Med. 93(5-6):100-101, June 1978.

Gleich, G. J. and Welsh, P. W.

Immunochemical and physicochemical properties of tobacco extracts.

Am. Rev. Respir. Dis. 120(5):995-1001, Nov. 1979.

Gloyna, E. F. and Taylor, R. D.

Los Alamos Life Sciences Symposium: Hazardous Solid Wastes and their Disposal. Elimination of the hazards from hazardous wastes.

Environ. Health Perspect. 27:323-335, Dec. 1978.

Godbold, Jr., J. H. and Tompkins, E. A.

A long-term mortality study of workers occupationally exposed to metallic nickel at the oak ridge gaseous diffusion plant.

JOM 21(12):799-806, Dec. 1979.

Godoy, H. M., et al.

Mechanism of dimethylnitrosamine metabolism and activation in rats.

JNCI 61(5):1285-1289, Nov. 1978.

Goedde, H. W.

Colloque International de Biologie Prospective: Genetic aspects in the metabolism of drugs and environmental agents.

Ann. Biol. Clin. (Paris) 36(3):181-189, 1978.

Goerttler, K., et al.

Systemic two-stage carcinogenesis in the epithelium of the forestomach of mice using 7,12-dimethylbenz(a)anthracene as initiator and the phorbol ester 12-O-tetradecanoylphorbol-13-acetate as promoter.

Cancer Res. 39(4):1293-1297, Apr. 1979.

Goerttler, K., et al.

Two-stage tumorigenesis of dermal melanocytes in the back skin of the Syrian goldern hamster using systemic initiation with 7,12-dimethylbenz(a) anthracene and topical promotion with 12-O-tetradecanoylphorbol-13-acetate.

Cancer Res. 40(1):155-161, Jan. 1980.

Goethe, C.-J.

Symposium om Diagnostik vid Bronkial-Cancer: Anamnes, roek anor, sjukdomsbakgrund. (Swed.)

Lakardtidningen 75(17):1725-1726, Apr. 26, 1978.

Going, R. E., et al.

Sugar and fluoride content of various forms of tobacco.

J. Am. Dent. Assoc. 100(1):27-33, Jan. 1980.

Gold, E., et al.

Risk factors for brain tumors in children.

Am. J. Epidemiol. 109(3):309-319, Mar. 1979.

Goldberg, J.

Lassen sich Rauchgewohnheiten Jugendlicher beeinflussen? Erster Erfahrungsbericht ueber einen Versuch der Reduzierung von Rauchgewohnheiten bei Oberschuelern. (Ger.)

Dtsch. Gesundheitswes. 32(38):1809-1812, 1977.

Goldberg, R., et al.

Length of time between hospital admission and ventricular fibrillation or cardiac arrest complicating acute myocardial infarction: Effect on prognosis.

Johns Hopkins Med. J. 145(5):187-191, Nov. 1979.

Goldberg, T., et al.

Time trends in prognosis of patients with myocardial infarction: A population-based study.

Johns Hopkins Med. J. 144(3):73-80, Mar. 1979.

Goldbourt, U. and Medalie, J. H.

High density lipoprotein cholesterol and incidence of coronary heart disease - The Israeli Ischemic Heart Disease Study.

Am. J. Epidemiol. 109(3):296-308, Mar. 1979.

Gontovnick, L. S., et al.

The irreversible binding of benzo[a]pyrene to rat liver macromolecules in vivo and in vitro: Effects of agents that influence benzo[a]pyrene metabolism.

Can. J. Physiol. Pharmacol. 57(11):1238-1245, Nov. 1979.

Gordon, R. S. (Editor)

From the NIH: Cause of diabetes... Helping patients stop smoking.

JAMA 242(10):1015-1016, Sept. 7, 1979.

Gordon, T., et al.

Predictability of coronary heart disease.

J. Chronic Dis. 32(6):427-440, 1979.

Gori, G. B.

Proceedings of the American Cancer Society and National Cancer Institute National Conference on Nutrition in Cancer: Dietary and nutritional implications in the multifactorial etiology of certain prevalent human cancers.

Cancer 43(5, Suppl.):2151-2161, May 1979.

Gori, G. B.

Workshop on Carbon Monoxide and Cardiovascular Disease: Summary of the workshop on carbon monoxide and cardiovascular disease, Berlin, October 10-12, 1978.

Prev. Med. 8(3):404-406, May 1979.

Gori, G. B. and Lynch, C. J.

Toward less hazardous cigarettes: Current advances.

JAMA 240(12):1255-1259, Sept. 15, 1978.

Gori, G. B. and Ellis, R. L.

Workshop on Carbon Monoxide and Cardiovascular Disease: Reduction of carbon monoxide in cigarette smoke.

Prev. Med. 8(3):358-368, May 1979.

Gould, L., et al.

Premature hair graying: A problem coronary risk factor.

Angiology 29(11):800-803, Nov. 1978.

Grab, D.J., et al.

Mechanism of inhibition of hepatic protein synthesis in rats by the carcinogen, methylazoxymethanol acetate.

Biochim. Biophys. Acta 563(1):240-252, June 20, 1979.

Gracey, M., et al.

The 1977 Busselton childrens survey.

Med. J. Aust. 2(5):265-267, Sept. 8, 1979.

Gram, L. F., et al.

d-Propoxyphene kinetics after single oral and intravenous doses in man.

Clin. Pharmacol. Ther. 26(4):473-482, Oct. 1979.

Grandjean, E., et al.

"Passivrauchen". (Ger.)

Bull. Schweiz. Akad. Med. Wiss. 35(1-3):99-109, Mar. 1979.

Granger, D. L., et al.

Injury of neoplastic cells by murine macrophages leads to inhibition of mitochondrial respiration.

J.Clin.Invest. 65(2):357-370, Feb. 1980.

Grant, E. C. G.

Oral contraceptives, smoking, migraine, and food allergy. (Letter to the Editor.)

Lancet 2(8089):581-582, Sept. 9, 1978.

Grant, E. C. G.

Food allergies and migraine.

Lancet 1(8123):966-969, May 5, 1979.

Grassi, C. and Rampulla, C.

La diagnosi precoce delle malattie ostruttive delle vie aeree: Possibilita e limiti dei tests funzionali. (Ital.)

Minerva Med. 69(2):85-110, Jan. 14, 1978.

Grebska, E.

Odwracalnosc zaburzen czynnosciowych oddychania po zaprzestaniu palenia papierosow. (Pol.)

Pneumonol. Pol. 46(10):707-711, Oct. 1978.

Grebska, E.

Zaburzenia czynnosciowe ukladu oddechowego u osob palacych papierosy. (Pol.)

Pneumonol. Pol. 46(10):697-706, Oct. 1978.

Gredler, B., et al.

Raunchen und Lungenkrebs"- Wissen, Einstellungne und" Meinungen der Bevoeklerung. (Ger.)

Prax. Klin. Pneumol. 34(1):45-53, Jan. 1980.

Green, A. F., et al.

Pharmacological Methods in Toxicology. Autonomic pharmacology: Report of the main working party.

Pharmacol. Ther. 5(1-3, Suppl.):9-48, 1979.

Green, A. R.

An updated assessment of the critical environmental factors involved in the prevention of allergic disease.

Ann. Allergy 42(6):372-383, June 1979.

Green, D. M. and Jaffe, N.

Wilm's tumor-Model of a curable pediatric malignant solid tumor.

Cancer Treat. Rev. 5(3):143-172, Sept. 1978.

Green, M. R., et al.

Elastolytic activity of alveolar macrophages in normal dogs and human subjects.

J. Lab. Clin. Med. 94(4):549-562, Oct. 1979.

Greenblatt, D. J., et al.

Diazepam disposition determinants.

Clin. Pharmacol. Ther. 27(3):301-312, Mar. 1980.

Greenblatt, D. J., et al.

Lorazepam kinetics in the elderly.

Clin. Pharmacol. Ther. 26(1):103-113, July 1979.

Greenburg, D. S.

Carter's purge: The Califano file.

N. Engl. J. Med. 301(8):451-452, Aug. 23, 1979.

Greene, E. J., et al.

In vitro mutagenicity and cell transformation screening of phenylglycidyl ether.

Mutat. Res. 67(1):9-19, May 1979.

Greene, F. E. and Jernstrom, B.

Epoxide hydratase and glutathione S-transferase activities in human lungs.

Cancer Lett. 8(3):235-239, Jan. 1980.

Greenland, S.

The interaction of nitrites with food, drugs, and contaminants.

J. Environ. Health 41(3):141-143, Nov.-Dec. 1978.

Greer, C. A. and Alpern, H. P.

Maturational changes related to dopamine in the effects of d-amphetamine, cocaine, nicotine, and strychnine on seizure susceptibility.

Psychopharmacology (Berlin) 64(3):255-260, Sept. 1979.

Greer, S.

Psychological enquiry: A contribution to cancer research.

Psychol. Med. 9(1):81-89, Feb. 1979.

Greiner, J. W., et al.

Detection of aryl hydrocarbon hydroxylase activity in normal and neoplastic human breast epithelium.

Life Sci. 26(4):313-319, Jan. 28, 1980.

Griciute, L.

Environmental Carcinogens - Selected Methods of Analysis, Vol. 1. Analysis of Volatile Nitrosamines in Food: Carcinogenicity of N-nitroso compounds and their possible role in the development of human cancer.

IARC Sci. Publ. No. 18:3-9, 1978.

Griffin, A. C.

Proceedings of a Conference on the Relationship between Environmental Chemicals and Cancer. Environmental cancer: Animal studies and assay procedures.

Tex. Rep. Biol. Med. 37:45-49, 1978.

Grimes, D. S. and Goddard, J.

Effect of cigarette smoking on gastric emptying.

Br. Med. J. 2(6135):460-461, Aug. 12, 1978.

Grinspan, D. and Abulafia, J.

Oral florid papillomatosis (verrucous carcinoma).

Int. J. Dermatol. 18(8):608-622, Oct. 1979.

Grisham, J. W., et al.

Proceedings of an International Workshop Meeting on Factors Influencing Metabolism and Toxicity of Metals. In vitro assay of cytotoxicity with cultured liver: Accomplishments and possibilities.

Environ. Health Perspect. 25:161-171, Aug. 1978.

Groenhagen-Riska, C.

Angiotensin-converting enzyme: I. Activity and correlation with serum lysozyme in sarcoidosis, other chest or lymph node diseases and healthy persons.

Scand. J. Respir. Dis. 60(2):83-93, Apr. 1979.

Gronow, M.

Nuclear proteins and chemical carcinogenesis.

Chem. Biol. Interact. 29(1):1-30, Jan. 1980.

Grosz, H. J.

Nicotine addiction: Treatment with medical hypnosis: Part 1.

J. Indiana State Med. Assoc. 71(11): 1074-1075, Nov. 1978.

Grosz, H. J.

Nicotine addiction: Treatment with medical hypnosis. Part 2.

J. Indiana State Med. Assoc. 71(12): 1136-1137, Dec. 1978.

Grosz, H. J.

Hypnotherapy in the management of terminally ill cancer patients.

J. Indiana State Med. Assoc. 72(2):126-129, Feb. 1979.

Gruenke, L. D., et al.

The determination of nicotine in biological fluids at picogram levels by selected ion recording.

Anal. Biochem. 94(2):411-416, Apr. 15, 1979.

Grunberger, D., et al.

Translation of globin messenger RNA modified by benzo[a]pyrene 7,8-dihydrodiol 9,10-oxide in a wheat germ cell-free system.

J. Biol. Chem. 255(2):390-394, Jan. 25, 1980.

Grundy, P. F.

Meeting of the Society for Social Medicine: Ten-year mortality follow-up of 5000 steelwokers in relation to lung functions, respiratory symptomatology, obesity, and smoking habit. (Abstr.)

J. Epidemiol. Commun. Health 33(2): 165, June 1979.

Grygiel, J. J., et al.

Effects of allopurinol on theophylline metabolism and clearance.

Clin. Pharmacol. Ther. 26(5):660-667, Nov. 1979.

Gsell, O., et al.

Rauchen und Mortalitaet der Schweizer Aerzte: Resultate nach 18 Jaehriger Beobachtung. (Ger.)

Bull. Schweiz. Akad. Med. Wiss. 35(1-3):71-82, Mar. 1979.

Gudbjarnason, S., et al.

Sudden Coronary Death: Myocardial membrane lipids in relation to cardiovascular disease.

Adv. Cardiol. 25:130-144, 1978.

Gudbjarnason, S., et al.

International Symposium on Prostaglandins: Docosahexaenoic acid in cardiac metabolism and function.

Acta Biol. Med. Ger. 37(5-6):777-784, 1978.

Guengerich, F. P.

Similarity of nuclear and microsomal cytochromes P-450 in the in vitro activation of aflatoxin B1.

Biochem. Pharmacol. 28(19):2883-2890, Oct. 1, 1979.

Guengerich, F. P., et al.

Rat and human liver microsomal epoxide hydratase: Purification and evidence for the existence multiple forms.

J. Biol. Chem. 254(23):12248-12254, Dec. 10, 1979.

Guengerich, F. P.

Isolation and purification of cytochrome P-450 and the existence of multiple forms.

Pharmacol. Ther. 6(1):99-121, 1979.

Guenthner, T. M., et al.

Effects of different cell constituents on metabolic activation and binding of benzo(a)pyrene to purified and nuclear DNA.

Biochem. Biophys. Res. Commun. 91(3):842-848, Dec. 14, 1979.

Guenthner, T. M., et al.

Nadph-cytochrome P-450 reductase: Preferential inhibition by ellipticine and other type II compounds having little effect on nadph-cytochrome c reductase.

Biochem. Pharmacol. 29(1):89-95, Jan. 1, 1980.

Guerin, M. R., et al.

Inhalation bioassay chemistry - Walton horizontal smoking machine for inhalation exposure of rodents to cigarette smoke.

JNCI 63(2):441-448, Aug. 1979.

Guerrero, R. R., et al.

Bioassay procedure for the detection of mutagenic metabolites in human urine with the use of sister chromatid exchange analysis.

JNCI 62(4):805-809, Apr. 1979.

Guidotti, T. L.

Coal workers' pneumoconiosis and medical aspects of coal mining.

South. Med. J. 72(4):456-466, Apr. 1979.

Guillot, C., et al.

Le pouvoir oxyphorique: Precision et variabilite de la mesure; influence du taux de carboxyhemoglobine. (Fr.)

Pathol. Biol. (Paris) 27(2):91-94, Feb. 1979.

Guirgis, H. A., et al.

Genetic and communicable effects on carcinoembryonic antigen expres sivity in the cancer family syndrome.

Cancer Res. 38(8):2523-2528, Aug. 1978.

Guirgis, H. A., et al.

Proceedings of the International Conference on the Clinical Uses of Carcinoembryonic Antigen: Carcinoembryonic antigen (CEA) in the cancer family syndrome.

Cancer 42(3, Suppl.):1574-1578, Sept. 1978.

Guirgis, H. A., et al.

Carcinoembryonic Proteins: Recent Progress. Immunochemical biological markers and hereditary cancer risk.

Scand. J. Immunol. 8(Supp. 8): 647-652, 1978.

Guize, L., et al.

L'obesite facteur de risque de l'atherosclerose. (Fr.)

Gaz. Med. Fr. 85(31):3593-3599, Oct. 13, 1978.

Gullestad, L., et al.

Roekevaner hos gravide i Troendelag. (Norw., Engl. Summary)

Tidsskr. Nor. Laegeforen. 99(12):575-579;596, Apr. 30, 1979.

Gulsvik, A. and Fagerhol, M. K.

Smoking and immunoglobulin levels. (Letter to the Editor.)

Lancet 1(8113):449, Feb. 24, 1979.

Guomundsson, S., et al.

Sjuklingar med kransaedastiflu a borgarspitala 1972-1975. (Ice.)

Laeknabladid 65(3):123-131, July 1979.

Gupta, P. K., et al.

Morphological identification of alpha-1-antitrypsin in pulmonary macrophages.

Hum. Pathol. 10(3):345-347, May 1979.

Gurtoo, H. L. and Dahms, R. P.

Effects of inducers and inhibitors on the metabolism of aflatoxin B1 by rat and mouse.

Biochem. Pharmacol. 28(23):3441-3449, Dec. 1, 1979.

Gurtoo, H. L., et al.

Cytochrome p-450 in a cultured human lymphocyte cell line.

Biochem. Pharmacol. 27(22):2659-2662, 1978.

Gurtoo, H. L., et al.

Induction, inhibition, and some enzymological properties of aryl hydrocarbon hydroxylase in fresh mitogen-activated human lymphocytes.

Cancer Res. 39(11):4620-4629, Nov. 1979.

Gutierrez, P. L., et al.

Paramagnetic changes in cancer: DMBA-induced tumours studied in non-lyophilized and lyophilized tissues.

Br. J. Cancer 39(3):330-336, Mar. 1979.

Gutner, R., et al.

Coronary artery aneurysms: Clinical angiographic, and therapeutic considerations.

Vasc. Surg. 12(6):392-409, Nov.-Dec. 1978.

Guttenplan, J. B.

Detection of trace amounts of dimethylnitrosamine in a modified salmonella/microsome assay.

Mutat. Res. 64(2):91-94, Apr. 1979.

Guzelian, P. S. and Elshourbagy, N. A.

Induction of hepatic heme oxygenase activity by bromobenzene.

Arch. Biochem. Biophys. 196(1):178-185, Aug. 1979.

Guzman Blanco, G.

Effet de la fumee du tabac sur le surfactant pulmonaire. (Fr.)

Bronchopneumologie 28(4):290-296, July-Aug. 1978.

Haack, D. G.

Interactions of risk factors for COPD. (Letter to the Editor.)

Am. Rev. Respir. Dis. 118(4):798-799, Oct. 1978.

Haag, W. M.

Workshop on Carbon Monoxide and Cardiovascular Disease: Methods to reduce carbon monoxide levels at the workplace.

Prev. Med. 8(3):369-378, May 1979.

Haas, J. F. and Schottenfeld, D.

Risks to the offspring from parental occupational exposures.

JOM 21(9):607-613, Sept. 1979.

Hacker, N. F. and Biggs, J. S. G.

Blood pressure changes when uterine stimulants are used after normal delivery.

Br. J. Obstet. Gynaecol. 86(8):633-636, Aug. 1979.

Hackett, D. R.

Smoking habits during pregnancy.

Ir. Med. J. 72(11):483-486, Nov. 30,. 1979.

Haenszel, W., et al.

A case-control study of large bowel cancer in Japan.

JNCI 64(1):17-22, Jan. 1980.

Hafermann, D. R., et al.

Effects of influenza vaccination on the peripheral airways of healthy human volunteers.

Chest 75(4):468-470, Apr. 1979.

Haft, J. I.

Role of blood platelets in coronary artery disease.

Am. J. Cardiol. 43(6):1197-1206, June 1979.

Haimes, A. P., et al.

Ethnic-group differences in serum levels of carcinoembryonic antigen. (Letter to the Editor.)

Lancet 2(8149):969, Nov. 3, 1979.

Haire, H. M., et al.

Smoking, hypertension, and mortality in a maintenance dialysis population.

Cardiovasc. Med. 3(11):1163-1168, Nov. 1978.

Hajeri, H., et al.

Smoking during pregnancy and maternal weight gain.

J. Perinat. Med. 7(1):33-38, 1979.

Hale, M.

Preventing toxic insult to fetus and newborn.

Contempt. Ob/Gyn 15(2):143-161, Feb. 1980.

Hall, J. H.

The case for health hazard appraisals: Which health-screening techniques are cost-effective?

Diagnosis 2(2):60-82, Feb. 1980.

Hall, W. J. and Hall, C. B.

Clinical significance of pulmonary function tests: Alterations in pulmonary function following respiratory viral infection.

Chest 76(4):458-465, Oct. 1979.

Halling, H.

Health Effects of Halogenated Aromatic Hydrocarbon: Suspected link between exposure to hexachlorophene and malformed infants.

Ann. NY Acad. Sci. 320:426-435, 1979.

Halperin, J. L. and Coffman, J. D.

Pathophysiology of Raynaud's disease.

Arch. Intern. Med. 139(1):89-92, Jan. 1979.

Halperin, M., et al.

Genesis and interpretation of differences in distribution of baseline characteristics between cases and non-cases in cohort studies.

J. Chron. Dis. 32(7):483-491, 1979.

Halpert, J., et al.

Isolation and incorporation of rabbit liver epoxide hydrase into phospholipid vesicles.

J. Biol. Chem. 254(15):7434-7441, Aug. 10, 1979.

Hamann, G. O. and Christensen, N. J.

Total serum-oestriol: Hojle kliniske data paa danske gravide kvinder. (Dan.)

Ugeskr. Laeger 141(6):360-362, Feb. 5, 1979.

Hamby, R. I. and Sherman, L.

Duration and treatment of diabetes: Relationship to severity of coronary artery disease.

NY State J. Med. 79(11):1683-1688, Oct. 1979.

Hammer, R. E. and Mitchell, J. A.

Nicotine reduces embryo growth, delays implantation and retards parturition in rats.

Proc. Soc. Exp. Biol. Med. 162(2): 333-336, Nov. 1979.

Hamosh, M., et al.

Effect of tobacco smoke on the metabolism of rat lung.

Arch. Environ. Health 34(1):17-23, Jan.-Feb. 1979.

Hanawalt, P. C., et al.

DNA repair in bacteria and mammalian cells.

Ann. Rev. Biochem. 48:783-836, 1979.

Handelsman, D. J. and Turtle, J. R.

Diabetes control: A changing scene.

Med. J. Aust. 1(13):607-611, June 30, 1979.

Hankinson, J. L., et al.

Pulmonary air space size in coal miners.

Am. Rev. Respir. Dis. 119(3):391-397, Mar. 1979.

Hankinson, O.

Single-step selection of clones of a mouse hepatoma line deficient in aryl hydrocarbon hydroxylase.

Proc. Natl. Acad. Sci. USA 76(1):373-376, Jan. 1979.

Hard, G. C.

Effect of age at treatment on incidence and type of renal neoplasm induced in the rat by a single dose of dimethylnitrosamine.

Cancer Res. 39(12):4965-4970, Dec. 1979.

Hard, G. C.

Definition of target cell populations in carcinogenesis.

Cancer Forum 16:194-197, Mar. 1979.

Hardell, L. and Sandstroem, A.

Case-control study: Soft-tissue sarcomas and exposure to phenoxyacetic acids or chlorophenols.

Br. J. Cancer 39(6):711-717, June 1979.

Harkey, M. R., et al.

Spectral studies on the interaction of dichloromethane with hemoglobin.

Mol. Pharmacol. 16(3):1065-1074, Nov. 1979.

Harlap, S., et al.

A prospective study of spontaneous fetal losses after induced abortions.

N. Engl. J. Med. 301(13):677-681, Sept. 27, 1979.

Harlem, O. K.

Ikke vaart bord? (Norw.)

Tidsskr. Nor. Laegeforen. 99(12):567-568, Apr. 30, 1979.

Harris, C. C., et al.

Metabolism of benzo(a)pyrene, N-nitrosodimethylamine, and N-nitrosopyrrolidine and identification of the major carcinogen-DNA adducts formed in cultured human esophagus.

Cancer Res. 39(11):4401-4406, Nov. 1979.

Harris, R. M., et al.

Interactions of retroviruses with chemical carcinogens: I. Noncovalent binding of unactivated polycyclic aromatic hydrocarbons.

Virology 97(1):42-54, Aug. 1979.

Harrison, A., et al.

Smoking and ulcer. (Letter to the Editor and Reply.)

Gastroenterology 75(6):1188-1189, Dec. 1978.

Harrison, G. N., et al.

Small airway disease: Comparison of tests in young smokers versus non-smokers.

South. Med. J. 71(9):1079-1081, Sept. 1978.

Harrison, G. N., et al.

Peripheral airway function in healthy young cigarette smokers.

Lung 156(3):205-215, 1979.

Harrup, T., et al.

Clinical methods in smoking cessation: Description and evaluation of a stop smoking clinic.

Am. J. Public Health 69(12):1226-1231, Dec. 1979.

Harshbarger, J. C. (Moderator), et al.

Aquatic Pollutants and Biologic Effects with Emphasis on Neoplasia. Neoplasms in Aquatic Animals: General discussion.

Ann. NY Acad. Sci. 298:463-481, Sept. 29, 1977.

Harshbarger, J. C.

Aquatic Pollutants and Biologic Effects with Emphasis on Neoplasia: Role of the Registry of Tumors in Lower Animals in the study of environmental carcinogenesis in aquatic animals.

Ann. NY Acad. Sci. 298:280-289, Sept. 29, 1977.

Hashimoto, Y. and Kitagawa, H. S.

Antigen characteristics of nitrosamine-induced urinary bladder cancer in rats.

Gan 70(3):305-314, June 1979.

Hasin, Y., et al.

Relationship between extent of coronary artery disease and correlative risk factors.

Am. Heart J. 98(5):555-561, Nov. 1979.

Haslam, P. L., et al.

Bronchoalveolar lavage in pulmonary fibrosis: Comparison of cells obtained with lung biopsy and clinical features.

Thorax 35(1):9-18, Jan. 1980.

Haslam, S. Z.

Age as a modifying factoe of 7,12-dimethylbenz(a)-anthracene-induced mammary carcinogenesis in the Lewis rat.

Int. J. Cancer 23(3):374-379, Mar. 15, 1979.

Haspels, A. A. and Kremer, J.

De anticonceptiepil. (Dut.)

Ned. Tijdschr. Geneeskd. 122(32): 1188-1190, Aug. 12, 1978.

Havlik, R. J., et al.

Blood pressure aggregation in families.

Am. J. Epidemiol. 110(3):304-312, Sept. 1979.

Hawthorne, V. M. and Gilmour, W. H.

Asymptomatic Hyperglycemia and Coronary Heart Disease: Relationship of glucose to prevalence of ECG abnormalities at baseline and to 6-yr mortality in Scottish males aged 45-64 yr.

J. Chronic Dis. 32(11/12):787-796, 1979.

Hay, D. R.

Cigarette smoking in New Zealand: Results from the 1976 population census.

NZ Med. J. 88(618):135-138, Aug. 23, 1978.

Hayashi, M., et al.

Morphometric analyses of tracheal gland secretion and hypertrophy in male and female rats after experimental exposure to tobacco smoke.

Am. Rev. Respir. Dis. 119(1):67-73, Jan. 1979.

Hayem, A., et al.

Composition proteique et enzymatique des liquides de lavage bronchique et broncho-alveolaire de six sujets normaux. (Fr.)

Bull. Eur. Physiopathol. Respir. 15(4): 611-624, 1978.

Hayes, D. A., et al.

Detection of respiratory mechanical dysfunction by forced random noise impedance parameters.

Am. Rev. Respir. Dis. 120(5):1095-1100, Nov. 1979.

Hecht, A.

Entspricht das Konzept zur Praevention der chronisch ischaemischen Herzkrankheit den gegenwaertigen Vorstellungen zur Aetiologie und Pathogenese der Arteriosklerose? (Ger.)

Z. Gesamte Inn. Med. 34(11):297-301, June 1, 1979.

Hecht, R. and Thielmann, H. W.

Purification and characterization of an endonuclease from Micrococcus luteus that acts on depurinated and carcinogen-modified DNA.

Eur. J. Biochem. 89(2):607-618, Sept. 1, 1978.

Hecht, S. S., et al.

Comparative tumor initiating activity of 10-methylbenzo[a]pyrene, 7,10-dimethylbenzo[a]pyrene and benzo[a]-pyrene.

Cancer Lett. 5(3):179-183, Sept. 1978.

Hecht, S. S., et al.

Environmental Aspects of N-Nitroso Compounds: Chemical studies on tobacco smoke LVI. Tobacco specific nitrosamines: Origins, carcinogenicity and metabolism.

IARC Sci. Publ. No. 19:395-413, 1978.

Hecht, S. S., et al.

Comparative carcinogenicity in F344 rats of the tobacco-specific nitrosamines, N'-nitrosonornicotine and 4 (N-methyl-N-nitrosamino)-1-(3-pyridyl)-1-butanone.

Cancer Res. 40(2):298-302, Feb. 1980.

Hecker, L. I., et al.

Metabolism of liver carcinogen N-nitrosopyrrolidine by rat liver microsomes.

Cancer Res. 39(7, Part 1):2679-2686, July 1979.

Hedenberg, L., et al.

Riktad haesoundersoekning av asbestexponderade. (Swed.)

Lakartidningen 75(45):4151-4152, Nov. 8, 1978.

Hedstrand, H., et al.

Roekavvaenjning bland 50-aariga maen. (Swed.)

Lakartidningen 75(41):3676-3678, Oct. 11, 1978.

Heino, M., et al.

Work conditions and health of locomotive engineers: I. Noise, vibration, thermal climate, diesel exhaust constituents, ergonomics.

Scand. J. Work Environ. Health. 4(Suppl. 3):3-14, 1978.

Heit, M. and Tan, Y. L.

The concentrations of selected polynuclear aromatic hydrocarbons in the surface sediments of some fresh and marine waters of the United States.

Environ. Meas. Lab. Environ. Q. No. 353:I-3-I-39, Apr. 1, 1979.

Heit, P. and GibsOn, J.

Treatment vs. prevention of smoking.

Health Educ. 9(3):8-9, May-June 1978.

Helsing, K. J., et al.

Comparison of three standardized questionnaires on respiratory symptoms.

Am. Rev. Respir. Dis. 120(6):1221-1231, Dec. 1979.

Hemminki, K. and Vainio, H.

Preferential binding of benzo[a]pyrene into nuclear matrix fraction.

Cancer Lett. 6(3):167-173, Mar. 1979.

Hemminki, K., et al.

Tyoeperaeinen syoepae - Haaste tutkimukselle ja sairauksien ehkaeisylle. (Finn.)

Suom. Laeaekaeril. 34(10):781-791, Apr. 2, 1979.

Henderson, B. E. and Louie, E.

Nasopharyngeal carcinoma: Etiology and Control. Discussion of risk factors for nasopharyngeal carcinoma.

IARC Sci. Publ. No. 20:251-260, 1978.

Hendtlass, J.

Survey of alcoholism treatment services in Victoria: Relationship of alcoholics' drug use to their use of medical facilities.

Med. J. Aust. 2(12):635-636, Dec. 15, 1979.

Henkes, H. E.

Stoornissen in het gezichstvermogen als gevolg van ethylalcoholgebruik. (Dut.)

Ned. Tijdschr. Geneeskd. 123(29):1260-1264, July 21, 1979.

Hennekens, C. H., et al.

Use of permanent hair dyes and cancer among registered nurses.

Lancet 1(8131):1390-1393, June 30, 1979.

Hennekens, C. H., et al.

Oral contraceptive use and fasting triglyceride, plasma cholesterol and HDL cholesterol.

Circulation 60(3):486-489, Sept. 1979.

Hennemann, H. H., et al.

Frueherkennung des Bronchial-karzinoms. (Ger.)

Med. Klin. 74(24):959-963, June 15, 1979.

Henry, R. C.

The transformation of laryngeal leucoplakia to cancer.

J. Laryngol. Otol. 93(5):447-459, May 1979.

Hepper, N. G. G., et al.

Chronic obstructive pulmonary disease: A community-oriented program including professional education and screening by a voluntary health agency.

Am. Rev. Respir. Dis. 121(1):97-104, Jan. 1980.

Herbert, V.

Facts and fictions about megavitamin therapy.

J. Fla. Med. Assoc. 66(4):475-481, Apr. 1979.

Hernandez Mijares, A., et al.

Valor del antigeno carcino-embrionario en el diagnostico del cancer. (Span.)

Rev. Clin. Esp. 152(4):291-294, Feb. 28, 1979.

Herrmann, H.

Tagungsbericht der Gesellschaft fuer Innere Medizin der DDR: Chronische Atemwegserkrankungen. (Ger.)

Z. Gesamte Inn. Med. 34(4):21-25, Feb. 15, 1979.

Herscowitz, H. B. and Cooper, R. B.

Effect of cigarette smoke exposure on maturation of the antibody response in spleens of newborn mice.

Pediatr. Res. 13(9):987-991, Sept. 1979.

Hersey, P.

Smoking and natural immunity to tumours.

Med. J. Aust. 2(5):233, Sept. 8, 1979.

Hertz, C. W.

Scandinavian Symposium on Chronic Obstructive Airways Disease: Historical aspects of anticholinergic treatment of obstructive airways disease.

Scand. J. Respir. Dis. Suppl. 103:105-109, 1979.

Hertzer, N. R., et al.

Routine coronary angiography prior to elective aortic reconstruction.

Arch. Surg. 114(11):1336-1344, Nov. 1979.

Herxheimer, A. (Editor)

Less dangerous smoking.

Drug Ther. Bull. 16(5):17-19, Mar. 3, 1978.

Herzog, Ch.

Ovulationshemmer: Kardiovaskulaere Komplikationen und zusaetzliche Risikofaktoren. (Ger.)

Praxis 68(41):1321-1329, Oct. 9, 1979.

Hess, P.

Modifications de l'epithelium bronchique en fonction du tabagisme en 1955-1960 et 1970-1977. (Fr.)

Med. Hyg. 37(1328):1336;1335, Apr. 11, 1979.

Hess, P.

Donnees nouvelles sur les consequences foetales du tabagisme maternel. (Fr.)

Med. Hyg. 37(1332):1744, May 9, 1979.

Hevelke, G.

Aetiologie und Therapie der Ateriosklerose. (Ger.)

Ther. Ggw. 117(12):1869-1889, Dec. 1978.

Hewer, T. et al.

Ingested mutagens from opium and tobacco pyrolysis products and cancer of the oesophagus.

Lancet 2(8088):494-496, Sept. 2, 1978.

Heyden, S., et al.

The combined effect of smoking and coffee drinding on LDL and HDL cholesterol.

Circulation 60(1):22-25, July 1979.

Heyden, S., et al.

Smoking and coffee consumption in three groups: Cancer deaths, cardio-vascular deaths and living controls. A prospective study in Evans County, Georgia.

J. Chronic Dis. 32(9-10):673-677, 1979.

Hickey, N., et al.

Asymptomatic Hyperglycemia and Coronary Heart Disease. The relationship between blood glucose and prevalence of coronary heart disease: A study in the Republic of Ireland.

J. Chronic Dis. 32(11/12):757-772, 1979.

Hicks, R. M.

Multistage carcinogenesis in the urinary bladder.

Br. Med. Bull. 36(1):39-46, Jan. 1980.

Hida, W., et al.

Inflection points of lung pressure-volume curves using a three balloon-catheter system.

J. Appl. Physiol. 47(5):931-937, Nov. 1979.

Higenbottam, T. and Dixon, J.

Chondritis associated with fatal intramural bronchial fibrosis.

Thorax 34(4):563-564, Aug. 1979.

Higenbottam, T. and Clark, T. J. H.

A method for standardizing airway resistance for variations in lung volume.

Clin. Sci. 57(5):397-400, Nov. 1979.

Higenbottam, T., et al.

Lung function and symptoms of cigarette smokers related to tar yield and number of cigarettes smoked.

Lancet 1(8165):409-412, Feb. 23, 1980.

Higenbottam, T., et al.

Acute effects of smoking a single cigarette on the airway resistance and the maximal and partial forced expiratory flow volume curves.

Br. J. Dis. Chest 74(1):37-46, Jan. 1980.

Higgins, P. J., et al.

Tissue distribution and biochemical properties of an interspecific tumour-associated gamma foetal antigen.

Br. J. Cancer 40(2):253-259, Aug. 1979.

Higginson, J.

New Concepts in Safety Evaluation, Part 2: Role of epidemiology in identifying environmental carcinogens.

Adv. Mod. Toxicol. 1(Part 2): 11-25, 1979.

Higginson, J.

International Cancer Congress, Part I. special lecture: Perspectives in environmental carcinogenesis.

Cancer Bull. 31(3):50-52, Mar.-Apr. 1979.

Higginson, J. and Muir, C. S.

Environmental carcinogenesis: Misconceptions and limitations to cancer control.

JNCI 63(6):1291-1298, Dec. 1979.

Higuchi, T., et al.

Microsomal enzymes in patients with gastric carcinoma as determined by plasma half-life of antipyrine.

Gann 69(6):753-756, Dec. 1978.

Hilado, C. J., et al.

Toxicity of pyrolysis gases from synthetic polymers.

Proc. West. Pharmacol. Soc. 22:209-211, 1979.

Hilado, C. J., et al.

Effect of char yield and chemical structure on toxicity of pyrolysis gases.

Proc. West. Pharmacol. Soc. 22:201-204, 1979.

Hill, D. L., et al.

Macromolecular binding and metabolism of the carcinogen 1,2-dibromoethane.

Cancer Res. 38(8):2438-2442, Aug. 1978.

Hill, D. L., et al.

Macromolecular binding and metabolism of the carcinogen 4-chloro-2-methylaniline.

Cancer Res. 39(7, Part 1):2528-2531, July 1979.

Hill, D., et al.

Smoking and impairment of performance.

Med. J. Aust. 2(2):60-63, July 15, 1978.

Hill, P. and Wynder, E. L.

Nicotine and cotinine in breast fluid.

Cancer Lett. 6(4-5):251-254, Apr. 1979.

Hill, R. M. and Stern, L.

Drugs in pregnancy: Effects on the fetus and newborn.

Curr. Ther. 20(2):131-150, Feb. 1979.

Hill, R. M. and Stern, L.

Drugs in pregnancy: Effects on the fetus and newborn.

Drugs 17(3):182-197, Mar. 1979.

Hillbom, M. and Kaste, M.

Does ethanol intoxication promote brain infarction in young adults?

Lancet 2(8101):1181-1183, Dec. 2, 1978.

Hillerdal, G. and Nou, E.

Occupation and bronchial carcinoma.

Scand. J. Resp. Dis. 60(2):76-82, Apr. 1979.

Hillman, R. W., et al.

Oral cytologic patterns and nutritional status: Some relationships in alcoholic subjects.

Oral Surg. 49(1):34-36, Jan. 1980.

Hills, E. A., et al.

Frequency dependence of dynamic compliance in patients with rheumatoid arthritis.

Thorax 34(6):755-761, Dec. 1979.

Himmelberger, D. U., et al.

Cigarette smoking during pregnancy and the occurrence of spontaneous abortion and congenital abnormality.

Am. J. Epidemiol. 108(6):470-479, Dec. 1978.

Hinds, M. W., et al.

Asbestos, dental X rays, tobacco, and alcohol in the epidemiology of laryngeal cancer.

Cancer 44(3):1114-1120, Sept. 1979.

Hinman, L. M., et al.

Angiotensin convertase activities in human alveolar macrophages: Effects of cigarette smoking and sarcoidosis.

Science 205(4402):202-203, July 13, 1979.

Hirakawa, T., et al.

Induction of enzyme-altered islands in rat liver by a single treatment with benzo(a)pyrene after partial hepatectomy.

Gan 70(3):393-394, June 1979.

Hirayama, T.

Nasopharyngeal carcinoma: Etiology and Control. Descriptive and analytical epidemiology of nasopharyngeal cancer.

IARC Sci. Publ. No. 20: 167-189, 1978.

Hirose, M., et al.

Carcinogenic effect of N-ethyl and N-amyl-N-nitrosourethans on female donryu rats.

Gan 70(5):653-652, Oct. 1979.

Hirota, N.

Intranuclear rodlets in undifferentiated carcinomas of salivary glands in strain A mice in a study involving a tobacco specific nitrosamine, n-nitrosonornicotine.

Cancer Lett. 6(6):365-369, May 1979.

Hirsch, A., et al.

Asbestos fibers in laryngeal tissues: Findings in two patients with asbestosis associated with laryngeal tumors.

Chest 76(6):697-699, Dec. 1979.

Hirvonen L. and Kaensaekoski, I.

Psykiatrisen sairaalan potilaiden ja henkiloekunnan tupakointi. (Finn.)

Suom. Laeaekaeril. 34(18):1473-1476, June 20, 1979.

Hitzemann, R. J., et al.

Effects of nicotine on brain 1-phosphatidylinositol-4-phosphate and 1-phosphatidylinositol-3,4-bisphosphate synthesis and metabolism - Possible relationship to nicotine-induced behaviors.

Biochem. Pharmacol. 27(21):2519-2523, 1978.

Hjalmarson, A.

Proceedings of a Symposium: Management of Ventricular Tachycardia - Role of Mexiletine. Prospects for the prevention of sudden death after myocardial infarction.

Int. Congr. Ser. No. 458:559-571, 1978.

Hjermann, I., et al.

Serum insulin response to oral glucose load during a dietary intervention trial in healthy coronary high risk men: The Olso study.

Scand. J. Clin. Lab. 40(1):89-94, Feb. 1980.

Hladovec, J.

Endothelial injury by nicotine and its prevention.

Experientia 34(12):1585-1586, Dec. 15, 1978.

Hlastala, M. P.

Physiological significance of the interaction of oxygen and carbon dioxide in blood.

Crit. Care Med. 7(9):374-379, Sept. 1979.

Ho, Y. L. and Ho, S. K.

The induction of a mutant prophage lambda in escherichia coli: A rapid screening test for carcinogens.

Virology 99(2):257-264, Dec. 1979.

Hocking, W. G. and Golde, D. W.

The pulmonary-alveolar macrophage. (First of two parts.)

N. Engl. J. Med. 301(11):580-587, Sept. 13, 1979.

Hocking, W. G. and Golde, D. W.

The pulmonary-alveolar marophage. (Second of two-parts.)

N. Engl. J .Med. 301(12):639-645, Sept. 20, 1979.

Hodara, D. and Roux, E.

Le cancer de l'oesophage, maladie nutritionelle. (Fr.)

Gaz. Med. Fr. 85(37):4497-4500, Nov. 24, 1978.

Hodara, D. and Roux, E.

Education nutritionnelle de l'enfant et tabac attention! attention! (Fr.)

Gaz. Med. Fr. 86(18):1913-1914, May 4, 1979.

Hoegetveit, A. Ch., et al.

Plasma nickel as a primary index of exposure in nickle refining.

Ann. Occup. Hyg. 21(2):113-120, Aug. 1978.

Hoffman, D., et al.

Assessment of tobacco-specific N-nitrosamines in tobacco products.

Cancer Res. 39(7, Part 1):2505-2509, July 1979.

Hoffman, G. S.

Raynaud's disease and phenomenon.

Am. Fam. Physician 21(1):91-97, Jan. 1980.

Hoffman, R. and Wasserman, L. R.

Natural history and management of polycythemia vera.

Adv. Intern. Med. 24:255-285, 1979.

Hoffmann, D., et al.

Model studies in tobacco carcinogenesis with the Syrian golden hamster.

Prog. Exp. Tumor Res. 24:370-390, 1979.

Hoffmann, D., et al.

Workshop on Carbon Monoxide and Cardiovascular Disease: Formation and analysis of carbon monoxide in cigarette mainstream and sidestream smoke.

Prev. Med. 8(3):344-350, May 1979.

Hofnung, M. J.

Mechanisms of DNA Repair: Introduction a l'etude des relations entre mutagenese et cancerogenese. (Fr.)

Biochimie 60(10):1151 1171, Oct. 1978.

Hoidal, J. R., et al.

Proceedings of the Aspen Lung Conference. Oxidative metabolism of alveolar macrophages from young asymptomatic cigarette smokers: Increased superoxide anion release and its potential consequences.

Chest 77(2, Suppl.):270-271, Feb. 1980.

Holden, W. E., et al.

Effect of static or slowly flowing blood on carbon monoxide diffusion in dog lungs.

J. Appl. Physiol. 46(5):992-997, May 1979.

Holland, J. M., et al.

Epidermal carcinogenicity of bis(2,3-epoxycyclopentyl)ether, 2,2-bis(p-glycidyloxyphenyl)propane, and m-phenylenediamine in male and female C3H and C57BL/6 mice.

Cancer Res. 39(5):1718-1725, May 1979.

Holland, W. W. and Wainwright, A.

Praevention und ihre Moeglichkeiten: Forum Davos 1978: Prevention - Everybody's responsibility.

Soz. Praventivmed. 23(5-6):313-326, Dec. 1978.

Holland, W. W., et al.

Health Effects of Particulate Pollution. Reappraising the Evidence. Exposure to particulate pollution: Mortality in adults.

Am. J. Epidemiol. 110(5):554-579, Nov. 1979.

Holland, W. W., et al.

Health Effects of Particulate Pollution: Reappraising the Evidence. Exposure to particulate pollution: Morbidity in adults.

Am. J. Epidemiol. 110(5):580-603, Nov. 1979.

Hollander, D. H., et al.

Sister chromatid exchanges in the peripheral blood of cigarette smokers and in lung cancer patients; and the effect of chemotherapy.

Hum. Genet. 44(2):165-171, Oct. 31, 1978.

Hollinshead, III, W. H.

The consequences of smoking in pregnancy: Decreased birth weight, spontaneous abortions, increased perinatal mortality, and slowed childhood development are demonstrable effects.

RI Med. J. 62(6):207-212, June 1979.

Hollnagel, H. and McCartney, P.

Asymptomatic Hyperglycemia and Coronary Heart Disease. Relationship of fasting and post-load serum glucose to prevalance of ECG abnormalities in forty-year-old men: From the glostrup population studies.

J. Chronic Dis. 32(11/12):709 719, 1979.

Hollo, I., et al.

Dohanyzas es osteoporosis. (Hung.)

Orv. Hetil. 120(11):641-643, Mar. 18, 1979.

Hollo, I., et al.

Influence of heavy smoking upon the bone mineral content of the radius of the aged and effect of tobacco smoke on the sensitivity to calcitonin of rats.

Aktuel. Gerontol. 9(8):365-368, Aug. 1979.

Holmes, I., et al.

Asphyxiation by combustion gases.

Environ. Health 87(2):25-28, Feb. 1979.

Holmstrup, P. and Pindborg, J. J.

Erythroplakic lesions in relation to oral lichen planus.

Acta Derm. Venereol. (Stockh.) 59(Suppl. 85):77-84, 1979.

Holt, P. G., et al.

Immunological function in mice chronically exposed to nitrogen oxides (NOx)

Environ. Res. 19(1):154-162, June 1979.

Holtz, B., et al.

Prediction of postoperative hypoxemia in smokers and non-smokers.

Acta Anaesthesiol. Scand. 23(5):411-418, Oct. 1979.

Holtzman, J. L.

The role of the stimulation of nadph-cytochrome P-450 reductase activity in hepatic, microsomal mixed function oxidase activity.

Pharmacol. Ther. 4(3):601-627, 1979.

Homburger, F.

Ocngenesis and Natural Immunity in Syrian Hamsters. Chemical carcinogenesis in Syrian hamsters: A review (through 1976.)

Prog. Exp. Tumor Res. 23:100-179, 1979.

Homburger, F., et al.

Socially tolerable cigarette smoke? (Letter to the Editor and Reply.)

JAMA 241(20):2142-2143, May 18, 1979.

Homburger, F., et al.

Animal model of human disease: Carcinoma of the larynx in hamster exposed to cigarette smoke.

Am. J. Pathol. 95(3):845-848, June 1979.

Hommes, F. A., et al.

The development of DT-daiphorase in rat liver and its induction by benzo(a)pyrene.

Biol. Neonate 34(5-6):248-252, 1978.

Hommes, F. A., et al.

Induction of DT-diaphorase by benzo(a)pyrene in rat liver: Relation to the cell cycle.

Arch. Biochem. Biophys. 197(1):236-243, Oct. 1, 1979.

Hope, W., et al.

Human beta-thromboglobulin inhibits PGI2 production and binds to a specific site in bovine aortic endothelial cells.

Nature 282(5735):210-212, Nov. 8, 1979.

Hopkin, J. M. and Evans, H. J.

Cigarette smoke condensates damage DNA in human lymphocytes.

Nature 279(5710):241-242, May 17, 1979.

Hopkin, J. M. and Evans, H. J.

Cigarette smoke-induced DNA damage and lung cancer risks.

Nature 283(5745):388-390, Jan. 24, 1980.

Hopkins, G. J. and Carroll, K. K.

Relationship between amount and type of dietary fat in promotion of mammary carcinogenesis induced by 7,12-dimethylbenz[a]anthracene.

JNCI 62(4):1009-1012, Apr. 1979.

Hopkins, J.

Foetal health warning.

Food Cosmet. Toxicol. 17(2):172-174, Apr. 1979.

Horan, J. J., et al.

Factors to consider when using expired air carbon monoxide in smoking assessment.

Addict. Behav. 3(1):25-28, 1978.

Horie, T., et al.

Annual Meeting Symposium on Smoking and Cardiopulmonary Function. Smoking and cardiopulmonary function. Vmax. (Jpn.)

Jpn. J. Thorac. Dis. 15(9):553-557, Sept. 1977.

Horn, D.

How much real progress have we made in the fight against smoking?

Am. Lung Assoc. Bull. 65(1):6-9, Jan.-Feb. 1979.

Horn, D.

Effectiveness of measures against smoking.

Bull. Schweiz. Akad. Med. Wiss. 35(1-3):131-136, Mar. 1979.

Horster, M., et al.

Nephron electrolyte transport and sodium-potassium adenosine triphosphatase activity: Influence of nicotine in rat and rabbit.

J. Physiol. (Lond.) 295:353-363, 1979.

Horwitz, D. L.

Cholesterol: Good and bad.

Compr. Ther. 6(1):3-4, Jan. 1980.

Hoshino, T.

Electron microscopic studies on changes of rat mammary tumor, bone-marrow and liver after ovariectomy or some anticancer agent treatments. (Jpn.)

J. Nagoya City Univ. Med. Sch. 28(2[1]):454-467, Aug. 1977.

Houston, C. S.

Proceedings of a Symposium. Acute Mountain Sickness. Introductory address: Lessons to be learned from high altitude.

Postgrad. Med. J. 55645):447-453, July 1979.

Howard, Jr., J. C., et al.

Effectiveness of antihistamines in the symptomatic management of the common cold.

JAMA 242(22):2414-2417, Nov. 30, 1979.

Howells, R. D., et al.

Benzodiazepine binding sites are present in retina.

Life Sci. 25(24-25):2131-2136, Dec. 10-17, 1979.

Howett, M. K., et al.

Enhancement of biochemical transformation of mammalian cells by herpes simplex virus following nitrosomethylurea treatment.

Cancer Res. 39(3):1041-1045, Mar. 1979.

Hoyumpa, Jr., A. M.

McLean Hospital Symposium: Minor Tranquilizers in Everyday Practice. Disposition and elimination of minor tranquilizers in the aged and in patients with liver disease.

South. Med. J. 71(Suppl. 2):23-28, Aug. 1978.

Hsu, I. C., et al.

Induction of ouabain-resistant mutation and sister chromatid exchanges in chinese hamster cells with chemical carcinogens mediated by human pulmonary macrophages.

J. Clin. Invest. 64(5):1245-1252, Nov. 1979.

Hsu, K. H. K., et al.

Ventilatory function of normal children and young adults - Mexican-American, white, and black. I. Spirometry.

J. Pediatr. 95(1):14-23, July 1979.

Hsu, W. T., et al.

Comparative reactivities of diolepoxide metabolites of carcinogenic hydrocarbons with OX174 viral DNA.

Biochem. Biophys. Res. Commun. 88(1): 251-257, May 14, 1979.

Huang, D. P., et al.

Nasopharyngeal Carcinoma: Etiology and Control. Analysis for volatile nitrosamines in salt-preserved foodstuffs traditionally consumed by southern Chinese.

IARC Sci. Publ. No. 20:309-314, 1978.

Huang, N. N.

Evaluation of recurrent respiratory tract infections.

Pediatr. Ann. 6(8):500-513, Aug. 1977.

Huang, S. L. and Whong, W-Z.

Induction of 6-thioguanine resistance in chinese hamster lung cells treated with dimethlynitrosamine'2-amino-anthracene or 7,12-dimethylbenz(A) anthracene in the presence of rat liver microsomes.

Toxicol. Lett. 3(4):209-214, Apr. 1979.

Huber, G. L., et al.

Proceedings of the Aspen Lung Conference: The alveolar macrophage as a mediator of tobacco-induced lung injury.

Chest 77(2 Suppl.):272, Feb. 1980.

Huber, S. and Lucas, Z. J.

A quantitative assay for tumor antigen based on inhibition of cytotoxicity of sensitized lymphocytes.

Int. J. Cancer 23(2):224-232, Feb. 15, 1979.

Huberman, E.

Mutagenesis and cell transformation of mammalian cells in culture by chemical carcinogens.

J. Environ. Pathol. Toxicol. 2(1):29-42, Sept.-Oct. 1978.

Huberman, E. and Slaga, T. J.

Mutagenicity and tumor-initiating activity of flourinated derivatives of 7,12-dimethylbenz(a)anthracene.

Cancer Res. 39(2, Part 1):411-414, Feb. 1979.

Hudgel, D. W., et al.

A community pulmonary disease screening effort: "Denver lung days."

Chest 74(6):619-623, Dec. 1978.

Hudson, R. D.

Central nervous system responses to cigarette smoke inhalation in the cat.

Arch. Int. Pharmacodyn. Ther. 237(2): 191-212, Feb. 1979.

Hugenholtz, P. G., et al.

De preventie van coronaire hartziekten. (Dut.)

Ned. Tijdschr. Geneeskd. 122(8):262-264, Feb. 25, 1978.

Hugod, C., et al.

Passivrygning - Eksposition for gasfase- og partikelgase- komponenter i cigaretroeg. (Dan.)

Ugeskr. Laeger 140(44):2707-2711, Oct. 30, 1978.

Hugod, C., et al.

Exposure of passive smokers to tobacco smoke constituents.

Int. Arch. Occup. Environ. Health 42(1): 21-29, Sept. 15, 1978.

Huhti, E., et al.

Chronic respiratory disease in rural women: An epidemiological survey at Hankasalmi Finland.

Ann. Clin. Res. 10(2):95-101, Apr. 1978.

Huhti, E., et al.

Chronic respiratory disease in rural men: An epidemiological survey at Hankasalmi, Finland.

Ann. Clin. Res. 10(2):87-94, Apr. 1978.

Hultin, T., et al.

RNA metabolism and poly(A) distribution in mouse liver following administration of dimethylnitrosamine.

Chem. Biol. Interact. 21(1):45-58, Apr. 1978.

Humes, H. D., et al.

The Kidney in Health and Disease: IX. Disorders of water balance.

Hosp. Pract. 14(3):133-145, Mar. 1979.

Humphries, S. V.

Cannabis - Its merits and hazards: Part I.

Cent. Afr. J. Med. 25(1):19-20, Jan. 1979.

Hunninghake, G. W., et al.

Inflammatory and immune processes in the human lung in health and disease: Evaluation by bronchoalveolar lavage.

Am. J. Pathol. 97(1):149-206, Oct. 1979.

Hunninghake, G., et al.

Proceedings of the Aspen Lung Conference: Mechanism by which cigarette smoke attracts polymorphonuclear leukocytes to lung.

Chest 77(2 Suppl.):273, Feb. 1980.

Hunter, K. I. and Linn, M. W.

Cultural and sex differences in dietary patterns of the urban elderly.

J. Am. Geriatr. Soc. 27(8):359-363, Aug. 1979.

Hurschman, L. G., et al.

The implications of sidestream cigarette smoke for cardiovascular health.

J. Environ. Health 41(3):145-149, Nov.-Dec. 1978.

Hurst, J. W. and King, III, S. B.

To what extent does bypass relieve pain and prolong life?

Med. Times 107(3):87-94, Mar. 1979.

Hurwich, B. J. and Nubani, N.

Blood pressures in a highly inbred community - Abu Ghosh, Israel. I. Original survey.

Isr. J. Med. Sci. 14(9):962-969, Sept. 1978.

Hurych, J. and Pisa, Z.

Problematika hypertenze a soucasny stav jeji kontroly ve svete. (Czech)

Cas. Lek. Cesk. 117(14):419-423, Apr. 7, 1978.

Husain, A. and Kashani, J.

Maternal medication and minimal brain dysfunction: A possible relationship.

Mo. Med. 75(10):508-511, Oct. 1978.

Hutt, M. S. R.

The geography of cancer.

Practitioner 222(1328):181-190, Feb. 1979.

Hutt, P. B.

Unresolved issues in the conflict between individual freedom and government control of food safety.

Ecotoxicol. Environ. Safety 2(3-4): 447-469, Dec., 1978.

Hutton, J. J., et al.

Comparison of the in vitro mutagenicity and metabolism of dimethylnitrosamine and benzo[a]pyrene in tissues from inbred mice treated with phenobarbital, 3-methylcholanthrene or polychlorinated biphenyls.

Mutat. Res. 66(1):75-94, Jan. 1979.

Huuskonen, M. S., et al.

Sputum cytology of asbestosis patients.

Scand. J. Work Environ. Health 4(4): 284-294, Dec. 1978.

Huuskonen, M. S.

Clinical features, mortality and survival of patients with asbestosis.

Scand. J. Work Environ. Health 4(4): 265-274, Dec. 1978.

Huuskonen, M. S., et al.

HLAB18 antigens and protection from pulmonary fibrosis in asbestos workers.

Br. J. Dis. Chest 73(3):253-259, July 1979.

Huuskonen, M. S., et al.

Asbestos exposure as a cause of immunological stimulation.

Scand. J. Respir. Dis. 59(6):326-332, 1978.

Hyden, S. P. and Springett, V. H.

An assessment of the place of follow-up in pulmonary tuberculosis.

Br. J. Dis. Chest 72(3):217-221, July 1978.

Ichikawa, Y. and Yamano, T.

Problems of reconstitution of the cytochrome P-450-linked mixed function oxidase system and trends in research on the mixed function oxidase system. (Jpn.)

Seikagaku 50(2):77-86, Feb. 1978.

Ichikawa, Y., et al.

Behaviors on NAD(P)H-reduction and their magnetic absorptions of multiple molecular forms of cytochromes P-450 and P-448.

Med. J. Osaka Univ. 28(3-4):205-214, Mar. 1978.

Ikegami, R., et al.

Prophylactic effect of BCG cell-wall skeleton on the tumor induction by 7,12-dimethylbenz[a]anthracene in mice: Strain difference.

Gann 70(1):101-107, Feb. 1979.

Ikeme, A. C., et al.

Cardiovascular status and blood pressure in a population sample in Ghana - The Mamprobi survey.

Trop. Geogr. Med. 30(3):313-324, Sept. 1978.

Imai, S. and Hiroishi, S.

Protease activity in relation to the stage of hepatocarcinogenesis in Wistar rats by 2-fluorenyl-acetamide.

J. Nara Med. Assoc. 28(6):891-897, Dec. 31, 1977.

Imamura, A., et al.

A molecular orbital study on the chemical reactivity and biolgical activity of polycyclic aromatic hydrocarbon diolepoxides in connection with bay region theory.

Gan 70(3):291-296, June 1979.

Indo, K. and Miyaji, H.

Qualitative changes in the biologic characteristics of cultured fetal rat keratinizing epidermal cells during the process of malignant transformation after benzo[a]pyrene treatment.

JNCI 63(4):1017-1027, Oct. 1979.

Indyke, D. and Ellis, Jr., B. H.

There's a leading role for physicians in helping smokers to quit.

Am. Lung Assoc. Bull. 66(2):2-6, Mar. 1980.

Ingenito, A. J.

Effects of cigarette smoke inhalation on the cat electroretinogram: Comparisons with nicotine and carbon monoxide.

J. Pharmacol. Exp. Ther. 211(3):647-655, Dec. 1979.

Ingento, A. J. and Durlacher, L.

Effects of carbon monoxide on the b-wave of the cat electroretinogram: Comparisons with nitrogen hypoxia, epinephrine, vasodilator drugs and changes in respiratory tidal volume.

J. Pharmacol. Exp. Ther. 211(3):638-646, Dec. 1979.

Ingram, R. and Goldstein, B.

Role of expectancy factors in behavioral self-control therapies: An experimental inquiry.

Psychol. Rep. 42(2):535-542, Apr. 1978.

Inman, W. H. W.

Oral contraceptives and fatal subarachnoid haemorrhage.

Br. Med. J. 2(6203):1468-1470, Dec. 8, 1979.

Ip, M. M., et al.

Characterization of androgen receptors in 7,12-dimethylbenz(a)anthracene-induced and transplantable rat mammary tumors.

Cancer Res. 38(9):2879-2885, Sept. 1978.

Irvine, D., et al.

Proceedings of the Aspen Lung Conference: The role of air pollution smoking and respiratory illness in childhood in the development of chronic bronchitis.

Chest 77(2 Suppl.):251-253, Feb. 1980.

Irvine, D., et al.

Meeting of the Society for Social Medicine: Repiratory symptoms and lung function among young adults in relation to smoking and air pollution. (Abstr.)

J. Epidemiol. Commun. Health 33(2): 165, June 1979.

Irving, C. C. et al.

Inhibition of N-n-butyl-N-(4-hydroxybutyl)nitrosamine-induced urinary bladder cancer in rats by administration of disulfiram in the diet.

Cancer Res. 39(8):3040-3043, Aug. 1979.

Ishii, Y., et al.

Quantitative assessment of ventilation perfusion mismatch by radioxenon imaging of lung. (Jpn.)

Nippon Acta Radiol. 38(11):1064-1072, Nov. 25, 1978.

Isles, C., et al.

Excess smoking in malignant-phase hypertension.

Br. Med. J. 1(6163):579-581, Mar. 3, 1979.

Itokawa, H., et al.

Radical methylation and radical hydroxymethylation of nicotine and quinine.

Chem. Pharm. Bull. 26(4):1295-1297, Apr. 1978.

Ivey, K. J. and Triggs, E. J.

Absorption of nicotine by the human stomach and its effect on gastric ion fluxes and potential difference.

Am. J. Dig. Dis. 23(9):809-814, Sept. 1978.

Iwata, H., et al.

Studies on the general pharmacological properties of guanazodine, [(octahydro-2-azocinyl) methyl] guanidine. (Jpn.)

Oyo Yakuri 14(2):235-249, 1977.

Izquierdo, I. and Elisabetsky, E.

Brain Mechanisms in Memory and Learning: From the Single Neuron to Man. Physiological and pharmacological dissection of the main factors in the acquisition and retention of shuttle behaviour.

IBRO Monogr. Ser. No. 74:227-248, 1979.

Jackson, D. L. and Menges, H.

Accidental carbon monoxide poisoning.

JAMA 243(8):772-774, Feb. 22/29. 1980.

Jackson, H.

Early chronic obstructive pulmonary disease: A clinical diagnosis.

J. La. State Med. Soc. 131(5):141-145, May 1979.

Jacob, J. and Grimmer, G.

Metabolitenprofile von polycyclischen aromatischen Kohlenwasserstoffen nach Vorbehandlung mit verschiedenen Induktoren mikrosomaler Monoxygenasen der Rattenleber. (Ger.)

Hoppe Seylers Z. Physiol. Chem. 360(1):1525-1534, Nov. 1979.

Jacobs, R., et al.

Nucleic acid metabolism in the rat following short-term and prolonged ingestion of chrysotile asbestos or cigarett-smoke condensate.

Br. J. Exp. Pathol. 59(6):594-600, Dec. 1978.

Jacobson, B.

Showing an example.

Nurs. Times 74(46):1877, Nov. 16, 1978.

Jacobson, M. K., et al.

Mutagenicity of the non-carcinogenic dibenzylnitrosamine and an alpha-acetoxy derivative.

Cancer Lett. 6(2):83-87, Feb. 1979.

Jafarey, N. A., et al.

Habits and dietary pattern of cases of carcinoma of the oral cavity and oropharynx.

JPMA 27(6):340-343, June 1977.

Jaffe, J. H.

Report of the Dahlem Workshop on the Bases of Addiction: Behavioral pharmacology of tobacco use.

Life Sci. Res. Rep. No. 8:175-198, 1978.

Jaffe, J. H., et al.

Inducing low tar/nicotine cigarette smoking in women.

Br. J. Addict. 73(3):271-281, Sept. 1978.

Jaggi, W., et al.

Comparative studies on the covalent binding of the carcinogen benzo(a)-pyrene to DNA in various model systems.

Experientia 35(5):631-632, May 15, 1979.

Jaillon, P. and Moreau, P.

Hyperviscosite sanguine et facteurs de risque cardio-vasculaire. (Fr.)

Gaz. Med. Fr. 84(28):3064-3074, Sept. 23, 1977.

James, O. F. W.

Neurological and Mental Disturbances in the Elderly. Proceedings of a Conference: Drug metabolism in the elderly.

Age Ageing 7(Suppl.):81-85, 1978.

James, W. E., et al.

Cardiac function in goats exposed to carbon monoxide.

J. Appl. Physiol. 47(2):429-434, Aug. 1979.

James, W. G.

Public Education about Cancer: A study of public school teachers' cigarette smoking attitudes and habits and their role in smoking education.

UICC Tech. Rep. Ser. 26:1-5, 1977.

Jamieson, G. A. (Editor)

Blood substitutes and plasma expanders: Discussion 1.

Prog. Clin. Biol. Res. 19:23-26, 1978.

Jamieson, G. A. (Editor)

Blood substitutes and plasma expanders: Discussion 5.

Prog. Clin. Biol. Res. 19:167-174, 1978.

Jamieson, M. P. G., et al.

Surgical management of bronchial carcinoma invading the chest wall.

Thorax 34(5):612-615, Oct. 1979.

Jammes, Y., et al.

The ventilatory pattern of conscious man according to age and morphology.

Bull. Eur. Physiopathol. Respir. 15(3):527-540, 1979.

Janka, H. U., et al.

Zur Epidemiologie der Hypertonie bei Diabetikern. (Ger.)

Dtsch. Med. Wochenschr. 103(40):1549-1555, Oct. 6, 1978.

Janoff, A., et al.

Lung injury induced by leukocytic proteases.

Am. J. Pathol. 97(1):111-135, Oct. 1979.

Janoff, A., et al.

Cigarette smoke inhalation decreases alpha1-antitrypsin activity in rat lung.

Science 206(4424):1313-1314, Dec. 14, 1979.

Jansen, H. M., et al.

The primary immune response of patients with different stages of squamous-cell bronchial carcinoma.

Thorax 33(6):755-760, Dec. 1978.

Jarman, C. M. B. and Kellett, J. M.

Alcoholism in the general hospital.

Br. Med. J. 2(6188):469-472, Aug. 25, 1979.

Jarrett, R. J. and Grabauskas, V.

The WHO multinational study of vascular disease in diabetes: 1. General Description.

Diabetes Care 2(2):175-186, Mar.-Apr. 1979.

Jarrett, R. J. and Keen, H.

The WHO multinational study of vascular disease in diabetes: 3. Microvascular disease.

Diabetes Care 2(2):196-201, Mar.-Apr. 1979.

Jarvik, M. E., et al.

Can cigarette size and nicotine content influence smoking and puffing rates?

Psychopharmacology 58(3):303-306, July 19, 1978.

Jatlow, P., et al.

Serum diazepam concentrations in overdose: Their significance.

Am. J. Clin. Pathol. 72(4):571-577, Oct. 1979.

Jay, S. J. and Hull, M. T.

Small airways disease: The bottom of the iceberg.

J. Indiana State Med. Assoc. 72(10): 753-760, Oct. 1979.

Jedrychowski, W.

Zmiennosc poziomu immunoglobulin IgG, IgA, IgM i IgD w zaleznosci od wieku i palenia tytoniu u zdrowych mezczyzn. (Pol.)

Patol. Pol. 29(2):153-163, Apr.-June 1978.

Jedrychowski, W. and Jaskolka, D.

Przedieg naturalnej historii przeleklego niezytu oskrzeli w obserwacji prospektywnej populacji prezemyslowej. (Pol.)

Pneumonol. Pol. 46(10):725-730, Oct. 1978.

Jedrychowski, W.

Zmiany czynnosci pluc w obserbacji prospektywnej w zaleznosci od wieku i palenia tytoniu oraz podatnosc osobnicza na zabutzenia wentylacyjne. (Pol.)

Pol. Tyg. Lek. 33(50):1913-1916, Dec. 11, 1978.

Jedrychowski, W.

A consideration of risk factors and development of chronic bronchitis in a five-year follow-up study of an industrial population.

J. Epidemiol. Commun. Health 33(3): 210-214, Sept.1979.

Jeffery, A. M., et al.

Benzo(a)pyrene-7,8-dihydrodiol 9,10-oxide adenosine and deoxyadenosine adducts: Structure and stereochemistry.

Science 206(4424):1309-1311, Dec. 14, 1979.

Jenkins, C. D.

National Conference on Emotional Stress and Heart Disease: Evidence for the relation of psychosocial factors to coronary heart disease.

J. SC. Med. Assoc. 75(11):537-547, Nov. 1979.

Jenkins, J. S.

Diabetes insipidus.

Practitioner 222(1329):312-316, Mar. 1979.

Jenkins, P. J., et al.

Severity of coronary atherosclerosis related to lipoprotein concentration.

Br. Med. J. 2(6134):388-391, Aug. 5, 1978.

Jenssen, D. and Ramel, C.

Factors affecting the induction of micronuclei at low doses of X-rays, MMS and dimethylnitrosamine in mouse erythroblasts.

Mutat. Res. 58(1):51-65, Sept. 1978.

Jernstroem, B., et al.

Formation of DNA-binding product from isolated benzo(a)pyrene metabolites in rat liver nuclei.

Chem. Biol. Interact. 20(3):311-321, Mar. 1978.

Jernstroem, B., et al.

Fluorescence study of DNA-binding metabolites of benzo(a)pyrene formed in hepatocytes isolated from 3-methylcholanthrene-treated rats.

Cancer Res. 38(8):2600-2607, Aug. 1978.

Jett, J. R., et al.

Macromolecular binding of 3H-benzo(a)pyrene metabolites and lymphocyte transformation in patients with lung cancer, and in smoking and nonsmoking control subjects.

Am. Rev. Respir. Dis. 120(2):369-375, Aug. 1979.

Jick, H., et al.

Myocardial infarction and other vascular diseases in young women: Role of estrogens and other factors.

JAMA 240(23):2548-2552, Dec. 1, 1978.

Jick, H., et al.

Lung cancer in young women.

Arch. Intern. Med. 139(7):745-746, July 1979.

Jienescu, Z., et al.

Ancheta epidemiologica privind tusea cronica si disfunctia ventilatorie obstructiva in mediul rural. (Rum.)

Rev. Ig. [Pneumoftiziol.] 26(4):207-209, Oct.-Dec. 1977.

Johansson-Brittebo, E. and Tjalve, H.

Studies on the distribution and metabolism of 14C-dimethylnitrosamine in foetal and young mice.

Acta Pharmacol. Toxicol. (Copenh.) 45(1):73-80, July 1979.

Johnson, E. F.

Isolation and characterization of a constitutive form of rabbit liver microsomal cytochrome P-450.

J. Biol. Chem. 255(1):304-309, Jan. 1980.

Johnson, G. T. (Editor)

The Surgeon General's Report - A response from the advisory board of the Harvard Medical School Health Letter.

Harv. Med. Health Lett. 4(6):6, Apr. 1979.

Johnson, G. T. (Editor)

Does it pay to quit?

Harv. Med. Sch. Health Lett. 4(7):5, May 1979.

Jolly, D. T.

Dyspnea in primary care.

Can. Fam. Physician 24:983-988, Oct. 1978.

Jolly, D. T.

Acute tonsillopharyngitis in native and white families.

Can. Fam. Physician 26:59-66, Jan. 1980.

Jones, J. G. and Minty, B. D.

Comparison of active and passive manoeuvres on the pattern of airway closure in man.

Br. J. Anaesth. 50(9):873-880, Sept. 1978.

Jones, J. G., et al.

Increased alveolar epithelial permeability in cigarette smokers.

Lancet 1(8159):66-67, Jan. 12, 1980.

Jones, J. W. and Bogat, G. A.

Air pollution and human aggression.

Psychol. Rep. 43(3, Part 1):721-722, Dec. 1978.

Jones, R. N., et al.

Mill effect and dose-response relationships in byssinosis.

Br. J. Ind. Med. 36(4):305-313, Nov. 1979.

Juaneda, A. and Ferrer, A.

Cancer de pulmon: Consideraciones generales.

Prensa Med. Argent. 65(15):553-555, 1978.

Juchau, M. R., et al.

A comparison of the capacity of fetal and adult liver, lung, and brain to convert polycyclic aromatic hydrocarbons to mutagenic and cytotoxic metabolites in mice and rats.

Toxicol. Appl. Pharmacol. 49(1): 171-178, June 15, 1979.

Jukes, T. H.

Carcinogens in food and the Delaney Clause.

JAMA 241(6):617-619, Feb. 9, 1979.

Junceda Avello, E.

Factores medico-sociales en maternologia y su repercusion perinatologica. (Span.)

Toko-Ginecol. Pract. 38(431):179-192, Mar. 31, 1979.

Jusko, W. J.

Drug Disposition in Man: Influence of cigarette smoking on drug metabolism in man.

Drug Metab. Rev. 9(2):221-236, 1979.

Jusko, W. J., et al.

Enhanced biotransformation of theophylline in marihuana and tobacco smokers.

Clin. Pharmacol. Ther. 24(4):406-410, Oct. 1978.

Jusko, W. J., et al.

Factors affecting theophylline clearances: Age, tobacco, marijuana, cirrhosis, congestive heart failure, obesity, oral contraceptives, benzodiazepines, barbiturates, and ethanol.

J. Pharm. Sci. 68(11):1358-1366, Nov. 1979.

Jussawalla, D. J.

Avenues leading to cancer control-the Indian scene.

Indian J. Cancer 15(2):1-5, June 1978.

Jussawalla, D. J. and Jain, D. K.

Lung cancer in greater Bombay: Correlations with religion and smoking habits.

Br. J. Cancer 40(3):437-448, Sept. 1979.

Juustila, H.

Medical, occupational and smoking characteristics related to ischemic heart disease in men and women.

Acta Med. Scand. Suppl. 613:1-120, 1977.

Kaden, D. A., et al.

Mutagenicity of soot and associated polycyclic aromatic hydrocarbons to Salmonella typhimurium.

Cancer Res. 39(10):4152-4159, Oct. 1979.

Kado, N. Y. and Wei, E. T.

Radioimmunoassay for benzo[a]-pyrene.

JNCI 61(1):221-225, July 1978.

Kaellen, B. and Winberg, J.

Dealing with suspicions of malformation frequency increase.

Acta Paediatr. Scand. [Suppl.] 275, 66-74, 1979.

Kagawa, J. and Itoh, H.

Inflamatory changes of chest roentgenogram by smoking habits and types of occupation. (Jpn. Eng. Summary)

Jpn. J. Ind. Health 20(2):105-109, Mar. 1978.

Kahl, R. and Wulff, U.

Induction of rat hepatic epoxide hydratase by dietary antioxidants.

Toxicol. Appl. Pharmacol. 47(2):217-227, Feb. 1979.

Kahl, R., et al.

Ethoxyquin feeding to rats increases liver microsome-catalyzed formation of benzo(a)pyrene diol epoxide - DNA adduct.

Biochem. Biophys. Res. Commun. 85(3): 938-945, Dec. 14, 1978.

Kahn, H.

Toxicity of oil shale chemical products: A review.

Scand. J. Work Environ. Health 5(1): 1-9, Mar. 1979.

Kahng, H. W., et al.

Induction and properties of aryl hydrocarbon hydroxylase in bovine pancreatic ducts.

JNCI 62(5):1251-1255, May 1979.

Kakande, I.

Primary lung carcinoma in Kenyatta national hospital Nairobi.

East Afr. Med. J. 56(7):325-330, July 1979.

Kakizoe, T., et al.

Volatile N-nitrosamines in the urine of normal donors and of bladder cancer patients.

Cancer Res. 39(3):829-832, Mar. 1979.

Kakizoe, T., et al.

Agglutination of bladder cells by concanavalin A during the early phase of treatment of rats with N-butyl-N-(4-hydroxybutyl)nitrosamine.

Cancer Res. 39(9):3353-3356, Sept. 1979.

Kalamegham, R., et al.

Metabolism of drugs and carcinogens in man: Antipyrine elimination as an indicator.

Clin. Pharmacol. Ther. 25(1):67-73, Jan. 1979.

Kallio, V., et al.

Reduction in sudden deaths by a multifactorial intervention programme after acute myocardial infarction.

Lancet 2(8152):1091-1094, Nov. 24, 1979.

Kalow, W.

Human Genetic Variation in Response to Medical and Environmental Agents: Pharmacogenetics and Ecogenetics. Assets and limitations of animal models.

Hum. Genet. Suppl. 1:79-80, 1978.

Kamikawa, Y. and Shimo, Y.

Cholinergic and adrenergic innervations of the muscularis mucosae in guinea-pig esophagus.

Arch. Int. Pharmacodyn. Ther. 238(2): 220-232, Apr. 1979.

Kampa, L. and Peisach, J.

Purification and characterization of hydroxyindole oxidase from the gills of Mytilus edulis.

J. Biol. Chem. 255(2):595-601, Jan. 1980.

Kane, P. A., et al.

Societe Medicale d'Afrique Noire de Langue Francaise. L'adeno-carcinome bronchique. (A propos de 3 cas apparemment primitifs). (Fr.)

Bull. Soc. Med. Afr. Noire Lang. Fr. 23(3):233-239, 1978.

Kaneko, A., et al.

A microsomal butyrylesterase appearing in rat livers during development, regeneration, and carcinogenesis, and after phenobarbital treatment.

JNCI 62(6):1489-1495, June 1979.

Kangas, L., et al.

Human pharmokinetics of nitrazepam: Effect of age and disease.

Eur. J. Clin. Pharmacol. 15(3):163-170, Apr. 17, 1979.

Kannel, W. B.

Mild Hypertension: To Treat or Not to Treat. Renin as a predictor of hypertensive complications: Discussion.

Ann. NY Acad. Sci. 304:161-164, 1978.

Kannel, W. B.

Mild Hypertension: To Treat or Not to Treat. Hypertension, blood lipids, and cigarette smoking as co-risk factors for coronary heart disease.

Ann. NY Acad. Sci. 304:128-139, 1978
1978.

Kannel, W. B. and McGee, D. L.

Diabetes and cardiovascular disease: The Framingham study.

JAMA 241(19):2035-2038, May 11, 1979.

Kannel, W. B. and McGee, D. L.

Diabetes and glucose tolerance as risk factors for cardiovascular disease: The Framingham study.

Diabetes Care 2(2):120-126, Mar.-Apr. 1979.

Kannel, W. B., et al.

Hypertension and cardiac impairments increase stroke risk.

Geriatrics 33(9):71-83, Sept. 1978.

Kannel, W. B., et al.

An investigation of coronary heart disease in families: The Framingham Offspring Study.

Am. J. Epidemiol. 110(3):281-290, Sept. 1979.

Kanner, R. E., et al.

Variables associated with changes in spirometry in patients with obstructive lung diseases.

Am. J. Med. 67(1):44-50, July 1979.

Kannerstein, M., et al.

Asbestos and mesothelioma: A review.

Pathol. Annu. 13(Part 1):81-129, 1978

Kantarev, N.

Influence of nicotine and chronic nicotine intoxication on the effects of some hypnotic drugs.

Folia Med. 19(2):93-100, 1977.

Kaplan, R. L. and Waite, D. H.

Progressive interstitial lung disease from prolonged methotrexate therapy.

Arch. Dermatol. 114(12):1800-1802, Dec. 1978.

Kappas, A., et al.

Proceedings of the International Symposium on Microsomes and Drug Oxidations: The regulation of human drug metabolism by nutritional factors.

Biochem. Pharmacol. Suppl.:703-708, 1977.

Karasick, D., et al.

Mucoid pseudotumors of the tracheobronchial tree in two cases.

AJR 132(3):459-460, Mar. 1979.

Karim, F., et al.

Responses of the heart to stimulation of aortic body chemoreceptors in dogs.

Circ. Res. 46(1):77 83, Jan. 1980.

Kato, M.

Annual Meeting Symposium on Smoking and Cardiopulmonary Function: Smoking and cardiopulmonary function: 5. VA/Q inequality in smokers. (Jpn.)

Jpn. J. Thorac. Dis. 15(9):580-588, Sept. 1977.

Kato, R.

Characteristics and differences in the hepatic mixed function oxidases of different species.

Pharmacol. Ther. 6(1):41-98, 1979.

Kauffmann, F.

Etude des facteurs de risque de la bronchite chronique obstructive par des enquetes epidemiologiques longitudinales. (Fr.)

Med. Hyg. 36(1301):3069-3073, Sept. 27, 1978.

Kauffmann, F., et al.

Evolution de VEMS en 12 ans et tabagisme chez 556 travailleurs de la region parisienne. (Fr.)

Bull. Eur. Physiopathol. Respir. 15(5):723-737, 1979.

Kavanagh, T., et al.

Prognostic indexes for patients with ischemic heart disease enrolled in an exercise-centered rehabilitation program.

Am. J. Cardiol. 44(7):1230-1240, Dec. 1979.

Kawasaki, H.

A study of cellular immunity in chorionic tumors and their prognosis. (Jpn.)

Acta Obstet. Gynaecol. Jpn. 29(9): 1127-1132, Sept. 1977.

Kawashiro, T.

Annual Meeting Symposium on Smoking and Cardiopulmonary Function: Respiratory function of blood. (Jpn.)

Jpn. J. Thorac. Dis. 15(9):589-594, Sept. 1977.

Kay, R. G. and Knight, G. S.

Blood selenium values in an adult Auckland population group.

NZ Med. J. 90(639):11-13, July 11, 1979.

Keen, H. and Jarrett, R. J.

The WHO multinational study of vascular disease in diabetes: 2. Macrovascular disease prevalence.

Diabetes Care 2(2):187-195, Mar.-Apr. 1979.

Kekki, P.

Kokemuksia keski-ikaeisten miesten seulontatutkimuksesta. (Finn.)

Soum. Laeaekaeril. 33(23):1759-1762, Aug. 10, 1978.

Kelada, F. and Euinton, L. E.

Health effects of long-term exposure to sodium sulfate dust.

JOM 20(12):812-814, Dec. 1978.

Keller, R. and Bohn, W.

Epidemiologie und sozialmedizinische Bedeutung von Erkrankungen der Atmungsorgane in der Schweiz. (Ger.)

Prax. Klin. Pneumol. 32(9):571-577, Sept. 1978.

Kellermann, G., et al.

Human Genetic Variation in Response to Medical and Environmental Agents: Pharmacogenetics and Ecogenetics. Aryl hydrocarbon hydroxylase in man and lung cancer.

Hum. Genet. Suppl. 1:161-168, 1978.

Kelly, H. B.

Routine examination of aircrew.

J. R. Soc. Med. 72(5):374-377, May 1979.

Kelman, G. R. and Davies, T. J.

Carboxyhaemoglobin levels in workers in Leicestershire garages.

Br. J. Ind. Med. 36(3):238-241, Aug. 1979.

Kemeny, M. M., et al.

Results of surgical treatment of carcinoma of the lung by stage and cell type.

Surg. Gynecol. Obstet. 147(5):865-871, Dec. 1978.

Kennedy, J. R. and Allen, P.

Effects of cigarette smoke residue on rabbit tracheal epithelium in organ culture.

Arch. Environ. Health 34(1):5-11, Jan.-Feb. 1979.

Kennedy, P. S., et al.

Adenocarcinoma of unknown origin: A rational approach to a diagnostic puzzle.

Postgrad. Med. 65(1):151-160, Jan. 1979.

Kent, S.

Vitamin C therapy: Colds, cancer, and cardiovascular disease.

Geriatrics 33(10):91-99, Oct. 1978.

Kerr, C.

New knowledge of mortality trends and oral contraceptives.

Bull. Postgrad. Comm. Med. Univ. Sydney 34(2):42-48, May 1978.

Keskinen, H., et al.

Occupational asthma in Finland.

Clin. Allergy 8(6):569-579, Nov. 1978.

Kessler, I. I.

Neurological Epidemiology: Principles and Clinical Applications. Parkinson's disease in epidemiologic perspective.

Adv. Neurol. 19:355-384, 1978.

Kesson, C. M. and Slater, S. D.

Smoking in diabetics. (Letter to the Editor.)

Lancet 1(8114):504-505, Mar. 3, 1979.

Ketkar, M., et al.

Investigations on the carcinogenic burden by air pollution in man. Intratracheal instillation studies with benzo[a]pyrene in a mixture of tris buffer and saline in syrian golden hamsters.

Cancer Lett. 6(4-5):279-284, Apr. 1979.

Ketterer, B., et al.

Glutathione adducts of N-methyl-4-aminoazobenzene formed in vivo and by reaction of N-benzoyloxy-N-mehyl-4-aminoazobenzene with glutathione.

Chem. Biol. Interact. 25(1):7-21, Apr. 1979.

Khadim, M. I.

The effects of Pan and its ingredients on oral mucosa.

JPMA 27(6):353-356, June 1977.

Khosla, T. and Campbell, H.

Mortality of male doctors and reductions in cigarette smoking. (Letter to the Editor.)

Br. Med. J. 280(6210):331, Feb. 2, 1980.

Khudoley, V. V. and Syrenko, O. A.

Tumor induction by N-nitroso compounds in bivalve mollusks Unio pictorum.

Cancer Lett. 4(6):349-354, June 1978.

Kieler, J., et al.

Comparative studies of two types of "spontaneous" malignant alteration of ST/a mouse lung fibroblasts propagated in vitro.

In Vitro 15(10):758-771, Oct. 1979.

Kimball, R. F.

The relation of repair phenomena to mutation induction in bacteria.

Mutat. Res. 55(2):85-120, 1978.

Kimbel, P.

Proceedings of the Aspen Lung Conference: Proteolytic lung damage.

Chest 77(2 Suppl.):274-276, Feb. 1980.

Kimura, N.

Smoking and cardiovascular disease.

Asian Med. J. 22(2):97-112, Feb. 1979.

Kinch, R. and Lough, J.

Transactions of the Annual Meeting of the American Gynecological Society: Local nodular hyperplasia of the liver and oral contraceptives.

Am. J. Obstet. Gynecol. 132(7):717-727, Dec. 1, 1978.

King, H. W. S., et al.

The identification of 3-methylcholanthrene-9,10-dihydrodiol as an intermediate in the binding of 3-methylcholanthrene to DNA in cells in culture.

Chem. Biol. Interact. 20(3):367-371, Mar. 1978.

King, H. W. S., et al.

The in vitro and in vivo reaction at the N7-position of guanine of the ultimate carcinogen derived from benzo[a]-pyrene.

Chem. Biol. Interact. 24(3):345-353, Mar. 1979.

King, M. M., et al.

Incidence and growth of mammary tumors induced by 7,12-dimethylbenz[a]anthracene as related to the dietary content of fat and antioxidant.

JNCI 63(3):557-563, Sept. 1979.

Kirkconnell, S. and Hegeman, G. D.

Mechanism of oxidation of carbon monoxide by bacteria.

Biochem. Biophys. Res. Commun. 83(4):1584-1587, Aug. 29, 1978.

Kirsh, M.M.

Clinical presentation and management of patients with carcinoma of the lung: A 14-year experience.

J. Fam. Pract. 8(6):1127-1131, June 1979.

Kishi, S., et al.

Follow up study on gastric ulcer.

Tokushima J. Exp. Med. 35(3-4):159-162, Dec. 1978.

Kitabgi, P. and Freychet, P.

Effects of neurotensin on isolated intestinal smooth muscles.

Eur. J. Pharmacol. 50(4):349-357, Aug. 15, 1978.

Kitagawa, T., et al.

Promotion by dietary phenobarbital of hepatocarcinogenesis by 2-methyl-N,N-dimethyl-4-aminoazobenzene in the rat.

Cancer Res. 39(1):112 115, Jan. 1979.

Kitagawa, Y. and Kuroiwa, Y.

Effect of phenobarbital and 3-methylcholanthrene on decrease in pH in liver induced by 3'-methyl-4-dimethylaminoazobenzene, of partial hepatectomy and hepatotoxic agents.

Chem. Pharm. Bull. (Tokyo) 27(3):586-591, 1979.

Kitson, T. M. and Fried, R.

Disulfiram and cigarettes. (Letter to the Editor and Reply.)

Alcoholism 2(4):396-398, Oct. 1978.

Kittel, F., et al.

Psycho-socio-biological correlates of moderate overweight in an industrial population.

J. Pschosom. Res. 22(3):145-158, 1978.

Kiviluoto, M., et al.

Effects of vanadium on the upper respiratory tract of workers in a vanadium factory: A macroscopic and microscopic study.

Scand. J. Environ. Health 5(1):50-58, Mar. 1979.

Kizilbash, M., et al.

Community cancer-screeening clinic: Evaluation of experiences.

NY State J. Med. 79(11):1703-1707 Oct. 1979.

Kjeldsen, J.

Hemodynamic Investigations During Labour and Delivery.

Acta Obstet. Gynecol. Scand. [Suppl.] 89:1-252, 1979.

Kjellstroem, T.

Exposure and accumulation of cadmium in populations from Japan, the United States, and Sweden.

Environ. Health Perspect. 28:169-197, Feb. 1979.

Klein-Szanto, A. J. P., et al.

Ultrastructural characteristics of carcinogen-induced nondysplastic changes in tracheal epithelium.

Am. J. Pathol. 98(1):61-82, Jan. 1980.

Klein-Szanto, A. J. P., et al.

Ultrastructural characteristics of carcinogen-induced dysplastic changes in tracheal epithelium.

Am. J. Pathol. 98(1):83-100, Jan. 1980.

Klein, A. E. and Gorrod, J. W.

Age as a factor in the metabolism of nicotine.

Eur. J. Drug Metab. Pharmacokinet. 3(1):51-58, 1978.

Klein, A. E. and Gorrod, J. W.

The metabolism of nicotine in cigarette smokers during pregnancy.

Eur. J. Drug Metab. Pharmacokinet. 3(2):87-93, Apr.-June 1978.

Kleinman, J. C., et al.

The effects of changes in smoking habits on coronary heart disease mortality.

Am. J. Public Health 69(8):795-802, Aug. 1979.

Kleinmann, D.

Sport und Ernaehrung. (Ger.)

ZFA (Stuttgart) 55(2):96-98, Jan. 20, 1979.

Klinger, W., et al.

The Induction of Drug Metabolism: Induction and its dependence on development.

Symp. Med. Hoechst 14:517-544, 1979.

Knoerr, K.

Der einfluss von Tabak und Alkohol auf Schwangerschaftsverlauf und Kindesentwicklung. (Ger.)

Bull. Schweiz. Akad. Med. Wiss. 35(1-3):137-146, Mar. 1979.

Knott, V. J. and Venables, P. H.

EEG alpha correlates of alcohol consumption in smokers and non-smokers: Effects of smoking and smoking deprivation.

J. Stud. Alcohol 40(3):247-257, Mar. 1979.

Knowles, M. A.

Effects of the tumor-promoting agent 12-O-tetradecanoylphorbol-13-acetate on normal and "preneoplastic" mouse submandibular gland epithelial cells in vitro.

JNCI 62(2):349-352, Feb. 1979.

Knox Ritchie, J. W.

Fetal breathing and generalized fetal movements in normal antenatal patients.

Br. J. Obstet. Gynaecol. 86(8):612-614, Aug. 1979.

Koch, A., et al.

Einfluss von Zigarettenrauchinhalation auf Kreislauf- und Stoffwechselgroessen. (Ger.)

Verh. Dtsch. Ges. Inn. Med. 84:1397-1400, 1978.

Kodama, M., et al.

Enzymic formation of free radical from anthanthrene and 10-aza-benzo[a]-pyrene lacking the bay region.

Gann 69(6):865-866, Dec. 1978.

Kodama, Y.

Benzo(a)pyrene in atmospheric environment. (Jpn.)

J. UOEH 1(3):383-391, Sept. 1, 1979.

Kohn, K. W.

Cancer Drug Development. Part A. DNA as a target in cancer chemotherapy: Measurement of macromolecular DNA damage produced in mammalian cells by anticancer agents and carcinogens.

Methods Cancer Res. 16:291-345, 1979.

Kollmorgen, G. M., et al.

Inhibition of lymphocyte function in rats fed high-fat diets.

Cancer Res. 39(9):3458-3462, Sept. 1979.

Kon, S. H.

Underestimation of chronic toxicities of food additives and chemicals: The bias of a phantom rule.

Med. Hypotheses 4(4):324-339, July-Aug. 1978.

Kondo, H.

A new experimental model for inducing lung cancer in rats - Lung carcinomas induced by oral administration of N-bis(2-hydroxypropyl) nitrosamine. (Jpn.)

J. Nara Med. Assoc. 28(3):418-434, June 30, 1977.

Konishi, Y., et al.

Induction of rat lung carcinoma by a single injection of N-bis(2-hydroxypropyl)nitrosamine.

Gann 69(6):855-856, Dec. 1978.

Konishi, Y., et al.

Carcinogenic effect of N-bis(2-hydroxypropyl)nitrosamine by a single administration in rats.

Cancer Lett. 6(2):115-119, Feb. 1979.

Konishi, Y., et al.

Heterotransplantation into nude mice of pancreatic carcinoma induced by N-bis(2-hydroxypropyl)nitrosamine in hamsters.

Cancer Lett. 5(6):333-337, Dec. 1978.

Kono, S. and Ikeda, M.

Correlation between cancer mortality and alcoholic beverage in Japan.

Br. J. Cancer 40(3):449-455, Sept. 1979.

Korfmacher, W. A., et al.

Oxidative transformations of polycyclic aromatic hydrocarbons absorbed on coal fly ash.

Science 207(4432):763-765, Feb. 15, 1980.

Kornitzer, M., et al.

The Belgian Heart Disease Prevention Project: Modification of the coronary risk profile in an industrial population.

Circulation 61(1):18-25, Jan. 1980.

Korsgaard, R.

Chaloner och lungcancer. (Swed.)

Kvartalsskrift (Stockh.) 73(3):89-98, 1978.

Korsgaard, R., et al.

Vad aer lungcancer? (Swed.)

Kvartalsskrift (Stockh.) 73(3):79-87, 1978.

Kosmider, S. and Wysocki, J.

Palanie papierosow a odpornosc. (Pol.)

Pol. Arch. Med. Wewn. 60(3):213-217, Sept. 1978.

Kotchen, J. M., et al.

Blood pressures of young mothers and their first children 3-6 years following hypertension during pregnancy.

J. Chronic Dis. 32(9-10):653-659, 1979.

Kouri, R. E., et al.

Biological activity of tobacco smoke and tobacco smoke-related chemicals.

Environ. Health Perspect. 29:63-69, Apr. 1979.

Kouri, R. E., et al.

2,3,7,8-tetrachlorodibenzo-p-dioxin as cocarcinogen causing 3-methylcholanthrene-initiated subcutaneous tumors in mice genetically 'nonresponsive' at Ah locus.

Cancer Res. 38(9):2777-2783, Sept. 1978.

Kovar, M. G.

Some indicators of health-related behavior among adolescents in the United States.

Public Health Rep. 94(2):109-118, Mar.-Apr. 1979.

Kozak, Jr., P. P.

Factors that influence theophylline metabolism.

West. J. Med. 131(4):319-320, Oct. 1979.

Kozlowski, L. T. and Kleiman, R. M.

Effects of oral pH on cigarette smoking.

Pharmacol. Biochem. Behav. 9(4):477-480, Oct. 1978.

Kramer, I. R. H.

Definition of leukoplakia and related lesions: An aid to studies on oral precancer. WHO Collaborating Centre for Oral Precancerous Lesions.

Oral Surg. 46(4):518-539, Oct. 1978.

Kramer, P.

Smoking and ulcers: True, true, and related? (Letter to the Editor.)

Gastroenterology 76(5, Part 1):1083-1084, May 1979.

Kramer, R. E., et al.

Requirement of the pituitary gland for gonadal hormone effects on hepatic drug metabolism in rats.

J. Pharmacol. Exp. Ther. 208(1):19-23, Jan. 1979.

Krantz, D. S., et al.

Psychological correlates of progression of atherosclerosis in men.

Psychosom. Med. 41(6):467-475, Oct. 1979.

Kraybill, H. F.

Aquatic Pollutants and Biologic Effects with Emphasis on Neoplasia: Global distribution of carcinogenic pollutants in water.

Ann. NY Acad. Sci. 298:80-89, Sept. 29, 1977.

Krebs, B. P., et al.

Clinical Application of Carcinoembryonic Antigen Assay: Carcinoembryonic antigen determinations in people submitted to cancer screening.

Int. Congr. Ser. No. 439:413-418, 1978.

Krempf, M., et al.

Societe Francaise de la Tuberculose et des Maladies Respiratoires: Etude comparative de differents tests fonctionnels de depistage de l'obstruction bronchique chez le tabagique jeune asymptomatique. (Fr.)

Rev. Fr. Mal. Respir. 6(5):547-548, Sept.-Oct. 1978.

Kreyberg, L.

Yrkesbetinget lungekreft: En vurdering. (Norw., Engl. Summary)

Tidsskr. Nor. Laegeforen. 99(12):570-574;596, Apr. 30, 1979.

Krishna, K.

Tobacco chewing in pregnancy.

Br. J. Obstet. Gynecol. 85(10):726-728, Oct. 1978.

Krishnaswamy, K.

Nutrition and drug metabolism.

Indian J. Med. Res. 68(Suppl.):109-120, Oct. 1978.

Kroeger-Koepke, M. B. and Michejda, C. J.

Evidence for several demethylase enzymes in the oxidation of dimethylnitrosamine and phenylmethylnitrosamine by rat liver fractions.

Cancer Res. 39(5):1587-1591, May 1979.

Krstic, M. K.

Cardiovascular response to intracerebroventricular administration of acetylcholine in rats treated with psysostigmine.

Neuropharmacology 17(12):1003-1008, Dec. 1978.

Krumpe, P. E., et al.

The search for expiratory obstruction in meat wrappers studied on the job.

Am. Rev. Respir. Dis. 119(4):611-618, Apr. 1979.

Kuba, K. and Koketsu, K.

Synaptic events in sympathetic ganglia.

Prog. Neurobiol. 11(2):77-169, 1978.

Kubel, M., et al.

Klinische Beurteilung des arteriellen Gefaesssystems bei Haemophiliepatienten als Modellfall einer Langzeitantikoagulierung. (Ger.)

Z. Gesamte Inn. Med. 33(16):550-552, Aug. 15, 1978.

Kubik, A.

Studies on smoking, chronic nonspecific respiratory diseases, and lung cancer in selected territories of Czechoslovakia.

Z. Erkr. Atmungsorgane 152(2):180-185, 1979.

Kubik, A.

Epidemiology of chronic non specific respiratory disease and the smoking-control program in young people.

Bronchopneumologie 24(3):255-260, 1979.

Kubik, M., et al.

Metoprolol with and without chlorthalidone in hypertension.

Clin. Pharmacol. Ther. 25(1):25-32, Jan. 1979.

Kubinyi, J., et al.

Reflexny bronchospazmus vyvolany cigaretovym dymom z hronych ciest u kralika. (Slov.)

Bratisl. Lek. Listy 71(3):340-347, Mar. 1979.

Kuhn, III, C. and Senior, R. M.

The role of elastases in the development of emphysema.

Lung 155(3):185-197, Oct. 3, 1978.

Kuhnert, B. R., et al.

Meperidine and normeperidine levels following meperidine administration during labor: I. Mother.

Am. J. Obstet. Gynecol. 133(8):904-908, Apr. 15, 1979.

Kuller, L. H.

Neurological Epidemiology: Principles and Clinical Applications. Epidemiology of stroke.

Adv. Neurol. 19:281-311, 1978.

Kuller, L. H.

National Conference on Emotional Stress and Heart Disease: Epidemiology of stress-related cardiovascular disease.

J. SC Med. Assoc. 75(11):521-531, Nov. 1979.

Kuller, L. H.

Prevention of cardiovascular disease and risk-factor intervention trials.

Circulation 61(1):26-28, Jan. 1980.

Kulpati, D. D. and Sharma, S. K.

Assessment of pulmonary functions in different pattern of smoking.

J. Assoc. Physicians India 26(8):677-681 Aug. 1978.

Kumakura, K., et al.

Modulation of nicotinic receptors by opiate receptor agonists in cultured adrenal chromaffin cells.

Nature 283(5746):489-492, Jan. 31, 1980.

Kumakura, K., et al.

Primary cultures of chromaffin cells: Molecular mechanisms for the induction of tyrosine hydroxylase mediated by 8-Br-cyclic AMP.

Mol. Pharmacol. 16(3):865-876, Nov. 1979.

Kunisake, N. and Hayashi, M.

Formation of N-nitrosamines from secondary amines and nitrite by resting cells of Escherichia coli B.

Appl. Environ. Microbiol. 37(2):279-282, Feb. 1979.

Kunze, M. and Vutuc, Ch.

Teer-exposition bei Tabak-assoziiertem Lungen- und Blasenkrebs.

MMW 121(32-33):1041-1042, Aug. 10, 1979.

Kurogochi, Y., et al.

An observation of nicotine metabolism in the dog.

J. Nara Med. Assoc. 29(4-5):669-676, Oct. 31, 1978.

Kurogochi, Y., et al.

Studies on nicotine metabolism in various animals (1) strains and species differences of drug metabolizing enzyme activities in male intact animals.

J. Nara Med. Assoc. 29(4-5):677-682, Oct. 31, 1978.

Kurt, T. L., et al.

Ambient carbon monoxide levels and acute cardiorespiratory complaints: An exploratory study.

Am. J. Public Health 69(4):360-363, Apr. 1979.

Kurt, T. L., et al.

Hemodynamic effects of cigarette smoking. (Letter to the Editor and Reply.)

Circulation 61(2):460, Feb. 1980.

Kwaan, H. C.

The Thrombotic Process in Atherogenesis: Possible effects of risk factors on fibrinolysis.

Adv. Exp. Med. Biol. 104:295-300, 1978.

Kyono, Y.

Temperature effects during and after the diethylnitrosamine treatment on liver tumorigenesis in the fish, Oryzias latipes.

Eur. J. Cancer 14(10):1089-1097, Oct. 1978.

Kyono, Y., et al

Changes in the labeling index and DNA content of liver cells during diethylnitrosamine-induced liver tumorigenesis in Oryzlas latipse.

JNCI 63(1):71-74, July 1979.

Laaser, U. and Schuett, A.

The cariovascular risk-profile of adolescents in Cologne: A representative study including 6302 pupils.

Z. Kardiol. 67(12):837-846, Dec. 1978.

Laduron, P. M., et al.

Stereospecific in vitro binding of [3H]-dexetimide to brain muscarinic receptors.

J. Neurochem. 32(2):421-427, Feb. 1979.

Lafarge-Frayssinet, C., et al.

Mise en evidence d'activites "hydroxylase" et "epoxyde hydrase" dan des preparations de nucleoles isoles a partir de foie de rat. (Fr.)

C.R. Acad. Sci. [D] (Paris) 289(11):777-780, Nov. 5, 1979.

Lagerson, J.

Pulmonary rehabilitation.

Crit. Care Q. 1(4):75-83, Mar. 1979.

Lagrue, G., et al.

Activites sportives et prevention des facteurs de risque vasculaire. (Fr.)

Sem. Hop. Paris 54(43-44):1385-1387, Dec. 8-15, 1978.

Lagrue, G., et al.

Deformabilite erythrocytaire: Influence du tabagisme et des facteurs de risque vasculaire. (Fr.)

Nouv. Presse Med. 8(50):4079-4081, Dec. 24, 1979.

Lai, D. Y., et al.

Factors influencing the microsome and mitochondria-catalyzed in vitro binding of diethylnitrosamine and n-nitrosopiperidine to deoxyribonucleic acid.

Biochem. Pharmacol. 28(24):3545-3550, Dec. 15, 1979.

Laitinen, L. A., et al.

Scandinavian Symposium on Chronic Obstructive Airways Disease: Comparison of ipratropium bromide and salbutamol in a long-term trial in asthmatic and bronchitic patients in a cold climate.

Scand. J. Respir. Dis. Suppl. 103:163-169, 1979.

Lakowicz, J. R. and Hylden, J. L.

Asbestos-mediated membrane uptake of benzo[a]pyrene observed by fluorescence spectroscopy.

Nature 275(5679):446-448, Oct. 5, 1978.

Lakowicz, J. R. and Bevan, D. R.

Effects of asbetos, iron oxide, silica, and carbon black on the microsomal availability of benzo[a]pyrene.

Biochemistry 18(23):5170-5176, Nov. 13, 1979.

Lakowicz, J. R. and Bevan, D. R.

Benzo[a]pyrene uptake into rat liver microsomes: Effects of adsorption of benzo[a]pyrene to asbetos and non-fibrous mineral particulates.

Chem. Biol. Interact. 29(2):129-138, Feb. 1980.

Lakowicz, J. R., et al.

Particle-enhanced membrane uptake of a polynuclear aromatic hyrocarbon: A possible role in cocarcinogenesis.

JNCI 61(4):1155-1159, Oct. 1978.

Lakowicz, J. R., et al.

Particulate enhanced membrane uptake of 1,2-benzanthracene observed by fluorescence spectroscopy: A possible role in co-carcinogenesis.

Biochem. Biophys. Acta 543(2):202-216, Oct. 3, 1978.

Lall, K. B., et al.

Probable tobacco addiction in a three-year old-child.

Clin. Pediatr. (Phila.) 19(1):56-58, Jan. 1980.

Lam, S., et al.

Nonspecific bronchial reactivity in occupational asthma.

J. Allergy Clin. Immunol. 63(1):28-34, Jan. 1979.

Lam, S., et al.

Neutrophil elastase and pulmonary function in subjects with intermediate alpha,-antitrypsin deficiency (MZ phenotype).

Am. Rev. Respir. Dis. 119(6):941-951, June 1979.

Lambert, B., et al.

Sister chromatid exchanges in lymphocyte cultures of patients receiving chemotherapy for malignant disorders.

Cancer Treat. Rep. 62(10):1413-1419, Oct. 1978.

Lambert, B., et al.

Prolonged increase of sister-chromatid exchanges in lymphocytes of melanoma patients after CCNU treatment.

Mutat. Res. 59(2):295-300, Feb. 1979.

Lambert, G. R., et al.

Duration of hydrogen formation by Anabaena cylindrica B629 in atmosphere of argon, air, and nitrogen.

Appl. Environ. Microbiol. 38(3):530-536, Sept. 1979.

Lambert, G. R., et al.

Effects of ammonium ions, oxygen, carbon monoxide, and acetylene on anaerobic and aerobic hydrogen formation by Anabaena cylindrica B629.

Appl. Environ. Microbiol. 38(3): 521-529, Sept. 1979.

Lambotte-Vandepaer, M., et al.

Styrene induced modifications of some rat liver enzymes involved in the activation and inactivation of xenobiotics.

Biochem. Pharmacol. 28(10): 1635-1659, May 15, 1979.

Lamontagne, Y., et al.

Thought-stopping, pocket timers and their combination, in the modification of smoking behaviour.

Br. J. Addict. 73(2):220-224, June 1978.

Landecker, K. D., et al.

Cimetidine and gastric ulcer healing: A double-blind controlled trial.

Med. J. Aust. 2(1):43-45, July 14, 1979.

Landolph, J. R. and Heidelberger, C.

Chemical carcinogens produce mutations to ouabain resistance in transformable C3H/10T1/2 Cl 8 mouse fibroblasts.

Proc. Natl. Acad. Sci. USA 76(2):930-934, Feb. 1979.

Lane, M.-A.

Muscarinic cholinergic activation of mouse spleen cells cytotoxic to tumor cells in vitro.

JNCI 61(3):923-926, Sept. 1978.

Langauer-Lewowicka, H.

Krioglobuliny, krioglobulinemia: Cryoglobulines and cryoglobulinemia. (Pol.)

Przegl. Lek. 36(2):275-278, 1979.

Lannerstad, O., et al.

Risk factors for premature death in men 56-60 years old: A prospective study of men born 1914, living in Malmoe, Sweden.

Scand. J. Soc. Med. 7(1):41-47, 1979.

LaPorte, R. E., et al.

The relationship of alcohol consumption to atherosclerotic heart disease.

Prev. Med. 9(1):22-40, Jan. 1980.

LaRiviere, W. and Pickett, A. B.

Clinical criteria in diagnosis of early squamous cell carcinoma of the lower lip.

J. Am. Dent. Assoc. 99(6):972-977, Dec. 1979.

Larsen, B. A. and Langnes, K. T.

Skadervirkninger ved snus og skraa. (Letter to the Editor.) (Norw.)

Tidsskr. Nor. Laegeforen. 98(11): 583, Apr. 20, 1978.

Larsson-Cohn, U.

Riskbedoemning vid preventivmedel-sraadgivning. (Swed.)

Lakartidningen 75(41):3670-3672, Oct. 11, 1978.

Lasagna, L.

The diseases and drug needs of the Third World.

J. Chronic Dis. 32(6):413-414, 1979.

Laties, V. G.

Symposium on Target Organ Toxicity: Nervous System. How operant conditioning can contribute to behavioral toxicology.

Environ. Health Perspect. 26:29-35, Oct. 1978.

Laties, V. G. and Merigan, W. H.

Behavioral effects of carbon monoxide on animals and man.

Annu. Rev. Pharmacol. Toxicol. 19:357-392, 1979.

Lattimer, G. L., et al.

International Symposium on Legionnaires' Disease. The Philadelphia epidemic of Legionnaires' disease: Clinical, pulmonary, and serologic findings two years later.

Ann. Intern. Med. 90(4):522-526, Apr. 1979.

Lau, P. P. and Luh, Y.

Effects of the comutagens, harman and norharman, on the interaction of a tryptophan product, 3-amino-1-methyl-5h-pyrido(4,3-b) indole with DNA.

Biochem. Biophys. Res. Commun. 89(1):188-194, July 12, 1979.

Lauridsen, K. N.

Kulilteforgiftning: To tilfaelde med et ejendommeligt forloeb. (Dan.)

Ugeskr. Laeger 141(12):796-797, Mar. 19, 1979.

Lauwerys, R. R., et al.

Investigations on the lung and kidney function in workers exposed to cadmium.

Environ. Health Perspect. 28:137-145, Feb. 1979.

Lawther, P. J., et al.

Respiratory function measurements in a cohort of medical students: A ten-year follow-up.

Thorax 33(6):773-778, Dec. 1978.

Laxenaire, M. C., et al.

Criteres d'evaluation du risque de decompensation respiratoire post-operatoire. (Fr.)

Anesth. Analg. (Paris) 35(4):613-624, July-Aug. 1978.

Le Bouffant, L., et al.

Action of intensive cigarette smoke inhalations on the rat lung. Role of particulate and gaseous cofactors.

JNCI 64(2):273-284, Feb. 1980.

Le Mesurier, S. M., et al.

Reduced yield of pulmonary surfactant: Patterns of response following administration of chemicals to rats by inhalation.

Toxicol. Lett. 5(1):89-93, Jan. 1980.

Le Mesurier, S. M., et al.

Pulmonary responses to atmospheric pollutants. II. Effect of petrol vapour inhalation on secretion of pulmonary surfactant.

Pathology 11(1):81-87, Jan. 1979.

Leaf, A., et al.

Neurology Forum: Neurogenic diabetes insipidus.

Kidney Int. 15(5):572-580, May 1979.

Leclerc, P.

Moyens de defense de la muqueuse bronchique. (Fr.)

Gaz. Med. (Fr.) 86(30):3331-3341, Oct. 5, 1979.

Leclercq, G. and Heuson, J. C.

Physiological and pharmacological effects of estrogens in breast cancer.

Biochim. Biophys. Acta 560(4):427-455, Dec. 19, 1979.

Leclercq, J. F., et al.

Enquete epidemiologique multicentrique sur les myocardiopathies primitives: A propos de 380 observations. (Fr.)

Arch. Mal. Coeur 72(12):1302-1310, Dec. 1979.

Lee, C., et al.

Lactate dehydrogenase in normal mammary glands and in 7,12-dimethylbenz[a]anthracene-induced mammary tumors in Sprague-Dawley rats.

JNCI 62(1):193-199, Jan. 1979.

Lee, H. K., et al.

Mechanism of antiemetic action of penfluridol in the dog.

Eur. J. Pharmacol. 53(1):29-38, Dec. 15, 1978.

Lee, I. P., et al.

Aryl hydrocarbon hydroxylase induction in rat lung, liver, and male reproductive organs following inhalation exposure to diesel emission.

Toxicol. Appl. Pharmacol. 52(1):181-184, Jan. 1980.

Lee, J. and Lauer, R. M.

Symposium on Pediatric Cardiology: Pediatric aspects of atherosclerosis and hypertension.

Pediatr. Clin. North Am. 25(4):909-929, Nov. 1978.

Lee, K.

Alcoholism and cerebrovascular thrombosis in the young.

Acta Neurol. Scand. 59(5):270-274, May 1979.

Lee, P. N.

Has the mortality of male doctors improved with the reductions in their cigarette smoking?

Br. Med. J. 2(6204):1538-1540, Dec. 15, 1979.

Lee, P. N.

Carbon monoxide yield of cigarettes. (Letter to the Editor.)

Br. Med. J. 2(6204):1584, Dec. 15, 1980.

Lee, R. A.

Febetron radiolysis of CO2 in the presence of oxygen and carbon monoxide.

Radiat. Res. 77(2):233-241, Feb. 1979.

Lee, S. M.

Diabetes and the kidney.

Ariz. Med. 36(2):134-137, Feb. 1979.

Lefevre, P. A.

Appendix IV: The degranulation test.

Br. J. Cancer 37(6):937-943, June 1978.

Leffell, M. S. and Coggin, Jr., J. H.

Increases and perturbations in thymocytes forming spontaneous rosettes during viral and chemical oncogenesis in hamsters.

Clin. Immunol. Immunopathol. 11(3): 275-287, Nov. 1978.

Leffingwell, C. M. and Low, R. B.

Cigarette smoke components and alveolar macrophage protein synthesis.

Arch. Environ. Health 34(2): 97-102, Mar.-Apr. 1979.

Leger, A. S. St., et al.

Factors associated with cardiac mortality in developed countries with particular reference to the consumption of wine.

Lancet 1(8124):1017-1020, May 12, 1979.

Legros, J. J.

Les neurophysines. (Fr.)

Ann. Endocrinol. (Paris) 39(4):319-339, July-Aug. 1978.

Lehrer, S. B., et al.

Immunogenic properties of tobacco smoke.

J. Allergy Clin. Immunol. 62(6):368-370, Dec. 1978.

Lehrer, S. B., et al.

IgE antibody response of smokers, nonsmokers, and "smoke-sensitive" persons to tobacco leaf and smoke antigens.

Am. Rev. Respir. Dis. 121(1):168-170, Jan. 1980.

Lehtovirta, P.

Tupakointi ja raskaus. (Finn.)

Duodecim 95(1):1-3, 1979.

Lehtovirta, P. and Forss, M.

The acute effect of smoking on intervillous blood flow of the placenta.

Br. J. Obstet. Gynecol. 85(10):729-731, Oct. 1978.

Lehtovirta, P. and Forss, M.

Die momentane Beeinflussung des intervilloesen Blutflusses der Plazenta durch Rauchen. (Ger.)

Gynaekol. Rundsch. 19(3):179-180, 1979.

Leitch, A. G. and Kay, A. B.

Aspen Lung Conference: Immunology of the Lung. Mediators of immediate type hypersensitivity in sputum from symptomatic young cigarette smokers.

Chest 75(2, Suppl.):223-224, Feb. 1979.

Lemoine J. M.

Reunion commune des groupes d'etudes sur les cancers bronchogeniques et sur les bronchites chroniques de L'A.I.B.P. a toulouse le 3-5-1978. (Fr.)

Bronchopneumologie 24(3):264-265, 1979.

Lemoine, J. M.

Le depistage presymptomatique des cancers bronchogeniques. (Fr.)

Rev. Med. Suisse Romande 99(4):203-204, Apr. 1979.

Lemoine, J. M.

Modalites de depistage presymptomatique des cancers bronchogeniques. (Fr.)

Bronchopneumologie 24(3):265-272, 1979.

Leonard, R. B.

Smoke inhalation.

NC Med. J. 40(10):628-630, Oct. 1979.

Leophonte, P., et al.

Resultats d'une enquete sur le tabagisme parmi les jeunes: Principe de lutte.

Rev. Med. Toulouse 15(3):123-127, Mar. 1979.

Leophonte, P., et al.

Premiers resultats d'une consultation d'aide medicale a la desintoxication tabagique. (Fr.)

Rev. Med. Toulouse 15(5):267-269, May 1979.

Leren, P., et al.

Hypertension Control in Scandinavia. Proceedings of a Dumex Symposium: Coronary risk and socio-economic status, the Oslo Study.

Acta Med. Scand. Suppl. 626: 33, 1979.

Lesca, P., et al.

Ellipticines as potent inhibitors of aryl hydrocarbon hydroxylase: Their binding to microsomal cytochromes P450 and protective effect against benzo(a)pyrene mutagenicity.

Biochem. Pharmacol. 27(8):1203-1209, Apr. 15, 1978.

Lesca, P., et al.

Symposium. Coordination Chemistry and Cancer Chemotherapy: Ellipticines as potent inhibitors of drug metabolism. Protective effect against chemical mutagenesis and carcinogenesis.

Biochimie 60(9):1011-1018, 1978.

Lester, D.

Proceedings of Alcohol and Cancer Workshop: Modes of alcohol administration appropriate for the study of the role of alcohol in carcinogenesis.

Cancer Res. 39(7, Part 2):2891-2893, July 1979.

Leu, R.

Praevention und ihre Moeglichkeiten: Betrachtungen zur Effizienz und Struktur des Gesundheitswesens. (Ger.)

Soz. Praventivmed. 23(5-6):335-340, Dec. 1978.

Leu, R.

Evaluation von Massnahmen zur Einschraenkung des Zigaretten-verbrauchs in der Schweiz. (Ger.)

Bull. Schweiz. Akad. Med. Wiss. 35(1-3):245-260, Mar. 1979.

Levin, W., et al.

Tumorigenic activity of 3-methyl-cholanthrene metabolites on mouse skin and in newborn mice.

Cancer Res. 39(9):3549-3553, Sept. 1979.

Levison, D. A.

Carcinoma of the pancreas.

J. Pathol. 129(4):203-223, Dec. 1979.

Levison, D. A., et al.

Carcinogenic effects of di(2-hydro-xypropyl)nitrosamine (DHPN) in male Wistar rats: Promotion of pancreatic cancer by a raw soya flour diet.

Scand. J. Gastroenterol. 14(2):217-224, 1979.

Levison, D. A., et al.

Oesophageal noeplasia in male Wistar rats due to parenteral di(2-hydroxy-propyl)-Nitrosamine (DHPN): A combined histopathological, histo-chemical and electron microscopic study.

J. Pathol. 129(1):31-36;Plate XVII-XXIV, Sept. 1979.

Levitt, R. C., et al.

Genetic differences in metabolism of polycyclic aromatic carcinogens and aromatic amines by mouse liver microsomes. Detection by DNA binding of metabolites and by mutagenicity in histidine-dependent Salmonella typhimurium in vitro.

JNCI 62(4):947-955, Apr. 1979.

Levy-Frebault, V and David, H. L.

Mutations affecting pigment synthesis in Mycobacterium aurum.

J. Gen. Microbiol. 115(2):317-323, Dec. 1979.

Levy, R. I.

Preventing the preventable.

Am. Pharm. NS20(2):19-24, Feb. 1980.

Lew, E. A. and Garfinkel, L.

Variations in mortality by weight among 750,000 men and women.

J. Chronic Dis. 32(8):563-576, 1979.

Lewak, N., et al.

Sudden Infant Death Syndrome risk factor: Prospective data review.

Clin. Pediatr. (Phila.) 18(7):404-411, July 1979.

Lewin, S., et al.

Legionnaires' disease: A cause of severe abscess-forming pneumonia.

Am. J. Med. 67(2):339-342, Aug. 1979.

Lewis, B.

Hypothesis into theory - The development of aetiological concepts of ischaemic heart disease: A review.

J. R. Soc. Med. 71(11):809-818, Nov. 1978.

Lewis, B. M. and Izbicki, R.

Routine pulmonary function tests during bleomycin therapy: Tests may be ineffective and potentially misleading.

JAMA 243(4):347-351, Jan. 25, 1980.

Lewis, B. V.

Drug therapy in pregnancy.

Practitioner 221(1326):866-873, Dec. 1978.

Lewis, D. J. and Prentice, D. E.

Effect of tobacco smoke on rat trachea and bronchus: A quantitative scanning electron microscopical study.

Toxicol. Lett. 3(1):1-6, Jan. 1979.

Lewis, D. J., et al.

A quantitative ultrastructural comparison of macrophages from rats exposed to smoke derived from conventional tobacco and a tobacco substitute.

Toxicol. Lett. 5(1):83-87, Jan. 1980.

Lewis, I. C. and Rayner, K.J.

The changing scene: Dieting, vitamins, analgesics, alcohol, smoking, and Hobart secondary school students.

Med. J. Aust. 2(14):632-635, Dec. 30, 1978.

Lewis, P. and Boylan, P.

Fetal breathing: A review.

Am. J. Obstet. Gynecol. 134(5):587-598, July 1, 1979.

Lichtenberg, F. W. and Dewitt, G. E.

The medical data base system of Owens-Corning fiberglass corporation.

Am. Ind. Hyg. Assoc. J. 41(2):103-112, Feb. 1980.

Lichtensteiger, W., et al.

Changes in the distribution of non-neuronal elements in rat median eminence and in anterior pituitary hormone secretion after activation of tuberoinfundibular dopamine neurons by brain stimulation or nicotine.

Brain Res. 157(1):73-88, Nov. 17, 1978.

Lieber, C. S., et al.

Proceedings of Alcohol and Cancer Workshop: Alcohol-related diseases and carcinogenesis.

Cancer Res. 39(7, Part 2): 2863-2886, July 1979.

Lieberman, B. A., et al.

The effects of maternally administered pethidine or epidural bupivacaine on the fetus and newborn.

Br. J. Obstet. Gynaecol. 86(8):598-606, Aug. 1979.

Lieberman, M. W.

Mutagenesis: DNA repair as it relates to mutagenesis and gene expression in mammalian cells and tissues.

Adv. Mod. Toxicol. 5:29-52, 1978.

Lijinsky, W.

Proceedings of Alcohol and Cancer Workshop: Current status of experimental chemical carcinogenesis and its applications to human cancer risk.

Cancer Res. 39(7, Part 2): 2887-2890, July 1979.

Lijinsky, W. and Taylor, H. W.

Relative carcinogenic effectiveness of derivatives of nitrosodiethylamine in rats.

Cancer Res. 38(8):2391-2394, Aug. 1978.

Lijinsky, W. and Taylor, H. W.

Comparison of bladder carcinogenesis by nitrosomethyldodecylamine in Sprague-Dawley and Fischer rats carrying transplanted bladder tissue.

Cancer Lett. 5(4):215-218, Oct. 1978.

Lijinsky, W. and Reuber, M. D.

Carcinogenicity in rats of nitrosomethylethylamines labeled with deuterium in several positions.

Cancer Res. 40(1):19-21, Jan. 1980.

Lijinsky, W., et al.

Carcinogenesis of nitrosomethylundecylamine in Fischer rats.

Cancer Lett. 5(4):209-213, Oct. 1978.

Lilienfeld, A. M. and Lilienfeld, D. E.

The Case Control Study: Consensus and Controversy. A century of case-control studies: Progress?

J. Chron. Dis. 32(1-2):5-13, 1979.

Lillehaug, J. R., et al.

Establishment of epithelial cell lines from adult mouse regenerating liver.

In Vitro 15(11):910-916, Nov. 1979.

Lindberg, U.

Hur tobaksinformationen i skolan paaverkar roekvanorna hos grundskoleelever. (Swed.)

Lakartidningen 75(34):2880-2882, Aug. 23, 1978.

Lindberg, U.

Tobaksinformationen i skolan: Tvaaaarsuppfoeljning av elevernas roekvanor. (Swed.)

Lakartidningen 76(17):1619-1620, Apr. 25, 1979.

Lindenschmidt, R. R. and Persaud, T. V. N.

Effect of ethanol and nicotine in the pregnant rat.

Res. Commun. Chem. Pathol. Pharmacol. 27(1):195-198, Jan. 1980.

Lindesmith, L. A.

Clean indoor air - A fight for rights for health - not unwarranted government intervention.

Wis. Med. J. 78(11):12-13, Nov. 1979.

Lindquist, O. and Bengtsson, C.

Menopausal age in relation to smoking.

Acta Med. Scand. 205(1-2):73-77, 1979.

Lindqvist, C.

Huulisyoepae ja sen riskitekijaet. (Finn.)

Duodecim 93(4):258-267, 1977.

Lindqvist, C.

Risk factors in lip cancer: A questionnaire survey.

Am. J. Epidemiol. 109(5):521-530, May 1979.

Lindqvist, C. and Teppo, L.

Epidemiological evaluation of sunlight as a risk factor of lip cancer.

Br. J. Cancer 37(6):983-989, June 1978.

Lipworth, L. L. and Rice, C. A.

Correlations in mortality data involving cancers of the colorectum and esophagus.

Cancer 43(5):1927-1933, May 1979.

Litterst, C. L.

In vitro hepatic drug metabolism and microsomal enzyme induction in genetically obese rat.

Biochem. Pharmacol. 29(3):289-296, Feb. 1, 1980.

Little, R. E. and Hook, E. B.

Maternal alcohol and tobacco consumption and their association with nausea and vomiting during pregnancy.

Acta Obstet. Gynecol. Scand. 58(1):15-17, 1979.

Litvitsky, P. F. and Kogan, A. Kh.

Nephrogenic hypertension and carcinogenesis. (Russ.)

Vopr. Onkol. 24(9):56-60, 1978.

Liu, K. and Dyer, A. R.

A rank statistic for assessing the amount of variation explained by risk factors in epidemiologic studies.

Am. J. Epidemiol. 109(5):597-606, May 1979.

Livett, B. G., et al.

Substance P inhibits nicotine activation of chromaffin cells.

Nature 278(5701):256-257, Mar. 15, 1979.

Livshits, N. A. and Korovina, O. V.

Chronic bronchitis and smoking. (Russ.)

Ter. Ark. 51(4):55-57, 1979.

Ljunggren, L.

Roekning och information. (Swed.)

Lakartidningen 75(45):4125-4126, Nov. 8, 1978.

Lob, M.

Maladies liees a l[asbeste. (Fr.)

Praxis 68(52):1717-1723, Dec. 27, 1979.

Loewhagen, O., et al.

Studies on histamine metabolism in intrinsic bronchial asthma.

Allergy 34(6):395-404, Dec. 1979.

Logan, R. L., et al.

Drugs, Lipid Metabolism, and Atherosclerosis. The Edinburgh-Stockholm study of coronary heart disease risk factors: A summary.

Adv. Exp. Med. Biol. 109:287-294, 1978.

Lomakin, M. S., et al.

Thermostable antigens of malignant tumours and normal tissues of experimental animals. (Russ.)

Biull. Eskp. Biol. Med. 85(6):726-728, June 1978.

London, S. W., et al.

Suppression of cancer chemotherapy-induced vomiting in the cat by nabilone, a synthetic cannabinoid.

Proc. Soc. Exp. Biol. Med. 160(4):437-440, Apr. 1979.

Longnecker, D. S., et al.

Focal acinar cell dysplasia in human pancreas.

Cancer 45(3):534-540, Feb. 1, 1980.

Longo, D. L. and Young, R. C.

Cosmetic talc and ovarian cancer.

Lancet 2(8138):349-351, Aug. 18, 1979.

Longstaff, E.

Appendix V: The sebaceous-gland test.

Br. J. Cancer 37(6):944-948, June 1978.

Longstaff, E.

Appendix VII: The implant test.

Br. J. Cancer 37(6):954-958, June 1978.

Lore, Jr., J. M., et al.

Sympossium on Malignant Disease of the Oral Cavity and Related Structures: Surgical management and epidemiology of lip cancer.

Otolaryngol. Clin. North Am. 12(1): 81-95, Feb. 1979.

Lorentzen, R. J., et al.

Toxicity of metabolic benzo(a)pyrenediones to cultured cells and the dependence upon molecular oxygen.

Cancer Res. 39(8):3194-3198, Aug. 1979.

Loss, R. W., et al.

Evaluation of early airway diseases in smokers: Cost effectiveness of pulmonary function testing.

Am. J. Med. Sci. 278(1):27-37, July-Aug. 1979.

Lotlikar, P. D., et al.

Effect of dimethylnitrosamine concentration on its demethylation by liver microsomes from control and 3-methylcolanthrene pretreated rats, hamsters and guinea pigs.

Cancer Lett. 4(6):355-361, June 1978.

Loudon, N. B.

Oral contraception.

Practitioner 223(1337):641-645, Nov. 1979.

Lovlin, R. E., et al.

Erythrocyte volume and count: A linear relation descriptive of population differences.

Scand. J. Haematol. 22(3):197-204, Mar. 1979.

Low, R. B., et al.

Biochemical analyses of bronchoalveolar lavage fluids of healthy human volunteer smokers and nonsmokers.

Am. Rev. Respir. Dis. 118(5):863-875, Nov. 1978.

Lowe, G. D. O., et al.

The effects of age and cigarette-smoking on blood and plasma viscosity in men.

Scott. Med. J. 25(1):13-17, Jan. 1980.

Lower, Jr., G. M., et al.

N-acetyltransferase phenotype and risk in urinary bladder cancer: Approaches in molecular epidemiology. Preliminary results in Sweden and Denmark.

Environ. Health Perspect. 29:71-79, Apr. 1979.

Lozzio, B. B., et al.

High incidence of mammary tumors in mice with inherited asplenia carriers for the nude gene.

Cancer Res. 39(5):1529-1533, May 1979.

Lubet, R. A., et al.

The metabolic activation of benzo (a)pyrene and 9-hydroxybenzo (a)pyrene by liver microsomal fractions.

Int. J. Cancer 23(3):353-357, Mar. 15, 1979.

Lufkin, E. G., et al.

Increased von Willebrand factor in diabetes mellitus.

Metabolism 28(1):63-66, Jan. 1979.

Lukas, R. J., et al.

Effects of thio-group modification and Ca-2-plus on agonist-specific state transitions of a central nicotinic acetylcholine receptor.

Biochemistry 18(11):2384-2395, May 29, 1979.

Lukasiewicz, R. J. and Bennett, E. L.

Alpha-bungarotoxin binding properties of a central nervous system nicotinic acetylcholine recpetor.

Biochim. Biophys. Acta. 544(2):294-308, Dec. 1, 1978.

Lundberg, G. D., et al.

Drugs (other than or in addition to ethyl alcohol) and driving behavior: A collaborative study of the California Association of Toxicologists.

J. Forensic Sci. 24(1):207-215, Jan. 1979.

Lundquist, P., et al.

Method for determining thiocyanate in serum and urine.

Clin. Chem. 25(5):678-681, May 1979.

Lundstroem, J.

Se upp foer hjaertinfarkt! (Swed.)

Svensk Farm. Tidskr. 82(5):206-209, May 1978.

Lundy, P. M.

The ganglionic blocking properties of the cholinesterase reactivator, HS-6.

Can. J. Physiol. Pharmacol. 56(5): 857-862, Oct. 1978.

Luria, S. N. and McKay, C. L.

Effects of low levels of carbon monoxide on visions of smokers and nonsmokers.

Arch. Environ. Health 34(1):38-44, Jan.-Feb. 1979.

Lurie, A. G. and Cutler, L. S.

Effects of low-level X-radiation on 7, 12-dimethylbenz(a)anthracene -induced lingual tumors in Syrian golden hamsters.

JNCI 63(1):147-152, July 1979.

Lutz, E. G.

Marihuana and paranoid disperception.

J. Med. Soc. NJ 76(4):253-259, Apr. 1979.

Lynch, H. T., et al.

Familial factors in bladder carcinoma.

J. Urol. 122(4):458-461, Oct. 1979.

Lynch, J., et al.

An association of upper respiratory cancer with exposure to diethyl sulfate.

JOM 21(5):333-341, May 1979.

Lyusov, V. A., et al.

Intravascular coagulation in chronic forms of ischemic heart disease (according to the data of radioisotopic studies). (Russ.)

Ter. Arkh. 50(9):128-131, 1978.

Mabuchi, K., et al.

Lung cancer among pesticide workers exposed to inorganic arsenicals.

Arch. Environ. Health 34(5):312-320, Sept.-Oct. 1979.

MacArthur, C. G. C., et al.

Ventilatory function in the Eisenmenger syndrome.

Thorax 34(3):348-353, June 1979.

Macfarlane, J. D., et al.

Pulmonary and pleural lesions in rheumatoid disease.

Br. J. Dis. Chest 72(4):288-300, Oct. 1978.

Mach, J.-P., et al.

Proceedings of the International Conference on the Clinical Uses of Carcinoembryonic Antigen: Long-term follow-up of colorectal carcinoma patients by repeated CEA radioimmunoassay.

Cancer 42(3, Suppl.):1439-1447, Sept. 1978.

Mach, J.-P., et al.

Interet et limites du dosage radio-immunologique de l'antigene carcinoembryonnaire (CEA) dans l'etablissment du pronostic et du traitement postoperatoire des malades atteints de carcinome du gros intestin. (Fr.)

Praxis 68(26):856-863, June 26, 1979.

Machalski, M., et al.

Wplyw palenia papierosow na niektore parametry hematologiczne. (Pol.)

Wiad. Lek. 32(1):11-14, Jan. 1, 1979.

Machol, L.

Smoking, estrogen replacement, and MI.

Contemp. Ob/Gyn 12(3):166, Sept. 1978.

Machol, L.

Environmental hazards: What they'll mean to your patients in the 1980's.

Contemp. Ob/Gyn. 15(1):22-48, Jan. 1980.

Machova, J. and Boska, D.

Production of decremental oscillations following spike potential by muscarinic drugs, histamine and bradykinin in cat sympathetic ganglion.

Neuropharmacology 18(4):355-360, Apr. 1979.

MacIntyre, D., et al.

Silver poisoning associated wih an anti-smoking lozenge.

Br. Med. J. 2(6154):1749-1750, Dec. 23-30, 1978.

Mackay, A. and Nias, B. C.

Strokes in the young and middle-aged: Consequences to the family and to society.

J. R. Coll. Physicians Lond. 13(2):106-112, Apr. 1979.

Mackay, A., et al.

Smoking and renal artery stenosis.

Br. Med. J. 2(6193):770, Sept. 29, 1979.

Mackay, I. R.

Clinical Application of Carcino-embryonic Antigen Assay: Use of carcinoembryonic antigen in screening an unselected population. A five year followup.

Int. Congr. Ser. No. 439:419-421, 1978.

Mackay, J. B.

Management of pneumonia.

NZ Med. J. 89(637):441-443, June 13, 1979.

Mackenzie, J. S. and Flower, R. L. P.

The effect of long term exposure to cigarette smoke on the height and specificity of the secondary immune response to influenza virus in a murine model system.

J. Hyg. (Lond.) 83(1):135-141, Aug. 1979.

MacLeod, M. C., et al.

Metabolism and macromolecular binding of the carcinogen benzo(a)pyrene and its relatively inert isomer benzo(e)pyrene by hamster embryo cells.

Cancer Res. 39(9):3463-3470, Sept. 1979.

Macnab, G. M., et al.

Carcinoembryonic antigen in hepatocellular cancer.

Br. J. Cancer 38(1):51-54, July 1978.

MacNicoll, A. D., et al.

The involvement of a non-'bay-region' diol-epoxide in the formation of benz(a)-anthracene-DNA adducts in a rat-liver microsomal system.

Biochem. Biophys. Res. Commun. 91(2):490-497, Nov. 28, 1979.

MacNicoll, A. D., et al.

The metabolism of a series of polycyclic hydrocarbons by mouse skin maintained in short-term organ culture.

Chem. Biol. Interact. 29(2):169-188, Feb. 1980.

MacVicar, J. and Kerr, M. M.

Maternal disease, infection, trauma rhesus isoimmunisation.

Lancet 2(8155):1284-1286, Dec. 15, 1979.

Madden, J. J., et al.

Effects of opiates and demographic factors on DNA repair synthesis in human leukocytes.

Proc. Natl. Acad. Sci. USA 76(11):5769-5773, Nov. 1979.

Maddox, W. L., et al.

A tobacco smoke inhalation exposure device for rodents.

Arch. Environ. Health 33(2):64-71, Mar.-Apr. 1978.

Madison, R., et al.

Proceedings of the Aspen Lung Conference: Inherited risk factors for chronic lung disease.

Chest 77(2 Suppl.):255-257, Feb. 1980.

Madsbad, S., et al.

Influence of smoking on insulin requirement and metabolic status in diabetes mellitus.

Diabetes Care 3(1):41-43, Jan.-Feb. 1980.

Maduagwu, E. N.

Microbial nitrosamine formation in palm wine: In vitro N-nitrosation by cell suspensions.

J. Environ. Pathol. Toxicol. 2(4):1183-1194, Mar.-Apr. 1979.

Maeda, K., et al.

Occupational cervicobrachial disorders of workwomen in assembly lines of a cigarette factory.

Jpn. J. Ind. Health 19(1):8-21, Jan. 1977.

Maerns, A. J. and Sherwood, M. J.

Aquatic Pollutants and Biologic Effects with Emphasis on Neoplasia: Distribution of neoplasms and other diseases in marine fishes relative to the discharge of waste water.

Ann. NY Acad. Sci. 298:210-224, Sept. 29, 1977.

Magee, P. N. (Chairman), et al.

Some N-Nitroso Compounds: N-nitrosomethylethylamine.

IARC Monogr. Eval. Carcinog. Risk Chem. Hum. 17:221-226, 1978.

Magee, P. N. (Chairman), et al.

Some N-Nitroso Compounds: N-nitrosodimethylamine.

IARC Monogr. Eval. Carcinog. Risk Chem. Hum. 17:125-175, 1978.

Magee, P. N. (Chairman), et al.

Some N-Nitroso Compounds: N'-nitrosonornicotine.

IARC Monogr. Eval. Carcinog. Risk Chem. Hum. 17:281-286, 1978.

Magee, P. N. (Chairman), et al.

Some N-Nitroso Compounds: N-nitrosodi-n-butylamine.

IRAC Monogr. Eval. Carcinog. Risk Chem. Hum. 17:51-75, 1978.

Magee, P. N. (Chairman), et al.

Some N-Nitroso Compounds: N-nitrosodiethanolamine.

IARC Monogr. Eval. Carcinog. Risk Chem. Hum. 17:77-82, 1978.

Magee, P. N. (Chairman), et al.

Some N-Nitroso Compounds: N-nitrosopyrrolidine.

IARC Monogr. Eval. Carcinog. Risk Chem. Hum. 17:313-326, 1978.

Magee, P. N. (Chairman), et al.

Some N-Nitroso Compounds: N-nitrosodiethylamine.

IARC Monogr. Eval. Carcinog. Risk Chem. Hum. 17:83-124, 1978.

Magnus, K., et al.

Walking, cycling, or gardening, with or without seasonal interruption, in relation to acute coronary events.

Am. J. Epidemiol. 110(6):724-733, Dec. 1979.

Maguire, M. G., et al.

Increased risk of thrombosis due to oral contraceptives: A further report.

Am. J. Epidemiol. 110(2):188-195, Aug. 1979.

Mahan, C. S.

Revolution in obstetrics: Pregnancy nutrition.

J. Fla. Med. Assoc. 66(4):367-372, Apr. 1979.

Mahendru, R. K., et al.

Smoking habits and emotional factors in coronary heart disease.

J. Assoc. Physicians India 26(10): 909-914, Oct. 1978.

Maiorana, A. and Gullino, P. M.

Acquisition of angiogenic capacity and neoplastic transformation in the rat mammary gland.

Cancer Res. 38(12):4409-4414, Dec. 1978.

Maiorana, A. and Gullino, P. M.

Acquisition of angiogenic capacity and neoplastic transformation in the rat mammary gland.

Cancer Res. 38(12):4409-4414, Dec. 1978.

Majewski, A.

Obraz kliniczny zatrucia nikotyna noworodkow karmionych piersia. (Pol.)

Wiad. Lek. 32(4):275-277, Feb. 15, 1979.

Malik, N., et al.

Induction of UDP-glucuronosyltransferase activity in the Reuber H-4-II-E hepatoma cell culture.

Mol. Pharmacol. 16(3):950-960, Nov. 1979.

Malik, S. K. and Singh, K.

Smoking habits, chronic bronchitis and ventilatory function in rural males.

Indian J. Chest Dis. Allied Sci. 20(2):73-79, Apr. 1978.

Malik, S. K. and Banga, N.

Peak expiratory flow rate in non-smoking rural males.

Indian J. Chest Dis. Allied Sci. 20(4): 183-186, Oct. 1978.

Malkova, J., et al.

Poruchy glycidoveho metabolismu a sekrece inzulinu ve vztahu k rizikovym faktorum ischemicke choroby srdecni. (Czech)

Cas. Lek. Listy 117(34):1044-1046, 1978.

Malmberg, P. O., et al.

Effect of increased blood-oxygen affinity on oxygen transport in hemorrhagic shock.

J. Appl. Physiol. 47(4):889-895, Oct. 1979.

Manciaux, M.

Developmental paediatrics.

Acta Paediatr. Scand. 68(4):469-473, July 1979.

Mandybur, T. I., et al.

Enhanced development of mammary tumors in rats following transplacental and neonatal exposure to elthylnitrosourea.

Cancer Res. 38(10):3182-3185, Oct. 1978.

Manger, W. M. and Gifford, Jr., R. W.

Pheochromocytoma: Diagnosis and management.

NY State J. Med. 80(2):216-226, Feb. 1980.

Manis, J. and Kim, G.

Introduction of iron transport by a potent inducer of aryl hydrocarbon hydroxylase, 2, 3, 7, 8-tetrachlorodibenzo-p-dixin.

Arch. Environ. Health 34(3):141-145, May-June 1979.

Manousos, O. N., et al.

A double-blind study of cimetidine in patients with duodenal or gastric ulcer in Greece.

J. Int. Med. Res. 6(5):381-383, 1978.

Marchandise, B., et al.

Platelet hyperreactivity to thrombin in patients with myocardial infarction and normal or slightly abnormal coronary arteries.

Clin. Invest. Med. 2(1):41-49, 1979.

Marcus, A. H. and Czajkowski, Jr., S.

First passage times as environmental safety indicators: Carboxyhemoglobin from cigarette smoke.

Biometrics 35(3):539-548, Sept. 1979.

Marcuson, R., et al.

Clinical importance of directional statistics for electrocardiographic differentiation of smoking habits.

J. Electrocardiol. 12(1):97-102, Jan. 1979.

Margison, G. P., et al.

Persistence of methylated bases in ribonucleic acid of Syrian golden hamster liver after administration of dimethylnitrosamine.

Biochem. J. 177(3):967-973, Mar. 1, 1979.

Margison, G. P., et al.

Effect of chronic N,N-diethylnitrosamine on the excision of O6-ethylguanine from rat liver DNA.

Br. J. Cancer 40(5):809-813, Nov. 1979.

Markiewicz, K. and Cholewa, M.

The influence of ethyl alcohol, coffee and tobacco on free fatty acid, triglyceride and glucose levels in serum during physical exercise and restitution.

Acta Med. Pol. 19(3):373-385, 1978.

Markiewicz, K., et al.

Influence of tobacco smoking on serum free fatty acid, triglyceride and glucose levels during physical training and post-exertional restitution.

Acta Med. Acad. Sci. Hung. 35(3-4): 225-232, 1978.

Markis, J. E., et al.

Sustained effect of orally administered isosorbide dinitrate on exercise performance of patients with angina pectoris.

Am. J. Cardiol. 43(2):265-271, Feb. 1979.

Markovits, P., et al.

Normal and benzo(a)pyrene-transformed fetal mouse brain cells. I. Tumorigenicity and immunochemical detection of glial fibrillary acidic protein.

Acta Neuropathol. (Berl.) 47(3): 197-203, Aug. 1979.

Marks, F., et al.

Ornithine decarboxylase activity, cell proliferation, and tumor promotion in mouse epidermis in vivo.

Cancer Res. 39(10):4183-4188, Oct. 1979.

Marks, I. N.

Healing of peptic ulcers on conventional antacid therapy with or without butriptyline.

S. Afr. Med. J. 55(9):331-334, Mar. 3, 1979.

Marks, V.

New developments in immunoassays for therapeutic drug monitoring.

Antibiot. Chemother. 26:16-26, 1979.

Marmot, M. G.

Epidemiological basis for the prevention of coronary heart disease.

Bull. WHO 57(3):331-347, 1979.

Marmot, M. G., et al.

Changing social-class distribution of heart disease.

Br. Med. J. 2(6145):1109-1112, Oct. 21, 1978.

Marquardt, H., et al.

Comparison of mutagenesis and malignant transformation by dihydrodiols from benz[a]antracene and 7,12-dimethylbenz[a]anthracene.

Br. J. Cancer 39(5):540-547, May 1979.

Marquis, J. K., et al.

Solubilization of cholinergic binding fractions from lobster axon membrane fragments.

Biochem. Pharmacol. 28(13):2094-2096, July 1, 1979.

Marsden, A.

Letter to the Editor.

J. R. Nav. Med. Serv. 64(3):185, Winter 1978.

Marselos, M., et al.

Comparison of phenobarbital- and carcinogen-induced aldehyde dehydrogenases in the rat.

Biochim. Biophys. Acta 583(1):110-118, Feb. 19, 1979.

Marsh, J. A., et al.

Do methoxyflurane an enflurane induce hepatic drug-metabolizing enzymes?

S. Afr. Med. J. 55(22):871-877, May 26, 1979.

Marshall, Jr., R. J.

Smoking in Rhode Island: The proportion of adult smokers in Rhode Island has apparently declined.

RI Med. J. 62(6):215-224, June 1979.

Marshall, M.

Atherogenese: Experimentelle Untersuchungen zur pathogenese obliterierender Arteriopathien am Miniaturschwein. (Ger.)

MMW 121(38):1211-1218, Sept. 21, 1979.

Marshall, M. V., et al.

Patterns of benzo[alpha]pyrene metabolism in normal human pulmonary alveolar macrophages.

Cancer Lett. 8(2):103-109, Dec. 1979.

Marshall, M., et al.

Experimentelle untersuchungen ueber den Risikofaktor Rauchen. (Ger.)

Vasa 7(4):389-397, 1978.

Martin, C. N., et al.

Testing of known carcinogens and noncarcinogens for their ability to induce unscheduled DNA synthesis in HeLa cells.

Cancer Res. 38(8):2621-2627, Aug. 1978.

Martin, E. and Mukkada, A. J.

Identification of the termnal respiratory chain in kinetoplast-mitochondrial complexes of Leishmania tropica promastigotes.

J. Biol. Chem. 254(23):12192-12198, Dec. 10, 1979.

Martin, J.

Praevention und ihre Moeglichkeiten. Legislation et prevention: Un cadre de reflexion. (Fr.)

Soz. Praventivmed. 23(5-6):405-411, Dec. 1978.

Martin, M.

Thrombolytic therapy in arterial thromboembolism.

Prog. Cardiovasc. Dis. 21(5):351-374, Mar.-Apr. 1979.

Martin, W. J., II and Taylor, J. C.

Abnormal interaction of alpha-antitrypsin and leukocyte elastolytic activity in patients with chronic obstructive pulmonary disease.

Am. Rev. Respir. Dis. 120(2):411-419, Aug. 1979.

Maruta, A., et al.

Mutagenicity of quercetin and kaempferol on cultured mammalian cells.

Gan 70(3):273-276, June 1979.

Marvit, R. C., et al.

A good neighbor policy: Controlled smoking areas and health department attitudes.

Hawaii Med. J. 39(1):7-10, Jan. 1980.

Masden, R. R. and Flowers, N. C.

Extension of experimental infarction with nicotine and estimates of infarct size.

Am. Heart J. 99(3):342-348, Mar. 1980.

Masi, A. T.

An holistic concept of health and illness: A tricentennial foal for medicine and public health. (Editorial)

J. Chronic Dis. 31(9-10):563-572, 1978.

Maskarinec, M. P., et al.

A novel method for the isolation and quantitative analysis of nicotine and cotinine in biological fluid.

J. Anal. Toxicol. 2(5):124-126, July-Aug. 1978.

Mass, M. J. and Kaufman, D. G.

Benzo(a)pyrene quinone metabolism in tracheal organ cultures.

Biochem. Biophys. Res. Commun. 89(3): 885-892, Aug. 13, 1979.

Masse, R. and Arnoux, B.

Mecanismes de la cancerisation bronchique. (Fr.)

Rev. Prat. 28(59):4679-4685, Nov.-Dec. 1978.

Massei, V., et al.

Distribuzione intrapolmonare delle costanti di tempo e frequenza-dipendenza della compliance. (Ital.)

Minerva Med. 69(13):911-913, Mar. 17, 1978.

Matejevic, D., et al.

Electrocardiographic changes in rats due to different nicotin doses. (Ser.)

Srp. Arh. Celok. Lek. 105(10):821-827, Oct. 1977.

Matroos, A., et al.

Fatal and nonfatal coronary attacks in relation to smoking in some Dutch communities.

Am. J. Epidemiol. 109(2):145-151, Feb. 1979.

Matsukura, S., et al.

Cotinine excretion and daily cigarette smoking in habituated smokers.

Clin. Pharm. Ther. 25(5, Part 1): 555-561, May 1979.

Matsukura, S., et al.

Effect of pH and urine flow on urinary nicotine excretion after smoking cigarettes.

Clin. Pharm. Ther. 25(5, Part 1): 549-554, May 1979.

Matsumoto, S., et al.

Effects of chemoreceptor stimulating agents on reflex bradycardia.

Arch. Int. Pharmacodyn. Ther. 239(2): 296-307, June 1979.

Matsumoto, T., et al.

Mutagenicities of the pyrolyzates of peptides and proteins.

Mutat. Res. 56(3):281-288, Jan. 1978.

Matsuoka, A., et al.

Chromosomal aberration tests on 29 chemicals combined with S9 mix in vitro.

Mutat. Res. 66(3):277-290, Mar. 1979.

Matsuzawa, A. and Yamamoto, T.

Regression of a pregnancy-dependent mouse mammary tumor (TPDMT-4) by the antiestrogen, tamoxifen.

Gan 70(3):387-388, June 1979.

Mattei, E., et al.

Protein synthesis inhibition induced by dimethylnitrosamine and diethylnitrosamine on isolated rat hepatocytes.

Experientia 35(9):1213-1215, 1979.

Matthay, R. A. and Depew, C. C.

Obstructive airway disease: Rational therapy with theophylline agents.

Geriatrics 35(2):65-77, Feb. 1980.

Mattheus, A. and Raetz, K.-H.

Die Bedeutung des Rhodanid in der Diagnostik von Fertilitaetsstoerungen: I. Zur Problematik der Bestimmungsmethode von Rhodanid und Ermittlung von Normativen im Blutserum und Ejakulat. (Ger.)

Andrologia 10(5):397-404, Sept.-Oct. 1978.

Mattila, M. J.

Laeaekeistae astmaatikoille aiheutuvat haitat. (Finn.)

Suom. Laeaekaeril. 34(20):391-400, June 1979.

Mattison, D. R. and Thorgeirsson, S. S.

Ovarian aryl hydrocarbon hydroxylase activity and primordial oocyte toxicity of polycyclic aromatic hydrocarbons in mice.

Cancer Res. 39(9):3471-3475, Sept. 1979.

Mattison, D. R., et al.

Differences in benzo(a)pyrene metabolic profile in rat and mouse ovary.

Biochem. Pharmacol. 28(13):2101-2104, July 1, 1979.

Matulionis, D. H.

Reaction of macrophages to cigarette smoke: I. Recruitment of pulmonary macrophages.

Arch. Environ. Health 34(5):293-297, Sept./Oct. 1979.

Matulionis, D. H.

Reaction of macrophages to cigarrette smoke: II. Immigration of macrophages to the lungs.

Arch. Environ. Health 34(5):298-301, Sept.-Oct. 1979.

May, J. F., et al.

Screeningsonderzoek naar cardiocasculaire risicofactoren met berekening van risicoscores. (Dut.)

Ned. Tijdschr. Geneeskd. 122(22):780-784, June 3, 1978.

Mazzocchi, G., et al.

High resolution autoradiographic investigations on the mechanism of the adrenolytic effect of 7,12-dimethylbenzanthracene on the inner layers of the rat adrenal cortex.

Virchows Arch. [Cell Pathol.] 28(2):97-104, Aug. 25, 1978.

McAllister, A. L., et al.

Adolescent smoking: Onset and prevention.

Pediatrics 63(4):650-658, Apr. 1979.

McAloon, E. J., et al.

Erythrocytosis associated with carboxyhemoglobineamia in smokers.

South. Med. J. 73(2):137-139, Feb. 1980.

McAvoy, S.

A 19th century perspective on the heatlh consequences of smoking.

J. Med. Assoc. Ga. 68(3):191, Mar. 1979.

McCann, J. and Ames, B. N.

Mutagenesis. The Salmonella/microsome mutagenicity test: Predictive value for animal carcinogenicity.

Adv. Mod. Toxicol. 5:87-108, 1978.

McCarthy, G. S. and Hedenstierna, G.

Arterial oxygenation during artificial ventilation: The effect of airway closure and of its prevention by positive end-expiratory pressure.

Acta Anaesthesiol. Scand. 22(6):563-569, 1978.

McCollum, C. N. and Campbell, I. T.

The value of measuring intravascular platelet aggregates in the prediction of postoperative pulmonary dysfunction.

Br. J. Surg. 66(10):703-707, Oct. 1979.

McCoy, G. D. and Wynder, E. L.

Proceedings of Alcohol and Cancer Workshop: Etiological and preventive implications in alcohol carcinogenesis.

Cancer Res. 39(7, Part 2):2344-2850, July 1979.

McCoy, G. D., et al.

Enhanced metabolism and mutagenesis of nitrosopyrrolidine in liver fractions isolated from chronic ethanol-consuming hamsters.

Cancer Res. 39(3):793-796, Mar. 1979.

McCredie, J. A., et al.

Effect of operation and radiotherapy on antibody-dependent cellular cytotoxicity.

Cancer 44(1):99-105, July 1979.

McDonagh, D. J., et al.

Assessment of alpha-1-antitrypsin deficiency heterozygosity as a risk factor in the etiology of emphysema: Physiological comparison of adult normal and heterozygous protease inhibitor phenotype subjects from a random population.

J. Clin. Invest. 63(2):299-309, Feb. 1979.

McDonald, M. J., et al.

Functional properties of the glycosylated minor components of human adult hemoglobin.

J. Biol. Chem. 254(3):702-707, Feb. 10, 1979.

McEwan, J.

The risks of oral contraception.

Br. J. Hosp. Med. 21(2):144-150, Feb. 1979.

McGill, Jr., H. C.

The Thrombotic Process in Atherogenesis: Risk factors for atherosclerosis.

Adv. Exp. Med. Biol. 104:273-280, 1978.

McGill, Jr., H. C.

Workshop on Carbon Monoxide and Cardiovascular Disease: Potential mechanisms for the augmentation of atherosclerosis and atherosclerotic disease by cigarette smoking.

Prev. Med. 8(3):390-403, May 1979.

McIntosh, H. D.

Jogging: Thou shall not kill (thyself).

JAMA 241(23):2547-2548, June 8, 1979.

McIntyre, K. M.

Prehospital cardiac arrest and resuscitation: Evaluation and alternative strategies.

JACEP 8(2):89-90, Feb. 1979.

McKee, R. H. and Tometsko, A. M.

Inhibition of promutagen activation by the antioxidants butylated hydroxyanisole and butylated hydroxytoluene.

JNCI 63(2):473-477, Aug. 1979.

McKenzie, M., et al.

A human plasma component that binds benzo(a)pyrene.

Cancer 42(6):2733-2737, Dec. 1978.

McKeown, K. C.

Carinoma of the oesophagus.

J. R. Coll. Surg. Edinb. 24(5):253-274, Sept. 1979.

McKinney, R. J. and Harris, E. A.

Instruments and techniques: Evaluation of the OSM2 hemoximeter.

Cardiovasc. Res. 12(10):630-634, Oct. 1979.

McLean, A. E. M.

Drug metabolising enzymes.

Nature 283(5744):245-246, Jan. 17, 1980.

McLinden, V. J. and Stenhouse, A. M.

A chromatography system for drug identification.

Forensic Sci. Int. 13(1):71-79, Jan./Feb. 1979.

Methaqualone is used as an example for a chromatography system for drug identification by using a drug data file.

McMahon, R. E., et al.

Assay of 855 test chemicals in ten tester strains using a new modification of the Ames test for bacterial mutagens.

Cancer Res. 39(3):682-693, Mar. 1979.

McMillan, G. H. G., et al.

A radiological follow-up study of the effect of asbestos in dockyard workers in Portsmouth.

J. R. Nav. Med. Serv. 65(2):63-74, Summer 1979.

McNair, P., et al.

Hypomagnesemia, a risk factor in diabetic retinopathy.

Diabetes 27(11):1075-1077, Nov. 1978.

McNeil, B. J., et al.

Fallacy of the five-year survival in lung cancer.

N. Engl. J. Med. 299(25):1397-1401, Dec. 21, 1978.

McQueen, E. G.

Hormonal steroid contraceptives: A further review of adverse reactions.

Curr. Ther. 19(10):176-200, Oct. 1978.

Meade, P. D., et al.

Influence of vitamin A on the laryngeal response of hamsters exposed to cigarette smoke.

Prog. Exp. Tumor Res. 24:320-329, 1979.

Meade, T. W., et al.

Ethnic group comparisons of variables associated with ischaemic heart disease.

Br. Heart J. 40(7):789-795, July 1978.

Meade, T. W., et al.

Characteristics affecting fibrinolytic activity and plasma fibrinogen concentrations.

Br. Med. J. 1(6157):153-156, Jan. 20, 1979.

Meadows, III, J. A., et al.

Density dependence of maximal expiratory flow in chronic obstructive pulmonary disease.

Am. Rev. Respir. Dis. 121(1):47-53, Jan. 1980.

Meberg, A. and Sande, H. A.

Roeking og graviditet. (Norw., Engl. Summary)

Tidsskr. Nor. Laegeforen. 99(12):580-582;596, Apr. 30, 1979.

Meberg, A., et al.

Erythroblastemia and thrombocytopenia in small for gestational age infants: Relation to intrauterine hypoxia, infections and maternal smoking.

Acta Paediatr. Belg. 31(4):213-218, 1978.

Meberg, A., et al.

Smoking during pregnancy - Effects on the fetus and on thiocyanate levels in mother and baby.

Acta Paediatr. Scand. 68(4):547-552, July 1979.

Meberg, A., et al.

Smoking during pregnancy - Hematological observations in the newborn.

Acta Paediatr. Scand. 68(5):731-734, Sept. 1979.

Medina, D.

Serial transplantation of chemical carcinogen-induced mouse mammary ductal dysplasias.

JNCI 62(2):397-405, Feb. 1979.

Meguro, T., et al.

Discriminant analysis of bronchial asthma by linear discriminant function with parameters of flow-volumes: Discriminant analysis of bronchial asthma in young male non-smokers.

Acta Med. Okayama 32(5):355-361, Oct. 1978.

Mehrotra, N. K. and Saxena, A. K.

Evaluation of carcinogenic effect of mineral oil used in the processing of jute fibers.

Br. J. Exp. Pathol. 60(5):518-525, Oct. 1979.

Mehta, R. and Cohen, G. M.

Major differences in the extent of conjugation with glucuronic acid and sulphate in human peripheral lung.

Biochem. Pharmacol. 28(16):2479-2484, Aug. 15, 1979.

Mehta, R. G., et al.

Distribution of retinoic acid-binding in normal and neoplastic mammary proteins tissues.

Cancer Res. 40(1):47-49, Jan. 1980.

Meire, F., et al.

Geneesmiddelengebruik tijdens de zwangerschap.(Dut.)

Ned. Tijdschr. Geneeskd. 123(17): 703-706, Apr. 28, 1979.

Melbostad, E.

Asbestose: Et klinisk materiale. (Norw., Engl. Abstr.)

Tidsskr. Nor. Laegeforen. 98(31):1561-1563;1574, Nov. 10, 1978.

Melbostad, E.

Asbesteksposisjon - Asbestskader: En kort oversikt. (Norw., Engl. Abstr.)

Tidsskr. Nor. Laegeforen. 98(31):1563-1564;1574, Nov. 10, 1978.

Melissinos, C. G., et al.

Time dependence of maximum flow as an index of nonuniform emptying.

Am. J. Phsyiol. 47(5):1043-1050, Nov. 1979.

Mello, N. K., et al.

Effect of alcohol and marihuana on tobacco smoking.

Clin. Pharmacol. Ther. 27(2):202-209, Feb. 1980.

Mello, N. K., et al.

Effects of heroin self-administration on cigarette smoking.

Psychopharmacology 67(1):45-52, Jan. 1980.

Melton, B.

Doctor, do you smoke?

Tex. Med. 75(5):69-70, May 1979.

Menard, R. H., et al.

Specificity of the in vitro destruction of adrenal and hepatic microsomal steroid hydroxylases by thiosteroids.

Mol. Pharmacol. 16(3):997-1010, Nov. 1979.

Mendez, L.

Aterosclerosis. (Span.)

Gac. Med. Mex. 114(7):307-311, July 1978.

Mendlewicz, J.

Perspectives in Psychopharmacotherapy: Perspectives and practical applications in psychopharmacogenetics.

Prog. Neuropsychopharmacol. 3(1-3): 155-163, 1979.

Mendoza-Figueroa, T., et al.

Dose-dependent DNA ruptures induced by the procarcinogen dimethylnitrosamine on primary rat liver cultures.

Cancer Res. 39(8):3254-3257, Aug. 1979.

Menon, M. A. and Saw, H.

Lung cancer in Malaysia.

Thorax 34(2):269-273, Apr. 1979.

Mergens, W. J., et al.

Environmental Aspects of N-Nitroso Compounds. Alpha-tocopherol: Uses in preventing nitrosamine formation.

IARC Sci. Publ. No. 19:199-212, 1978.

Mertens, H. M., et al.

Nichtinvasive Untersuchung ueber den Einfluss von Zigarettenrauchen auf den normalen linken Ventrikel in Ruhe und unter Belastung. (Ger.)

Z. Kardiol. 68(6):375-381, June 1979.

Messerli, F. H. and Frolich, E. D.

Management principles for borderline hypertension.

Contin. Educ. Fam. Physician 9(2):44-49, Aug. 1978.

Metcalfe, J., et al.

Hen's eggs with retarded gas exchange. I. Chorioallantoic capillary growth.

Respir. Physiol. 36(2):97-101, Feb. 1979.

Mettlin, C. and Graham, S.

Dietary risk factors in human bladder cancer.

Am. J. Epidemiol. 110(3):255-263, Sept. 1979.

Meyer, M. B.

Breast-feeding and smoking. (Letter to the Editor.)

Lancet 1(8123):975-976, May 5, 1979.

Meyer, O. and Schlegel, H. G.

Oxidation of carbon monoxide in cell extracts of Pseudomonas carboxydovorans.

J. Bacteriol. 137(2):811-817, Feb. 1979.

Michael, L. W.

Workshop on Carbon Monoxide and Cardiovascular Disease: Comliance with the carbon monoxide standard in the workplace.

Prev. Med. 8(3):289-294, May 1979.

Michaels, R., et al.

Elastic recoil of the lung in cigarette smokers: The effect of nebulized bronchodilator and cessation of smoking.

Am. Rev. Respir. Dis. 119(5):707-716, May 1979.

Michal, V., et al.

Phalloarteriography in the diagnosis of erectile impotence.

World J. Surg. 2(2):239-248, Mar. 1978.

Michel, F.-B. and Bousquet, J.

Pathologie respiratoire genetique. (Fr.)

Rev. Prat. 28(59):4701-4710, Dec. 21, 1978.

Micillo, E., et al.

Action du tabagisme sur des sujets exposes a l'action d'autres facteurs de pollution aerienne. (Fr.)

Bronchopneumologie 28(4):267-271, July-Aug. 1978.

Mikhail, M. M., et al.

Effect of chronic exposure to tobacco smoke on some blood lipids and coagulation parameters in the rat.

Pharmazie 34(2):95-96, Feb. 1979.

Miller, F. R. and Blazkovec, A. A.

Guinea pig cell-mediated tumor immunity: The chromium release assay detects both cytolysis and serum blocking for syngeneic chemically-induced tumors.

Immunol. Commun. 8(1):31-47, 1979.

Miller, G. H.

The filter cigareet controversy.

J. Indiana State Med. Assoc. 72(12):903-905, Dec. 1979.

Miller, G. H., et al.

Less hazardous cigarette debated. (Letter to the Editor and Reply.)

JAMA 242(10):1029-1031, Sept. 7, 1979.

Miller, M. and Hales, C. A.

Role of Cytochrome P-450 in alveolar hypoxic pulmonary vasoconsriction in dogs.

J. Clin. Invest. 64(2):666-673, Aug. 1979.

Miller, R. D., et al.

Immunoglobulin concentrations in serum and nasal secretions in chronic obstructive pulmonary disease: A matched-pair study.

Am. Rev. Respir. Dis. 119(2):229-238, Feb. 1979.

Miller, R. R. and Fox, E. R. W.

On smoking and advertising. (Letter to the Editor and Reply.)

West. J. Med. 131(4):334, Oct. 1979.

Mills, D., et al.

Smoking cessation in high school.

Health Educ. 9(3):5-7, May-June 1978.

Milne, J. S.

Longitudinal respiratory studies in older people.

Thorax 33(5):547-554, Oct. 1978.

Milne, J. S. and Lauder, I. J.

Factors associated with mortallity in older people.

Age Ageing 7(3):129-137, Aug. 1978.

Milon, H. and Froment, A.

Les facteurs de risque de l'infarctus du myocarde. (Fr.)

Cah. Med. 4(2):71-80, Sept. 15, 1978.

Milstein, S. and Guttenplan, J. B.

Near quantitative production of molecular nitrogen from metabolism of dimethylnitrosamine.

Biochem. Biophys. Res. Commun. 87(1): 337-342, Mar. 15, 1979.

Milvy, P.

The Marathon: Physiological, Medical, Epidemiological, and Psychological Studies. Statistical analysis of deaths from coronary heart disease anticipated in a cohort of marathon runners.

Ann. NY Acad. Sci. 301:620-625, 1977.

Mimica, M., et al.

Nasa ispitivanja navici pusenja. (Croat.)

Arh. Hig. Rada Toksikol. 29(3):209-218, 1978.

Mimica, M., et al.

Pusenje duhana kao uzrok kronicne nespecificne bolesti pluca. (Croat.)

Arh. Hig. Rada. Toksikol. 29(4):289-304, 1978.

Minh, V.-D., et al.

Entretiens de Physiopathologie Respiratoire: Relation of Vo2max. to cardiopulmonary function in patients with chronic obstructive lung disease.

Bull. Eur. Physiopathol. Respir. 15(2):359-377, 1979.

Minick, C. R., et al.

Atheroarteriosclerosis induced by infection with a herpesvirus.

Am. J. Pathol. 96(3):673-706, Sept. 1979.

Miranda, C. L., et al.

Effects of vitamin A deficiency on hepatic and extrahepatic mixed-function oxidase and epoxide-metabolizing enzymes in guinea pig and rabbit.

Biochem. Pharmacol. 28(18):2713-2716, Sept. 15, 1979.

Miskowiak, J.

How thge lower oesophageal sphincter affects submucosal oesophageal varices.

Lancet 2(8103):1284-1285, Dec. 16, 1978.

Mitchell, C. and Stuart, R. B.

Weight control and smoking reduction: Friends or enemies?

Can. J. Public Health 70(6):399-404, Nov.-Dec. 1979.

Mitchell, D. S., et al.

Effects of ethanol and carbon monoxide on two measures of behavioral incapacitation of rats.

Proc. West. Pharmacol. Soc. 21:427-431, 1978.

Mitchell, M. K., et al.

Smoking, carboxyhemoglobin, and oxygen therapy. (Letters to the Editor.)

Chest 75(3):407-408, Mar. 1979.

Mitchell, R. S., et al.

Health effects of urban air pollution: Special consideration of areas at 1,500m and above.

JAMA 242(11):1163-1168, Sept. 14, 1979.

Mitra, G., et al.

Effect of tobacco-leaf extract administration on liver, lung, intestine, and serum enzymes.

Toxicol. Appl. Pharmacol. 52(2):262-266, Feb. 1980.

Mittman, C.

Antitrypsin deficiency: A model to illustrate the pathogenesis of emphysema. (Jpn.)

Jpn. J. Thorac. Dis. 16(6):369-382, June 1978.

Mittman, C., et al.

The respiratory disease questionnaire: Use of a self-administered version.

Arch. Environ. Health 34(3):151-157, May-June 1979.

Miyata, Y., et al.

Effect of vitamin A acetate on urinary bladder carcinogenesis induced by N-butyl-N-(4-hydroxybutyl)nitrosamine in rats.

Gann 69(6):845-848, Dec. 1978.

Mizuguchi, T., et al.

Memory test under NLA and modified NLA. (Jpn.)

Jpn. J. Anesthesiol. 27(6):592-599, June 1978.

Moberger, G., et al.

Etiologi, diagnostik och behandling. (Swed.)

Lakartidningen 75(35):2947-2951, Aug. 30, 1978.

Mochizuki, M., et al.

Syntheses of N-(omega-acetoxyalkyl and omega-carbomethoxyalkyl)-N-(alpha-acetoxyalkyl)nitrosamines, model compounds for possible metabolically activated N,N-dialkylnitrosamines.

Chem. Pharm. Bull. (Tokyo) 26(12):3914-3919, Dec. 1978.

Mochizuki, M., et al.

Syntheses of N-alkyl-N-(alpha-acetoxyalkyl)nitrosamines, model compounds for metabolically activated N,N-dialkylnitrosamines.

Chem. Pharm. Bull. (Tokyo) 26(12):3905-3908, Dec. 1978.

Mochizuki, M., et al.

Synthesis and mutagenicity of 4-(N-Butylnitrosamino)-4-hydroxybutyric acid lactone, a possible activated metabolite of the proximate bladder carcinogen N-butyl-N-(3-carboxypropyl) nitrosamine.

Cancer Res. 40(1):162-165, Jan. 1980.

Mochizuki, M., et al.

Mutagenic and DNA-damaging effects of N-alkyl-N-(alpha-acetoxyalkyl)nitrosamines, models for metabolically activated N,N-dialkylnitrosamines.

Gan 70(5):663-670, Oct. 1979.

Moffat, K., et al.

A structural model for the kinetic behavior of hemoglobin.

Science 206(4422):1035-1042, Nov. 30, 1979.

Moga, A., et al.

Factori de risc pentru ateroscleroza la copii. (Rum.)

Rev. Med. Intern. [Med. Intern.] 30(2): 105-112, Mar.-Apr. 1978.

Moghissi, K. S.

Basic Concepts in Infertility: Basic work-up evaluation of infertile couples.

Clin. Obstet. Gynecol. 22(1):11-25, Mar. 1979.

Mohan, D., et al.

Prevalence of drug abuse in young rural males in Punjab.

Indian J. Med. Res. 68:689-694, Oct. 1978.

Mohn, G. R.

Human Genetic Variation in Response to Medical and Environmental Agents: Pharmacogenetics and Ecogenetics. An overview of animal and microbial test systems for carcinogenesis and mutagenesis: Problems with human variation.

Hum. Genet. Suppl. 1:169-176, 1978.

Mohr, U.

Toxicologic and pathologic data on polycyclic aromatic hydrocarbons and automobile exhaust condensate.

Ecotoxicol. Environ. Safety 2(3-4): 267-276, Dec. 1978.

Mohsenifar, Z. and Tashkin, D. P.

Effect of carboxyhemoglobin on the single breath diffusing capacity: Derivation of an empirical correction factor.

Respiration 37(4):185-191, 1979.

Moncada, S. and Vane, J. R.

Arachidonic acid metabolites and the interactions between platelets and blood-vessel walls.

N. Engl. J. Med. 300(20):1142-1147, May 17, 1979.

Monji, N. and Castro, A.

Plasma nicotine pharmacokinetics in dogs after intravenous administration: Determination by radioimmunoassay.

Res. Commun. Chem. Pathol. Pharmacol. 23(2):267-277, Feb. 1979.

Montesano, R., et al.

Increased excision of O6-methylguanine from rat liver DNA after chronic administration of dimethylnitrosamine.

Cancer Res. 39(5):1798-1802, May 1979.

Mookherjee, S., et al.

Improvement in arterial oxygenation by saralasin infusion in man.

Chest 75(4):492-494, Apr. 1979.

Moolten, F., et al.

Reduction of respiratory tract binding of benzo[a]pyrene in mice by immunization.

JNCI 61(5):1347-1349, Nov. 1978.

Moore, B. P. and Cohen, G. M.

Metabolism of benzo(a)pyrene and its major metabolites to ethyl acetate-soluble and water-soluble metabolites by cultured rodent trachea.

Cancer Res. 38(9):3066-3075, Sept. 1978.

Moore, J. N., et al.

A case of pituitary adrenocorticotropin-dependent Cushing's syndrome in the horse.

Endocrinology 104(3):576-582, Mar. 1979.

Moore, M. R. and Meredith, P. A.

The effect of carbon monoxide upon erythrocyte gamma-aminolevulinicacid dehydratase activity.

Arch. Environ. Health 34(3):158-161, May-June 1979.

Morgan, W. D.

New ways of measuring cadmium in man.

Nature 282(5740):673-674, Dec. 13, 1979.

Morgan, W. K. C.

Screening for occupational cancer of the lung. (Editorial.)

Chest 74(3):239-241, Sept. 1978.

Morgan, W. W. and Pfeil, K. A.

Macamylamine blockade of nicotine enhanced noradrenaline turnover in rat brain.

Life Sci. 24(5):417-420, Jan. 29, 1979.

Mori, Y., et al.

Analysis of biliary and urinary metabolites of 3'-methyl-4-(dimethylamino) azobenzene in rats.

Gann 69(6):757-762, Dec. 1978.

Morreal, C. E., et al.

Estrogenic properties of 3,9-dihydroxy-7,12-dimethylbenz[a]anthracene in rats.

JNCI 62(6):1585-1588, June 1979.

Morris, G. K.

Transactions of the Annual Meeting of the International Committee on Thrombosis and Haemostasis: Preoperative prediction of postoperative deep vein thrombosis.

Thromb. Haemost. 40(1):27-31, Feb. 28, 1979.

Morrison, A. S.

Prostatic hypertrophy in greater Boston.

J. Chronic Dis. 31(5):357-362, 1978.

Morrison, A. S.

Urinary Bladder Cancer: Public health value of using epidemiologic information to identify high-risk groups for bladder cancer screening.

Semin. Oncol. 6(2):184-188, June 1979.

Morrison, A. S. and Buring, J. E.

Artifical sweeteners and cancer of the lower urinary tract.

N. Engl. J. Med. 302(10):537-541, Mar. 6, 1980.

Morrison, J. A., et al.

Cigarette smoking, alcohol intake, and oral contraceptives: Relationship to lipids and lipoproteins in adolescent school-children.

Metabolism 28(11):1166-1170, Nov. 1979.

Morse, J. O.

Alpha1-antitrypsin deficiency. (Second of two parts.)

N. Engl. J. Med. 299(20):1099-1105, Nov. 16, 1978.

Mosadomi, A., et al.

Effects of tobacco smoking and age on the keratinization of palatal mucosa: A cytologic study.

Oral Surg. 46(3):413-417, Sept. 1978.

Moss, A. J., et al.

Ventricular ectopic beats and their relation to sudden and nonsudden cardiac death after myocardial infarction.

Circulation 60(5):998-1003, Nov. 1979.

Mossanda, K., et al.

Detection of mutagenic polycyclic aromatic hydrocarbons in African smoked fish.

Food Cosmet. Toxicol. 17(2):141-143, Apr. 1979.

Moulin, M.-A., et al.

Les embryopathies medicamenteuses. (Fr.)

Ouest Med. 32(10):651-658, May, 10, 1979.

Mowe, G.

Undersoekelse av kjemiske arbeidsmiljoeproblemer. (Norw.)

Tidsskr. Nor Laegenforen. 98(17-18): 885-886, June 20, 1978.

Mueller-Salamin, L., et al.

Interaction of retinoic acid and 3-methylcholanthrene on the fine structure of mouse prostate epithelium in vitro.

JNCI 63(2):485-495, Aug. 1979.

Mueller, R.

Soziokulturelle Voraussetzungen von Alkohol - Und Tabakerziehungsmassnahmen. (Ger.)

Bull. Schweiz. Akad. Med. Wiss. 35(1-3):237-244, Mar. 1979.

Mueting, D.

Stoffwechsel-Risikofaktoren und ihr Umfeld. Haeufigkeit und Therapie von Hypertonie, Hyperurikaemie, Hyperlipidaemie, Diabetes mellitus, Nikotin- und Alkohol-Abusus sowie Uebergewicht: Bericht ueber das V. Internationale Kissinger Kolloquium, 21.-22. 4. 1978. (Ger.)

Fortschr. Med. 96(25):1319-1322, July 6, 1978.

Muiesan, G.

Proceedings of a Symposium on Hypertension. Risk Factors and Recent Advances in Treatment with Tienilic Acid: Risk factors in hypertension and ischaemic heart disease.

Postgrad. Med. J. 55(Suppl. 3):15-18, 1979.

Mukhopadhyay, A. K. and Kunnemann, M.

Mechanism of lower esophageal sphincter stimulation by bombesin in the opossum.

Gastroenterology 76(6):1409-1414, June 1979.

Mule, S. J., et al.

Radioimmunoassay of methaqualone in human urine compared with chromatographic methods.

Clin. Chem. 24(9):1473-1476, Sept. 1978.

Mull, R. L., et al.

Hexachlorobenzene II. Effects on growing lambs of prolonged low-level oral exposure to hexachlorobenzene (HCB).

J. Environ. Pathol. Toxicol. 1(6):927-938, July-Aug. 1978.

Mull, R. L., et al.

Hexachlorobenzene I. Uptake, distribution and excretion of hexachlorobenzene (HCB) in growing lambs.

J. Environ. Pathol. Toxicol. 1(6):865-878, July-Aug. 1978.

Muraki, T., et al.

Inhibition of cholinergic agonists of the prolactin release induced by morphine.

Naunyn Schmiedebergs Arch. Pharmacol. 308(3):249-254, Sept. 1979.

Muramatsu, I., et al.

Effects of loperamide on the guinea pig taenia coli.

Eur. J. Pharmacol. 55(2):181-187, Apr. 15, 1979.

Murphy, H. B. M.

Historic changes in the sex ratios for different disorders.

Soc. Sci. Med. 12(3B):143-149, July 1978.

Murphy, J. B. and Giunta, J. L.

The effect of dinitrochlorobenzene (DNCB) on dimethylbenzathracene (DMBA) carcinogenesis on hamster buccal pouch.

Oral Surg. 46(5):669-675, Nov. 1978.

Murphy, Jr., R. L. H., et al.

Diagnosis of 'asbestosis': Observations from a longitudinal survey of shipyard pipe coverers.

Am. J. Med. 65(3):488-498, Se pt. 1978.

Murphy, M. J., et al.

The role of cytochrome P-450-inducing agents in potentiating the toxicity of fluroxene (2,2,2,-trifluoroethyl) vinyl ether)1.

Toxicol. Appl. Pharmacol. 52(1):69-81, Jan. 1980.

Murray, M., et al.

Meeting of the Society for Social Medicine: Can we predict children's smoking from their attiudes? (Abstr.)

J. Epidemiol. Commun. Health 33(2):167-168, June 1979.

Mushinski, M. H. and Stellman, S. D.

Impact of new smoking trends on women's occupational health.

Prev. Med. 7(3):349-365, Sept. 1978.

Musk, A. W., et al.

Respiratory function and the chest radiograph: An epidemiological study of the significance of minor radiographic abnormalities.

Aust. NZ J. Med. 8(1):7-13, Feb. 1978.

Musk, A. W., et al.

Entretiens de Physiopathologie Respiratoire: Factors contributing to the clinical grade of breathlessness of coalworkers with pneumoconiosis.

Bull. Eur. Physiopathol. Respir. 15(2):343-355, 1979.

Musson, D. G. and Sternson, L. A.

Analysis of nitrosamines in aqueous and biological fluids based on measure ment of photochemically liberated nitrate.

J. Pharm. Sci. 68(9):1159-1162, Sept. 1979.

Mustard, J. F., et al.

Thrombosis: Animal and Clinical Models. Platelets and thrombosis in the development of atherosclerosis and its complications.

Adv. Exp. Med. Biol. 102:7-30, 1978.

Mustard, J. F., et al.

The Thrombotic Process in Atherogenesis: Platelets, thrombosis and atherosclerosis.

Adv. Exp. Med. Biol. 104:127-144, 1978.

Nachbur, B. and Studer, U.

Der heutige Stand des Bronchialkarzinoms aus chirurgischer Sicht. (Ger.)

Praxis 68(24):772-781, June 12, 1979.

Nadjari, Y.

Les risques des petits fumeurs. (Fr.)

Concours Med. 101(18):3007-3008, May 5, 1979.

Naess, K.

Polycytemi, kronisk CO-forgiftning og roeking. (Norw.)

Tidsskr. Nor Laegeforen. 98(14):751, May 20, 1978.

Naeye, R. L.

Effects of maternal cigarette smoking on the fetus and placenta.

Br. J. Obstet. Gynecol. 85(10):732-737, Oct. 1978.

Nagahama, F., et al.

Clinical and statistic study of the relationship between primary lung cancer and smoking. (Jpn.; Engl. Abstr.)

Iryo 31(6):511-516; 494, June 1977.

Nagao, M., et al.

Mutagenicity of optically pure (-)trans-7,8-dihydroxy-dihydrobenzo[a]pyrene.

Mutat. Res. 58(2-3):361-365, Nov. 1978.

Nagasawa, H.

Prolactin: Its role in the development of mammary tumours.

Med. Hypotheses 5(10):1117-1121, Oct. 1979.

Nagasubramanian, S.

Proceedings of the William Mackenzie Memorial Symposium: Role of pituitary vasopressin in the formation and dynamics of aqueous humour.

Trans. Ophthalmol. Soc. UK 97(4):686-701, Sept. 1977.

Naik, R. S., et al.

Buerger's disease versus adrenalectomy and sympathectomy.

J. Indian Med. Assoc. 71(8):199-202, Oct. 16, 1978.

Nakamura, H., et al.

Combined effect of aminopyrine with phenopyrazone on analgesic, anti-pyretic and anti-inflammatory activities in experimental animals.

J. Pharm. Soc. Jpn. 98(6):679-688, June 1978.

Nakamura, J.

The effect of neuroleptics on the dopaminergic and cholinergic systems in sympathetic ganglia.

Kurume Med. J. 25(4):241-253, 1978.

Nakayama, H.

A comparison of the effects of Kanechlor 400, phenobarbital, and 3,4-benzpyrene pretreatment on liver microsomal enzymes in the rat.

Kumamoto Med. J. 31(3):89-97, Sept. 30, 1978.

Nakayama, H., et al.

Studies of induction and in vitro inhibition in microsomal drug-metabolizing enzymes from the rat livers. (Jpn.)

J. Kumamoto Med. Soc. 52(4):131-138, July 25, 1978.

Namba, M., et al.

Effect of Nocardia rubra cell-wall skeleton on the induction of lung cancer in ACI/N rats.

Gann 70(1):55-62, Feb. 1979.

Napalkov, N. P. and Petrov, N. N.

Advances in Tumour Prevention, Detec tion and Characterization, Vol. 4. Characterization and Treatment of Human Tumours: Carcinogenic hazards from prenatal exposure to environmental chemicals.

Int. Congr. Ser. No. 420:63-71, 1978.

Naquira, D. and Arqueros, L.

Water intake in rats affected by addition of nicotine to drinking water.

Acta Physiol. Lat. Am. 28(1):73-76, 1978.

Nardizzi, L. R.

Computerized tomographic correlate of carbon monixide poisoning.

Arch. Neurol. 36(1):38-39, Jan. 1979.

Navin, T. R. and Hager, W. D.

Creatine kinase MB isoenzyme in the evaluation of myocardial infarction.

Curr. Probl. Cardiol. 3(12):1-32, Mar. 1979.

Nebert, D. W.

Symposium. Coordination Chemistry and Cancer Chemotherapy: Genetic control of carcinogen metabolism leading to individual differences in cancer risk.

Biochimie 60(9):1019 1029, 1978.

Nebert, D. W.

Multiple forms of inducible drug-metabolizing enzymes: A reasonable mechanism by which any organism can cope with adversity.

Mol. Cell. Biochem. 27(1):27-46, Sept. 28, 1979.

Nebert, D. W.

The Induction of Drug Metabolism: Genetic aspects of enzyme induction by drugs and chemical carcinogens.

Symp. Med. Hoechst 14:419-452, 1979.

Nebert, D. W.

Genetic differences in the induction of monooxygenase activities by polycyclic aromatic compounds.

Pharmacol. Ther. 6(2):395-417, 1979.

Nebert, D. W. and Atlas, S. A.

Human Genetic Variation in Response to Medical and Environmental Agents: Pharmacogenetics and Ecogenetics. The Ah locus: Aromatic hydrocarbon responsiveness...of mice and men.

Hum. Genet. Suppl. 1:149-160, 1978.

Nebert, D. W., et al.

Pyrolysis products from amino acids and protein: Highest mutagenicity requires cytochrome P1-450.

Proc. Natl. Acad. Sci. USA 76(11):5929-5933, Nov. 1979.

Neff, T. A.

When the X-ray shows a "spot" on the lung.

Resident Staff Physician 24(11):89-101, Nov. 1978.

Negishi, M. and Nebert, D. W.

Structural gene products of the Ah locus: Genetic and immunochemical evidence for two forms of mouse liver cytochrome P-450 induced by 3-methylcholanthrene.

J. Biol. Chem. 254(21):11015-11023, Nov. 10, 1979.

Nelems, J. M. B., et al.

Detection, localization, and treatment of occult bronchogenic carcinoma in nickel workers.

J. Thorac. Cardiovasc. Surg. 77(4):522-525, Apr. 1979.

Nemoto, N., et al.

Glucuronidation of benzo[a]pyrene in hamster embryo cells.

Chem. Biol. Interact. 22(1):1-14, July 1978.

Nemoto, N., et al.

Sulfate conjugation of benzo[a]pyrene metabolites and derivatives.

Chem. Biol. Interact. 23(1):19-30, Oct. 1978.

Nemoto, N., et al.

Modification of the mutagenicity of benzo(a)pyrene on bacteria by substrates of enzymes producing water soluble conjugates.

Toxicol. Lett. 2(4):205-211, Oct. 1978.

Nesnow, S. and Bergman, H.

1,2-Naphthoquinone: A mediator of non-enzymatic benzo(a)pyrene oxidation.

Life Sci. 25(24-25):2099-2104, Dec. 10-17, 1979.

Nespor, K.

Joga a prevence kardiovaskularnich chorob.(Czech.)

Cas. Lek. Cesk. 118(11):333-335, 1979.

Nestmann, E. R., et al.

Detection of the mutagenic activity of lead chromate using a battery of microbial tests.

Mutat. Res. 66(4):357-365, Apr. 1979.

Nettesheim, P., et al.

Vitamin A and the susceptibility of respiratory tract tissues to carcinogdn| cnsult.

Environ. Health Perspect. 29:89-93, Apr. 1979.

Neutra, R. R. and Drolette, M. E.

Estimating exposure-specific disease rates from case-control studies using Bayes' theorem.

Am. J. Epidemiol. 108(3):214-222, Sept. 1978.

Newberne, P. M., et al.

Effects of dietary fat on hepatic mixed-function oxidases and hepatocellular carcinoma induced by aflatoxin B1 in rats.

Cancer Res. 39(10):3986-3991, Oct. 1979.

Newsome, Jr, H. H.

Symposium on Hypertension, Steroid and Mineral Metabolism. Vasopressin: Deficiency, excess and syndrome of inappropriate antidiuretic hormone secretion.

Nephron 23(2-3):125-129, 1979.

Nguyen, T.-L., et al.

Metabolic oxidation of nicotine to chemically reactive intermediates.

J. Med. Chem. 22(3):259-263, Mar. 1979.

Nicholls, P.

Effects of inhibitory ligands on the aerobic carbon monoxide complex of cytochrome c oxidase.

Biochem. J. 183(3):519-529, Dec. 1, 1979.

Nichols, D., et al.

Acute and chronic pulmonary function changes in allergic bronchopulmonary aspergillosis.

Am. J. Med. 67(4):631-637, Oct. 1979.

Nicholson, J., et al.

Lipid and lipoprotein distributions in octo- and nonagenarians.

Metabolism 28(1):51-55, Jan. 1979.

Nicolle, P.

Un precurseur de la lutte contre le tabagisme. (Fr.)

Hist. Sci. Med. 12(2):143-144, 1978.

Nielsen, M. M. and Hjoellund, E.

Smoking and diabetic microangiopathy. (Letter to the Editor.)

Lancet 2(8088):533-534, Sept. 2, 1978.

Nielsen, P. E., et al.

Aendring i danskernes rygevaner 1958-1976. (Dan.)

Ugeskr. Laeger 140(41):2528-2532, Oct. 9, 1978.

Nieman, G. F., et al.

The effect of smoke inhalation on pulmonary surfactant.

Ann. Surg. 191(2):171-181, Feb. 1980.

Nieuw Amerongen, A. V., et al.

Comparison of adenylate cyclase activity and in vitro secretion in the parotid and sublingual glands of the mouse.

J. Physiol. (Lond.) 283:211-221, 1978.

Nilan, R. A.

Potential of plant genetic systems for monitoring and screening mutagens.

Environ. Health Perspect. 27:181-196, Dec. 1978.

Nishijima, T.

Studies on the immunological response in rats with experimental urinary bladder carcinoma. (Jpn.)

Jpn. J. Urol. 69(8):1044-1054, Aug. 1978.

Nishimoto, Y.

Annual Meeting Symposium on Smoking and Cardiopulmonary Function: Special comment (2). Smoking effects on cardiopulmonary function. (Abstr.) (Jpn.)

Jpn. J. Thorac. Dis. 15(9):614, Sept. 1977.

Nolewajka, A. J., et al.

Exercise and human collateralization: An angiographic and scintigraphic assessment.

Circulation 60(1):114-121, July 1979.

Nora, J. J., et al.

Genetic-epidemiologic study of early onset ischemic heart disease.

Circulation 61(3):503-508, Mar. 1980.

Norden, A.

Nutrition of Old Age: Ageing.

Scand. J. Gastroenterol. 14(Suppl. 52): 15-21, 1979.

Nordenskjoeld, M., et al.

Differences in the repair of DNA strand breaks induced by 9-hydroxy-benzo(a)-pyrene and trans-7,8-dihydro-7,8-dihydroxy-benzo(a)pyrene in cultured human fibroblasts.

Biochem. Biophys. Res. Commun. 85(4): 1535-1541, Dec. 29, 1978.

Norman, R. L., et al.

The role of cytochrome P-450 forms in 2-aminoanthracene and benz [a] pyrene mutagenesis.

Biochem. Biophys. Res. Commun. 89(1):195-201, July 12, 1979.

Normann, S. J. and Cornelius, J.

Concurrent depression of tumor macrophage infiltration and systemic inflammation by progressive cancer growth.

Cancer Res. 38(10):3453-3459, Oct. 1978.

Novak, R. F., et al.

Characterization of the interaction of the aromatic hydrocarbons benzene and toluene with human hemoglobin.

Mol. Pharmacol. 16(3):1046-1058, Nov. 1979.

Novros, J. S., et al.

Improved method for accurate quantitation of total and conjugated bilirubin in serum.

Clin. Chem. 25(11):1891-1899, Nov. 1979.

Moya, N. D.

The International Challenge of Drug Abuse. Coca and cocaine: A perspective from Bolivia.

Natl. Inst. Drug Abuse Res. Monogr. Ser. 19:82-90, 1978.

Numazawa, M., et al.

Properties of estradiol 2-hydroxylase and 2-hydroxy-3-deoxyestradiol 3-hydroxylase in rat liver.

J. Steroid Biochem. 10(2):227-233, Feb. 1979.

Nunnink, J. C., et al.

The ontogeny of nuclear aryl hydrocarbon hydroxylase.

Chem. Biol. Interact. 22(2-3):225-230, Sept. 1978.

Nupuf, M. S. and Sutherland, W. H. F.

High density lipoprotein levels in children of young men with ischaemic heart disease.

Atherosclerosis 33(3):365-370, July 1979.

Nygaard, O. and Hultin, T.

Early effects of dimethylnitrosamine on protein chain initiation and post-microsomal polyadenylic acid-containing RNA content in mouse liver.

Cancer Res. 39(9):3349-3352, Sept. 1979.

Nyqvist, B.

Luftvaegssymtom hos asfaltarbetare - ytterligare en yrkesbronkit? (Swed.)

Lakartidningen 75(12):1173-1175, Mar. 22, 1978.

O'Brien, E.

Some medical problems in pregnancy.

Practitioner 221(1326):857-862, Dec. 1978.

O'Brien, I. M., et al.

Toluene di-isocyanate-induced asthma: II. Inhalation challenge tests and bronchial reactivity studies.

Clin. Allergy 9(1):7-15, Jan. 1979.

O'Cain, C. F., et al.

Pattern and mechanism of airway response to hypocapnia in normal subjects.

J. Appl. Physiol. 47(1):8-12, July 1979.

O'Connell, M. J., et al.

A comparative clinical and immunological assessment of methanol extraction residue of Bacillus Calmette-Guerin versus placebo in patients with advanced cancer.

Cancer Res. 39(9):3720-3724, Sept. 1979.

O'Connor, S. A., et al.

Changes in pulmonary function after naturally acquired respiratory infection in normal persons.

Am. Rev. Respir. Dis. 120(5):1087-1093, Nov. 1979.

O'Donell, Jr., T. F.

Diagnosis of deep venous thrombosis in the outpatient by venography.

Surg. Gyencol. Obstet. 150(1):69-74, Jan. 1980.

Oerlander, J., et al.

Skeletal muscle metabolism, morphology and function in sedentary smokers and nonsmokers.

Acta Physiol. Scand. 107(1):39-46, Sept. 1979.

Oestergaard, K.

Renal cadmium concentration in relation to smoking habits and blood pressure.

Acta Med. Scand. 203(5):379-383, 1978.

Ogiu, T.

Hematological and histopathological characteristics of leukemias induced by 1-alkyl-1-nitrosoureas in Donryu rats.

Gann 69(6):781-791, Dec. 1978.

Okada, M., et al.

Syntheses of N-alkyl-N-(omega-carboxyalkyl)nitrosamines related to N-butyl-N-(3-carboxypropyl)nitrosamines, principal urinary metabolite of a (4-hydroxybutyl)nitrosamine.

Chem. Pharm. Bull. (Tokyo) 26(12):3909-3913, Dec. 1978.

Okada, M., et al.

Syntheses of N-alkyl-N-(hydroxy- or oxo-alkyl)nitrosamines related to N-butyl-N-(4-hydroxybutyl)nitroamine, a potent bladder carcinogen.

Chem. Pharm. Bull. (Tokyo) 26(12):3891-3896, Dec. 1978.

Okamoto, M., et al.

An NADPH-induced change in lipid bilayer of rat liver microsomes as observed by spin-labeled phosphatidylcholine.

Biochem. Biophys. Res. Commun. 87(1): 300-307, Mar. 15, 1979.

Okano, P., et al.

Comparison of benzol(a)pyrene and trans-7,8-dihydroxy-7,8- dihydrobenzo(a)pyrene metabolism in human blood monocytes and lymphocytes.

Cancer Res. 39(8):3184-3193, Aug. 1979.

Okita, R. T., et al.

Lauric acid hydroxylation in human liver and kidney cortex microsomes.

Biochem. Pharmacol. 28(23):3385-3390, Dec. 1, 1979.

Olajos, E. J. and Coulston, F.

Comparative toxicology of n-nitroso compounds and their carcinogenic potential to man.

Ecotoxicol. Environ. Safety 2(3-4): 317-367, Dec. 1978.

Oldenburg, Jr., F. A., et al.

Effects of postural drainage, exercise and cough on mucus clearance in chronic bronchitis.

Am. Rev. Respir. Dis. 120(4):739-745, Oct. 1979.

Olsen, J. S. and Neufeld, A. H.

The rabbit cornea lacks cholinergic receptors.

Invest. Ophthalmol. Vis. Sci. 18(12): 1216-1225, Dec. 1979.

Olsen, N. and Nielsen, S. L.

Prevalence of primary Raynaud phenomena in young females.

Scand. J. Clin. Lab. Invest. 38(8):761-764, Dec. 1978.

Olson, J. W. and Russell, D. H.

Prolonged induction of hepatic ornithine decarboxylase and its relation to cyclic adenosine 3': 5'-monophosphate-dependent protein kinase activation after a single administration of diethylnitrosamine.

Cancer Res. 39(8):3074-3079, Aug. 1979.

Omelka, F. and Bystry, J.

Problems of cholesterolemia in childhood and adolescence.

Scr. Med. (Brno) 52(5):289-291, 1979.

Omura, T.

The Induction of Drug Metabolism: Biosynthesis and drug-induced increase of microsomal enzymes.

Symp. Med. Hoechst 14:162-175, 1979.

Onari, K., et al.

Immunological study on cigarette smokers: Part I. Serum protein pattern in smokers.

Hiroshima J. Med. Sci. 27(2):113-118, June 1978.

Opdyke, D. L. J.

Monographs on Fragrance Raw Materials: Tobacco leaf absolute.

Food Cosmet. Toxicol. 16(Suppl. 1): 875, Dec. 1978.

Opherk, D., et al.

Beziehungen von "Risikofactoren" der Arteriosklerose zum Schweregrad der angiographisch nachweisbaren Koronarsklerose. (Ger.)

Z. Kardiol. 68(6):369-374, June 1979.

Orr, W. C., et al.

Hypersomnolent and nonhypersomnolent patients with upper airway obstruction during sleep.

Chest 75(4):418-422, Apr. 1979.

Orrenius, S.

The Induction of Drug Metabolism. Chairman's introductory statement: Effects o carcinogens on enzyme synthesis.

Symp. Med. Hoechst 14:417-418, 1979.

Oshiro, Y., et al.

Deuterium isotope effect on rat liver DNA damage in vivo by dimethylnitrosamine.

Chem. Biol. Interact. 23(2):263-266, Nov. 1978.

Oswald, R. E. and Freeman, J. A.

Characterization of the nicotinic acetylcholine receptor isolated from goldfish brain.

J. Biol. Chem. 254(9):3419-3426, May 10, 1979.

Otto, D. A., et al.

Carbon monoxide and human time discrimination: Failure to replicate Beard-Wertheim experiments.

Aviat. Space Environ. Med. 50(1):40-43, Jan. 1979.

Ouellet, B. L., et al.

Premature mortality attributable to smoking and hazardous drinking in Canada.

Am. J. Epidemiol. 109(4):451-463, Apr. 1979.

Overton, D. A.

Drug discrimination training with progressively lowered doses.

Science 205(4407):720-721, Aug. 17, 1979.

Owen, D. A., et al.

Progressive loss of consciousness in a 78-year old man with long-standing dyspnea.

Can. Med. Assoc. J. 121(6):727-735, Sept. 22, 1979.

Owens, I. S., et al.

Deoxyribonucleic acid binding of 3-hydroxy-and 9-hydroxy-benzo(a)pyrene following further metabolism by mouse liver microsomal cytochrome P1-450.

Biochem. Pharmacol. 28(10):1623-1629, May 15, 1979.

Oxhoj, H., et al.

Effects of electric arc welding on ventilatory lung function.

Arch. Environ. Health 34(4):211-217, July/Aug. 1979.

Ozgen, G., et al.

Brons kanserlerinin teshis ve tedavi yonunden degerlendirilmesi. (Turk.)

Tip Fak. Mecm. 30(1):207-218, 1977.

Pachman, J. S. and Frederiksen, L. W.

"Yes I do mind"; Social skills training for non-smokers.

Addict. Behav. 4(1):75-81, 1979.

Paffenbarger, Jr., R. S., et al.

Physical activity as an index of heart attack risk in college alumni.

Am. J. Epidemiol. 108(3):161-175, Sept. 1978.

Paganelli, R., et al.

Maternal smoking and cord blood immunity function.

Clin. Exp. Immunol. 36(2):256-259, May 1979.

Paigen, B., et al.

Proceedings of the International Symposium on Microsomes and Drug Oxidations: Aryl hydrocarbon hydroxylase in cultured human lymphocytes.

Biochem. Pharmacol. Suppl.:418-425, 1977.

Paigen, B., et al.

Aryl hydrocarbon hydroxylase inducibility is not altered in bladder cancer patients or their progeny.

Int. J. Cancer 23(3):312-315, Mar. 15, 1979.

Paiva, M. and Engel, L. A.

Pulmonary interdependence of gas transport.

J. Appl. Physiol. 47(2):296-305, Aug. 1979.

Pal, K., et al.

The induction of sister chromatid exchanges by dihydrodiols derived from 7,12-dimethylbenz[a]anthracene and 3-methylcholanthrene.

Cancer Lett. 7(1):45-49, June 1979.

Palmer, A., et al.

Respiratory disease prevalence in cosmetologists and its relationship to aerosol sprays.

Environ. Res. 19(1):136-153, June 1979.

Pantuck, E. J., et al.

Stimulatory effect of brussels sprouts and cabbage on human drug metabolism.

Clin. Pharmacol. Ther. 25(1):88-95, Jan. 1979.

Parent, R. A. and Casto, B. C.

Effect of acrylonitrile on primary Syrian golden hamster embryo cells in culture: Transformation and DNA fragmentation.

JNCI 62(4):1025-1029, Apr. 1979.

Park, K. K. and Archer, M. C.

Metabolism of N-nitroso-2-oxopropyl-propylamine by rat liver: Formation of products resulting from both oxidation and reduction.

Cancer Biochem. Biophys. 3(1):37-40, 1978.

Park, S.-M.

Fluorescence and electrogenerated chemiluminescence studies of several dimethyl-substituted benzo[a]pyrenes.

Photochem. Photobiol. 28(1): 83-90, July 1978.

Parke, D. V.

The interactions of food and 'foreign' substances: The effects of diet and nutrition on the metabolism of drugs.

R. Soc. Health J. 98(6):256-261, Dec. 1978.

Parke, D. V.

The Induction of Drug Metabolism: The responsiveness of cells to various drug inducers.

Symp. Med. Hoechst 14:101-111, 1979.

Parkinson, A., et al.

Induction of both-3-methylcholanthrene- and phenobarbitone-type microsomal enzyme activity by a single polychlorinated biphenyl isomer.

Biochem. Pharmacol. 29(2):259-262, Jan. 15, 1980.

Partridge, M. R., et al.

Topography of ventilation-perfusion ratios in obesity. (Fr.)

Bull. Eur. Physiopathol. Respir. 14(6): 765-773, Nov.-Dec. 1978.

Partridge, M. R., et al.

Effect of hyperlipidaemia on pulmonary diffusing capacity for carbon monoxide.

Thorax 34(2):265-268, Apr. 1979.

Pasotti, C., et al.

NAB 365 (clenbuterol) and salbutamol in asthmatics: A double-blind clinical trial.

Int. J. Clin. Pharmacol. Biopharm. 17(4):176-180, Apr. 1979.

Paterson, M. E. L., et al.

The effect of menopausal status and sequential mestranol and norethisterone on serum cholesterol, triglyceride and electrophoretic lipoprotein patterns.

Br. J. Obstet. Gynaecol. 86(10):810-815, Oct. 1979.

Pavia, D., et al.

Effect of ipratropium bromide on mucociliary clearance and pulmonary function in reversible airways obstruction.

Thorax 34(4):501-507, Aug. 1979.

Pavlik, I., et al.

Ucinnost cigaretoveho filtra in vitro pri arteficialnom fajceni. (Czech)

Cas. Lek. Cesk. 117(29-30):918-921, July 28, 1978.

Pawsey, S. A., et al.

Clinical, genetic and DNA repair studies on a consecutive series of patients with xeroderma pigmentosum.

Q. J. Med. 48(190):179-210, Apr. 1979.

Pearlman, A. L.

Cell cycle effects and dependency of a carcinogenic metabolite of benzo[a]pyrene.

Lawrence Berkeley Lab. Rep. No. 8169:162-185, Aug. 1978.

Pearlman, A. L.

Background to the cell cycle studies on effects of B[a]P diol epoxide upon NMuLi cells.

Lawrence Berkeley Lab. Rep. No. 8169:152-159, Aug. 1978.

Pearson, R. and Richardson, K.

The smoking habits of 16-year-olds in the National Child Development Study.

Public Health 92(3):136-144, May 1978.

Pedersen, E. B. and Hagn-Meincke, F.

Epidemiologi og prognose for patienter medkronisk bronchitis og asthma bronchiale: En praeliminaer analyse fra et dansk amt. (Dan.)

Ugeskr. Laeger 140(9):492-497, Feb. 27, 1978.

Pegg, A. E.

Dimethylnitrosamine inhibits enzymatic removal of O6-methylguanine from DNA.

Nature 174(5667):182-184, July 13, 1978.

Pegg, A. E.

Effect of pretreatment with other dialkylnitrosamines on excision from hepatic DNA of O6-methylguanine produced by dimethylnitrosamine.

Chem. Biol. Interact. 22(1):109-116, July 1978.

Pegg, A. E. and Hui, G.

Formation and subsequent removal of O6-methylguanine form deoxyribonucleic acid in rat liver and kidney after small doses of dimethylnitrosamine.

Biochem. J. 173(3):739-748, Sept. 1, 1978.

Pegg, A. E. and Balog, B.

Formation and subsequent excision of O6-ethylguanine from DNA of rat liver following adminstration of diethylnitrosamine.

Cancer Res. 39(12):5003-5009, Dec. 1979.

Pegg, A. E. and Swann, P. F.

Metabolism of O6-alkyldeoxyguanosines and their effect on removal of O6-methylguanine from rat liver DNA.

Biochim. Biophys. Acta 565(2):241-252, Dec. 17, 1979.

Pelkonen, O.

The Induction of Drug Metabolism: Prenatal and neonatal development of drug and carcinogen metabolism.

Symp. Med. Hoechst 14:507-516, 1979.

Pelkonen, O. and Korhonen, P.

Proceedings of the International Symposium on Microsomes and Drug Oxidations: The metabolism of benzo[a]pyrene in cell cultures and homogenates from different human fetal tissues.

Biochem. Pharmacol. Suppl.:411-417, 1977.

Pelkonen, O. and Moilanen, M.-L.

The specificity and multiplicity of human placental xenobiotic-metabolizing monooxygenase system studied by potential substrates, inhibitors and gel electrophoresis.

Med. Biol. 57(5):306-312, Oct. 1979.

Pelkonen, O., et al.

Genetic differences in the metabolic activation of benzo[a]pyrene in mice: Attempts to correlate tumorigenesis with binding of reactive intermediates to DNA and with mutagenesis in vitro.

Pharmacology 18(6):281-293, 1979.

Penney, D. G. and Bishop, P. A.

Hematologic changes in the rat during and after exposure to carbon monoxide.

J. Environ Pathol. Toxicol. 2(2):407-415, Nov.-Dec. 1978.

Penney, D. G., et al.

Cardiodynamic changes during prolonged carbon monoxide exposure in the rat.

Toxicol. Appl. Pharmacol. 50(2): 213-218, Sept. 15, 1979.

Pentecost, B. L.

Coronary care: Aftercare of acute myocardial infarction.

Br. J. Hosp. Med. 20(3):252-259, Sept. 1978.

Pentecost, B. L.

Preventing the second infarct.

J. R. Coll. Physicians Lond. 14(1):22-25, Jan. 1980.

Peraino, C., et al.

Annual Report. Carcinogenesis and cocarcinogenesis: Initiation, promotion, and synergistic activity among environmental pollutants in the production of tumors.

Argonne Natl. Lab. Div. Biol. Med. Res. ANL-78-90:51-57, 1977 (Publ. 1978).

Pereira, M. A., et al.

Dose response for benzo(a)pyrene adducts in mouse epidermal DNA.

Cancer Res. 39(7, Part 1):2556-2559, July 1979.

Perin-Roussel, O., et al.

Binding of dibenzo(a,e)fluoranthene, a carcinogenic, polycyclic hydrocarbon without K-region, to nucleic acids in a subcellular microsomal system.

Cancer Res. 38(10):3499-3504, Oct. 1978.

Peristianis, G. C., et al.

An ultrastructural investigation of nephrotoxicity in rats induced by feeding cultures of Penicillium verrucosum var. Cyclopium.

Virchows Arch. [Cell Pathol.] 28(4): 321-337, Nov. 6, 1978.

Pero, R. W., et al.

Polycyclic hydrocarbon-induced rat sarcomas correlated to disturbances in the deoxyadenylate regions of the tumor DNAs.

Eur. J. Cancer 14(9):961-969, Sept. 1978.

Perrault, J. L., et al.

Alpha1-antitrypsin deficiency: Genetic, clinical and functional correlations in a three generation family.

Respiration 37(5):291-300, 1979.

Perrin, Cl., et al.

La kinesitherapie respiatoire dans la chirurgie majeure des voies aeriennes superieures. (Fr.)

Ann. Med. Nancy 22:735-746, May 15, 1978.

Persky, V. W., et al.

Racial patterns of heart rate in employed adult population.

Am. J. Epidemiol. 110(3):274-280, Sept. 1979.

Persson, P.-H., et al.

A study of smoking and pRegnancy with special reference to fetal growth.

Acta Obstet. Gynecol. Scand. Suppl. 78: 33-39, 1978.

Pertynski, T., et al.

The influence of chemotherapy on the distribution of 57Co-bleomycin in chemically induced squamous cell carcinoma of mouse skin.

Eur. J. Nucl. Med. 4(1):55-59, Feb. 1, 1979.

Peter, T., et al.

Effect on survival after myocardial infarction of long-term treatment with phenytoin.

Br. Heart J. 40(12):1356-1360, Dec. 1978.

Petering, H. G., et al.

Some effects of oral ingestion of cadmium on zinc, copper, and iron metabolism.

Environ. Health Perspect. 28:97-106, Feb. 1979.

Peters, G., et al.

Pharmacological Methods in Toxicology: Effects of drugs on ingestive behavior.

Pharmacol. Ther. 5(1-3, Suppl.):485-503, 1979.

Peters, R. W., et al.

Prophylactic permanent pacemakers for patients with chronic bundle branch block.

Am. J. Med. 66(6):978-985, June 1979.

Petersen, G.

Laegemidler og graviditet. (Dan.)

Maanedsskr. Prakt. Laegeg. 57(3): 125-146, Mar. 1979.

Peterson, J. K.

Tobaksrygning og mudhulen. (Dan.)

Arch. Pharm. Chem. 85(15):781-790, July 22, 1978.

Petitti, D. B., et al.

Oral contraceptives, smoking, and other factors in relation to risk of venous thromboembolic disease.

Am. J. Epidemiol. 108(6):480-485, Dec. 1978.

Petitti, D. B., et al.

Risk of vascular disease in women: Smoking, oral contraceptives, noncontraceptive estrogens, and other factors.

JAMA 242(11):1150-1154, Sept. 14, 1979.

Petkov, V., et al.

Comparative studies of colon reactivity of healthy and ionization-radiated guinea-pigs to com spasmogens and their antogonists.

Acta Physiol. Pharmacol. Bulg. 4(1):26-37, 1978.

Peto, J.

Editorial: A question of morality.

Thorax 33(4):409-410, Aug. 1978.

Petrzlkova, A., et al.

Vyskyt akutni koronarni prihody v populaci Praha 4. (Czech.)

Cas. Lek. Cesk. 118(11):328-333, 1979.

Pettersson, B.

Isolated hamster brown fat cells: A bioassay for toxicity tests at the cellular level. Effect of cigarette smoke condensates from high and low tar yield cigarettes.

Chem. Biol. Interact. 29(1):95-102, Jan. 1980.

Petty, T. L.

Chronic obstructive pulmonary disease.

Resident Staff Physician 24(11):53-59, Nov. 1978.

Pezzagno, G., et al.

Habitude de fumer, empoussierage atmospherique et risques respiratoires professionnels: Enquete chez les foundeurs. (Fr.)

Bronchopneumologie 28(3):186-194, May-June 1978.

Pfaeffli, P., et al.

Proceedings of the International Symposium on Styrene Occupational and Toxicological Aspects: Thermal degradation products of homopolymer polystyrene in air.

Scand. J. Work Environ. Health 4(Suppl. 2):22-27, Apr. 17-19, 1978.

Pfeffer, R. I., et al.

Estrogen use and blood pressure in later life.

Am. J. Epidemiol. 110(4):469-478, Oct. 1979.

Phelan, J. P.

Diminished fetal reactivity with smoking.

Am. J. Obstet. Gynecol. 136(2):230-233, Jan. 15, 1980.

Phillips, D. H., et al.

The covalent binding of polycyclic hydrocarbons to DNA in the skin of mice of different strains.

Int. J. Cancer 22(4):487-494, Oct. 15, 1978.

Phillips, D. H., et al.

A quantitative determination of the covalent binding of as series of polycylic hydrocarbons to DNA in mouse skin.

Int. J. Cancer 23(2):201-208, Feb. 15, 1979.

Phillips, J. C., et al.

The effect of ethoxyquin on the hepatotoxicity of dimethylnitrosamine and carbon tetrachloride in the rat.

Biochem. Soc. Trans. 6(6):1244-1246, 1978.

Piantadosi, F. R., et al.

Arteriopatia periferica diabetica e fattori di rischio ad essa correlati. (Ital.)

Rass. Int. Clin. Ter. 58(19):1345-1350, Oct. 15, 1978.

Pickup, J. C., et al.

Treatment of Early Diabetes: Metabolic fate, vascular outcome and the effect of treatment in borderline diabetics.

Adv. Exp. Med. Biol. 119:407-410, 1979.

Piehler, J. M. and Crichlow, R. W.

Primary carcinoma of the gallbladder.

Surg. Gynecol. Obstet. 147(6):929-942, Dec. 1978.

Pinney, J. M.

The largest preventable cause of death in the United States.

Public Health Rep. 94(2):107-108, Mar.-Apr. 1979.

Piper, D. W., et al.

A review of observations on chronic gastric ulcer patients in Australia.

Aust. NZ J. Surg. 49(1):19-23, Feb. 1979.

Pirani, B. B. K. and MacGillivray, I.

Smoking during pregnancy: Its effect on maternal metabolism and fetoplacental function.

Obstet. Gynecol. 52(3):257-263, Sept. 1978.

Pitot, H. C.

Interactions in the natural history of aging and carcinogenesis.

Fed. Proc. 37(14):2841-2847, Dec. 1978.

Pitot, H. C.

The Induction of Drug Metabolism: Drugs as promoters of carcinogenesis.

Symp. Med. Hoechst 14:471-483, 1979.

Pitt, B. R., et al.

Interaction of carbon monoxide and cyanide on cerebral circulation and metabolism.

Arch. Environ. Health 34(5):354-359, Sept.-Oct. 1979.

Pizer, M. E. and Dubois, D. D

An assessment of toluidine blue for the diagnosis of lip lesions.

Va. Med. 106(11):860-862, Nov. 1979.

Plamenac, P., et al.

Cytology of the respiratory tract in asbestos miners.

Acta Med Iugosl. 32(4):297-309, 1978.

Plamenac, P., et al.

Cytologic changes in the respiratory tract in children smokers.

Acta Cytol. (Baltimore) 23(5):389-391, Sept.-Oct. 1979.

Plamenac, P., et al.

Cytologic changes of the respiratory tract as a consequence of air pollution and smoking.

Acta Cytol. (Baltimore) 23(6):449-453, Nov.-Dec. 1979.

Platt, H. M. and Mackie, P. R.

Analysis of aliphatic and aromatic hydrocarbons in Antartic marine sediment layers.

Nature 280(5723):576-578, Aug. 1979.

Pleban, P. A. and Pearson, K. H.

Determination of manganese in whole blood and serum.

Clin. Chem. 25(11):1915-1918, Nov. 1979.

Pleban, P. A. and Pearson, K. H.

Determination of cadmium in whole blood and urine by Zeeman atomic absorption spectroscopy.

Clin. Chim. Acta 99(3):267-277, Dec. 17, 1979.

Pleuvry, B. J. and Maddison, S. E.

A sex difference in the effects of oral codeine and promethazine on the ventilatory response to carbon dioxide in human volunteers.

Br. J. Pharmacol. 9(2):159-164, Feb. 1980.

Pliss, G. B.

Modern concepts of the mechanisms of chemical carcinogenesis. (Russ.)

Vopr. Onkol. 24(9):95-107, 1978.

Plumlee, L.

Panel discussion: Role of high risk groups in the derivation of environmental health standards.

Environ. Health Perspect. 29:155-159, Apr. 1979.

Pohle, W., e tal.

Medikamenteneinnahme und endoskopischer Befund. (Ger.)

Med. Welt. 29(50):1968-1969, Dec. 15, 1978.

Poiley, J. A., et al.

Use of hamster hepatocytes to metabolize carcinogens in an in vitro bioassay.

JNCI 63(2):519-524, Aug. 1979.

Poirier, L. A. and de Serres, F. J.

Initial National Cancer Institute studies on mutagenesis as a prescreen for chemical carcinogens: An appraisal.

JNCI 62(4):919-926, Apr. 1979.

Poirier, L. A. and Weisburger, E. K.

Selection of carcinogens and related compounds tested for mutagenic activity.

JNCI 62(4):833-840, Apr. 1979.

Poirier, M. C., et al.

Quantitation of benzo(a)pyrene-deoxyguanosine adducts by radio-immunoassay.

Cancer Res. 40(2):412-416, Feb. 1980.

Poirier, R., et al.

La tabagisme scolaire a Marseille. (Fr.)

Med. Hyg. 36(1311):4054-4056, Dec. 6, 1978.

Poirier, R., et al.

Le tabagisme scolaire: Premiers resultats d'une enquete realisee dans l'agglomeration marseillaise. (Fr.)

Poumon Coeur 35(1):13-16, Jan.-Feb. 1979.

Poklis, A. and Whyatt, P. L.

Current trends in the abuse of pentazocine and tripelennamine: The metropolitan St. Louis experience.

J. Forensic Sci. 25(1):72-78, Jan. 1980.

Pollard, M. R. and Brennan, Jr., J. T.

Ethical Issues in Public Health Policy: Health Education and Life-Style Interventions. Disease prevention and health promotion initiatives: Some legal considerations.

Health Educ. Monogr. 6(2):211-222, Summer 1978.

Polsky, R. H. and Chance, M. R. A.

An ethological perspective on social behavior in long stay hospitalized psychiatric patients.

J. Nerv. Ment. Dis. 167(11):658-668, Nov. 1979.

Pomerleau, O., et al.

Predictors of outcome and recidivism in smoking cessation treatment.

Addict. Behav. 3(2):65-70, 1978.

Pomeroy, T. C.

Combined Effects of Chemotherapy and Radiotherapy on Normal Tissue Tolerance. Carcinogenesis effects of combined treatment: Immunologic factors.

Front. Radiat. Ther. Oncol. 13:194-214, 1979.

Pompecki, R.

Analysis of human sera for carcino-embryonic antigen (CEA)nes.

Eur. J. Cancer 15(4):499-507, Apr. 1979.

Ponteva, M., et al.

Blood cadmium and plasma zinc measurements in acute myocardial infarction.

Eur. J. Cardiol. 9(5):370-391, May 1979.

Pool, J. L.

Youth perspectives: Smoking and health.

Chest 76(5):500, Nov. 1979.

Poss, R., et al.

Methylmethacrylate is a mutagen for Salmonella typhimurium.

J. Bone Joint Surg. 61-A(8):1203-1207, Dec. 1979.

Post, C.

Studies on the Pharmacokinetic Function of the Lung with Special Reference to Lidocaine.

Acta Pharmacol. Toxicol. (Copenh.) 44(Suppl. 1):1-53, 1979.

Poston, R. N.

Immunological aspects of atheroma: A review.

J. R. Soc. Med. 72(9):674-682, Sept. 1979.

Potts, D. M. and Edelman, D. A.

Reproductive mortality: (Letter to the Editor.)

Br. Med. J. 2(6201):1362, Nov. 24, 1979.

Prasad, R., et al.

Aryl hydrocarbon hydroxylase inducibility and lymphoblast formation in lung cancer patients.

Int. J. Cancer 23(3):316-320, Mar. 15, 1979.

Prashad, J., et al.

Respiratory effects of a single, moderately acute, smoke inhalation episode.

J. Natl. Med. Assoc. 71(3):251-255, Mar. 1979.

Pratt, P. C., et al.

Proceedings of the Aspen Lung Conference: Prevalence and severity of morphologic emphysema and bronchitis in non-textile and cotton-textile workers.

Chest 77(2 Suppl.):323-325, Feb. 1980.

Pregowski, W.

Walka z paleniem tytoniu na swiecie. (Pol.)

Pneumonol. Pol. 47(2):77-80, 1979.

Pregowski, W. and Cesarz-Fronczyk, M.

Zakonna opatreni a boj proti koureni v Polsku. (Czech)

Stud. Pneumol. Phtiseol. Cech. 38(8): 558-560, Oct. 1978.

Prescott, R. J., et al.

Smoking and risk factors in deep vein thrombosis.

Thromb. Haemostas. 40(1):128-133, Aug. 31, 1978.

Preussmann, R., et al.

Carcinogenicity and mutagenicity testing of three isomeric N-nitroso-N-methylaminopyridines in rats.

JNCI 62(1):153-156, Jan. 1979.

Pride, N. B., et al.

Proceedings of the Aspen Lung Conference: Peripheral lung function and spirometry in male smokers and exsmokers.

Chest 77(2 Suppl.):289-290, Feb. 1980.

Pride, N. B., et al.

Proceedings of the Aspen Lung Conference: Lung distensibility and airway function in intermediate alpha-antitrypsin deficiency (PiMZ).

Chest 77(2 Suppl.):253-255, Feb. 1980.

Priest, M. F., et al.

American Heart Association Monograph No. 59. Cardiovascular Surgery 1977: Changes in left ventricular segmental wall motion following randomization to medicine or surgery in patients with unstable angina.

Circulation 58(3, Suppl. 1):I-62-I-68, Sept. 1978.

Protas, L. L. and Muske, G. A.

The effects of some transmitter substances on the tube foot muscles of the starfish, Asterias amurensis (Luetken).

Gen. Pharmacol. 11(1):113-118, 1980.

Prough, R. A., et al.

Characteristics of benzo(a)pyrene metabolism by kidney, liver, and lung microsomal fractions from rodents and humans.

Cancer Res. 39(4):1199-1206, Apr. 1979.

Pruitt, Jr., B. A.

The burn patient: I. Initial care.

Curr. Probl. Surg. 16(4):1-62, Apr. 1979.

Puchmayer, V. and Bulvas, M.

Positive family history as a risk factor of obliterative atherosclerosis.

Cor Vasa 20(4):283-291, 1978.

Puchmayer, V., et al.

Kouri - Jeden z rizikovych cinitelu pro vznik uzaverove choroby. (Czech)

Vnitr. Lek. 25(3):225-234, Mar. 1979.

Pugh, T. D. and Goldfarb, S.

Quantitative histochemical and autoradiographic studies of hepatocarcinogenesis in rats fed 2-acetylaminofluorene followed by phenobarbital.

Cancer Res. 38(12):4450-4457, Dec. 1978.

Pullan, P. T., et al.

Plasma vasopressin and human neurophysins in physiological and pathological states associated with changes in vasopressin secretion.

J. Clin. Endocrinol. Metab. 49(4): 580-587, Oct. 1979.

Purchase, I. F. H., et al.

An evaluation of 6 short-term tests for detecting organic chemical carcinogens.

Br. J. Cancer 37(6):873-903, June 1978.

Purnell, D. M.

The relationship of terminal duct hyperplasia to mammary carcinoma in 7,12-dimethylbenz(alpha)anthracene-treated LEW/Mai rats.

Am. J. Pathol. 98(2):311-324, Feb. 1980.

Puska, P., et al.

Suomalaisen aikuisvaeestoen terveyskaeyttaeytyminen kevaeaellae 1978.

Suom. Laeaekaeril. 34(11):856-862, Apr. 10, 1979.

Puska, P., et al.

Changes in coronary risk factors during comprehensive five-year community programme to control cardiovascular diseases (North Karelia project.)

Br. Med. J. 2(6199):1173-1178, Nov. 10, 1979.

Pyoeraelae, K.

Relationship of glucose tolerance and plasma insulin to the incidence of coronary heart disease: Result from two population studies in Finland.

Diabetes Care 2(2):131-141, Mar.-Apr. 1979.

Pyoeraelae, K., et al.

Asymptomatic Hyperglycemia and Coronary Heart Disease. Glucose tolerance and coronary heart disease: Helsinki policemen study.

J. Chronic Dis. 32(11/12):729-745, 1979.

Pyoernilae, A., et al.

The influence of intrahypothalamically injected cholinergic agents on temperature regulation in the pigeon at ambient temperatures of 20 degrees, 32 degrees and 38 degrees C.

Neuropharmacology 18(5):503-510, May 1979.

Quarles, J. M., et al.

Transformation of hamster fetal cells by nitrosated pesticides in a transplacental assay.

Cancer Res. 39(11):4525-4533, Nov. 1979.

Quast, U., et al.

Ligand-induced changes in membrane-bound acetylcholine receptor observed by ethidium fluorescence. 2. Stopped-flow studies with agonists and antagonists.

Biochemistry 18(10):1891-1901, May 15, 1979.

Queval, P. and Beaumatin, J.

Etude complementaire de l'action inductrice de la benzo-5.6 flavone sur l'activite benzopyrene mono-oxydase pulmonaire.Comparaison avec d'autres agents chimiques ou physiques. (Fr.)

C. R. Acad. Sci. [D] (Paris) 288(15):1215-1217, Apr. 23, 1979.

Queval, P., et al.

Inducibility of microsomal enzymes in normal and pre-cancerous lung tissue. Synergistic action of 5-6 benzoflavon or methyl-cholanthrene in radiation induced carcinogenesis.

Biomedicine 31(6):182-186, Oct. 1979.

Quick, C. A., et al.

Frequency and significance of epithelial atypia in laryngeal papillomatosis.

Laryngoscope 89(4):550-560, Apr. 1979.

Quigley, M. E., et al.

Effects of maternal smoking on circulating catecholamine levels and fetal heart rates.

Am. J. Obstet. Gynecol. 133(6):685-690, Mar. 15, 1979.

Rabes, H. M. and Szymkowiak, R.

Cell kinetics of hepatocytes during the preneoplastic period of diethylnitrosamine-induced liver carcinogenesis.

Cancer Res. 39(4):1298-1304, Apr. 1979.

Rabes, H. M., et al.

Alkylation of DNA and RNA by 14C dimetheylnitrosamine in hydroxyurea-synchronized regenerating rat liver.

Cancer Res. 39(10):4228-4236, Oct. 1979.

Rabinowitz, B. D., et al.

Acute hemodynamic effects of cigarette smoking in man assessed by systolic time intervals and endocardiography.

Circulation 60(4):752-760, Oct. 1979.

Radford, E. P.

Inner-city housing and respiratory disease in children: A pilot study.

Arch. Environ. Health 34(1):23-30, Jan.-Feb. 1979.

Raeder, E. A., et al.

Effects of smoking and inhalation of carbon monoxide on systolic time intervals and blood pressure: Differences between two types of cigarettes and a cigar.

Chest 75(2):136-140, Feb. 1979.

Raftell, M. and Blomberg, K.

Immunochemical studies on two DT diaphorase active antigens isolated from rat liver cytosol by affinity chromotography.

Arch. Biochem. Biophys. 199(1):165-171, Jan. 1980.

Raftery, E. B.

Hypertension - day by day.

Practitioner 223(1334):166-175, Aug. 1979.

Raisfeld, I. H. and Lin, C.

Nitrosamine formation from interaction of isosorbide dinitrate and hydroxyzine HCl, a tertiary amine.

Biochem. Pharmacol. 28(23):3451-3455, Dec. 1, 1979.

Ramaciotti, D., et al.

Niveau pollution par le SO2 et prevalence de la bronchite. (Fr.)

Soz. Praventivmed. 22(4):189-190, July-Aug. 1977.

Rambaldi, M., et al.

Misura del closing volume con la tecnica di un gas residente (O2). Osservazioni personali. (Ital.)

Arch. Monaldi 32(4):243-260, July-Aug. 1977.

Ramoino, R.

Congresso Nazionale Associazione Italiana Dottoresse in Medicina e Chirurgia: Il fumo e l'apparato respiratorio nell' adolescente. (Ital.)

Minerva Med. 69(45):3054-3055, Sept. 29, 1978.

Ramsay, L. E.

Alcohol and myocardial infarction in hypertensive men.

Am. Heart J. 98(3):402-404, SEpt. 1979.

Ramsay, L. E.

Intermittent claudication in hypertensive men.

J. R. Coll. Physicians Lond. 13(2):100-102, Apr. 1979.

Rana, S. V. S., et al.

Tracheal phosphatases after a long term CO poisoning in Indian palm squirrels. A histochemical study.

Curr. Sci. (Bangalore) 47(20):751-753, Oct. 20, 1978.

Rana, S. V. S., et al.

Certain biochemical changes in the trachea, lungs, and heart of squirrels exposed to three principal air pollutants.

Arch. Environ. Contam. Toxicol. 8(2):231-239, 1979.

Ranga, V. and Kleinerman, J.

Structure and function of small airways in health and disease.

Arch. Pathol. Lab. Med. 102(12):609-617, Dec. 1978.

Rao, G. J., et al.

Studies on 2,3-diphosphoglycerate levels in blood.

Indian J. Med. Res. 70:483-486, Sept. 1979.

Rao, L. G. S.

Intrauterine growth retardation. (Letter to the Editor.)

Lancet 1(8123):976, May 5, 1979.

Rao, T. K., et al.

Metagenicity of aliphatic nitrosamines in Salmonella typhimurium.

Mutat. Res. 66(1):1-7, Jan. 1979.

Rao, T. K., et al.

Mutagenicity of cyclic nitrosamines in Salmonella typbimurium: Effect of ring size.

Mutat. Res. 67(1):21-26, May 1979.

Rappe, C.

Kemisk carcinogenes och laekemedel. (Swed.)

Sven. Farm. Tidskr. 83(5):186-190, Apr. 9, 1979.

Rasmussen, F. V., et al.

Scandinavian Symposium on Chronic Obstructive Airways Disease: Combined effect of an anticholinergic drug ipratropium bromide and disodium cromoglycate in exercise induced asthma.

Scand. J. Respir. Dis. Suppl. 103:159-162, 1979.

Rasmussen, F. V., et al.

Associations between housing conditions, smoking habits and ventilatory lung function in men with clean jobs.

Scand. J. Respir. Dis. 59(5):264-276, Oct. 1978.

Rasp, F. L., et al.

Reversible impairment of the adherance of alveolar macrophages from cigarette smokers.

Am. Rev. Respir. Dis. 118(6):979-986, Dec. 1978.

Raunio, H. and Pelkonen, O.

The inhibition of induction of microsomal monooxygenase activity by 1,3-diamino-2-propanol, an inhibitor of ornithine decarboxylase.

Biochem. Biophys. Res. Commun. 91(2):658-664, Nov. 28, 1979.

Rawbone, R. G.

Self-titration by cigarette smokers. (Letter to the Editor.)

Br. Med. J. 2(6192):731-732, Sept. 22, 1979.

Raybourn, M. S., et al.

An in vitro electrophysiological assessment of the direct cellular toxicity of carbon monoxide.

Toxicol. Appl. Pharmacol. 46(3):769-779, Dec. 1978.

Rayner, V.

Characteristics of the internal anal sphincter and the rectum of the vervet monkey.

J. Physiol. (Lond.) 286:383-399, 1979.

Rebel-de Vries, H. A. and Bruschke, A. V. G.

Coronaria-angiografische bevindingen bij vrouwen in de vruchtbare levensfase; het verband tussen klinische verschijnselen en risicofactoren. (Dut.)

Ned. Tijdschr. Geneeskd. 123(28):1202-1206, July 14, 1979.

Reddy, J. K. and Rao, M. S.

Enhancement by WY-14,643, a hepatic peroxisome proliferator, of diethylnitrosamine-initiated hepatic tumorigenesis in the rat.

Br. J. Cancer 38(4):537-543, Oct. 1978.

Reddy, M. S., et al.

Effect of chronic tobacco-betel-lime "quid" chewing on human salivary secretions.

Am. J. Clin. Nutr. 33(1):77-80, Jan. 1980.

Redon, A., et al.

Adenopathies cervicales sans primitif connu. (Fr.)

J. Radiol. 60(5):343-349, May 1979.

Rees, P. J., et al.

Evaluation of methods used to estimate inhaled dose of carbon monoxide.

Thorax 35(1):47-51, Jan. 1980.

Regan, J. D., et al.

Repair of DNA damaged by mutagenic metabolites of benzo(a)pyrene in human cells.

Chem. Biol. Interact. 20(3):279-287, Mar. 1978.

Regan, T. J.

Of beverages, cigarettes and cardiac arrhythmias.

N. Engl. J. Med. 301(19):1060-1062, Nov. 8, 1979.

Reginster-Haneuse, G. and Hullebroeck, G.

Enquetes aupres d'adolescents belges: Resultats et conclusions pour l'education sanitaire. (Fr.)

Arch. Belg. Med. Soc. 36(5):296-301, May 1978.

Reid, L. M.

Introductory remarks: Session on disease conditions predisposing afflicted individuals to the toxic effects of pollutants.

Environ. Health Perspect. 29:127-129, Apr. 1979.

Reidy, M. A.

Arterial endothelium around rabbit aortic ostia: A SEM study using vascular casts.

Exp. Mol. Pathol. 30(3):327-336, June 1979.

Reines, H. D. and Yardbrough, D. R.

Respiratory complications in patients with severe burns.

J. SC Med. Assoc. 76(1):14-16, Jan. 1980.

Remmer, H., et al.

The Induction of Drug Metabolism: Pharmacological consequences of induction of drug metabolizing enzymes.

Symp. Med. Hoechst 14:555-581, 1979.

Renaud, S., et al.

Platelet functions in relation to dietary fats in farmers from two regions of France.

Thromb. Haemost. 40(3):518-531, Feb. 15, 1979.

Renik-Schueller, H. M. and Tomaszewski, J. E.

Binding of radioactivity after transplacental administration of tritlated N-nitrosodiethylamine to Syrian golden hamsters.

JNCI 64(2):373-375, Feb. 1980.

Renshaw, D. C.

Sex and drugs.

S. Afr. Med. J. 54(8):322-326, Aug. 19, 1978.

Resnik, R., et al.

Catecholamine-mediated reduction in uterine blood flow after nicotine infusion in the pregnant ewe.

J. Clin. Invest. 63(6):1133-1136, June 1979.

Reunanen, A., et al.

Asymptomatic Hyperglycemia and Coronary Heart Disease. Glucose tolerance and coronary heart disease in middle-aged Finnish men: Social insurance institution's coronary heart disease study.

J. Chronic Dis. 32(11/12):747-758, 1979.

Rey, P.

Relations entre la consommation de cigarettes et les symptomes respiratoires chroniques. (Fr.)

Bull. Schweiz. Akad. Med. Wiss. 35(1-3):33-50, Mar. 1979.

Reynolds, H. Y.

The importance of lymphocytes in pulmonary health and disease.

Lung 155(3):225-242, Oct. 3, 1978.

Reynolds, H. Y., et al.

Secretory Immunity and Infection: Immunoglobulin A in secretions from the lower human respiratory tract.

Adv. Exp. Med. Biol. 107:553-564, 1978.

Reynolds, Jr., W. C. and Shapiro, I.

Retrobulbar neuritis with neuroretinal edema as a delayed manifestation of carbon monoxide poisoning: Case report.

Milit. Med. 144(7):472-473, July 1979.

Reznik-Schueller, H.

Veraenderungen des APUD-Zellsystems waehrend der Nitrosamin-induzierten Lungencarcinogenese beim Syrischen Goldhamster. (Ger.)

Vehr. Dtsch. Ges. Pathol. 61:136-138, 1977.

Reznik-Schueller, H.

Ultrastructure of nitrosoheptamethyleneimine-induced lung tumors in European hamsters.

Am. J. Pathol. 93(1):45-52, Oct. 1978.

Reznik-Schueller, H. and Lijinsky, W.

In vivo autoradiography and nitrosoheptamethyleneimine carcinogenesis in hamsters.

Cancer Res. 39(1):72-74, Jan. 1979.

Reznik, G.

Diisopropanolnitrosamin-induzierte Schilddruesentumoren bei Sprague-Dawley-Ratten. (Ger.)

Verh. Dtsch. Ges. Pathol. 61:299-302, 1977.

Rezaik, G. et al.

Renal carcinogenic and nephrotoxic effects of the flame retardant Tris (2,3-dibromopropyl) phosphate in F344 rats and (C57Bl/6N X C3H/HeN) F mice.

JNCI 63(1):205-212, July 1979.

Richard, J. L., et al.

Tabac, mortalite et incidence des maladies cardiovasculaires par atherosclerose - L'etude prospective parisienne. (Fr.)

Bull. Schweiz. Akad. Med. Wiss. 35(1-3):51-69, Mar. 1979.

Richardson, D. R. and Morton, R. F.

Differential effects of chronic nicotine and tobacco smoke administration on iliac vascular resistance in the rat.

Proc. Soc. Exp. Biol. Med. 161(3): 386-390, July 1979.

Richmond, J. B.

Physician advisory: Health effects of asbestos.

Prev. Med. 7(4):641-642, Dec. 1978.

Richmond, J. B.

Physician advisory-Health effects of asbestos.

Clin. Toxicol. 13(5):641-643, 1978.

Rico, A., et al.

Toxicite des gaz de combustion. (Fr.)

C. R. Acad. Sci.[D] 288(19): 1493-1496, May 21, 1979.

Riegelman, R.

Verifying the validity of outcome.

Postgrad. Med. 65(6):149-153, June 1979.

Rifkind, A. B., et al.

Equality of the rates of mixed function oxidation in livers of male and female chick embryos.

Biochem. Pharmacol. 28(10): 1681-1683, May 15, 1979.

Rillema, J. A., et al.

Phospholipase A2-activity in 9,10-dimethyl-1,2-benzanthracene-induced mammary tumors of rats.

Biochim. Biophys. Acta 617(1): 150-155, Jan. 18, 1979.

Rimpelae, M.

Hintapolitiikan vaikutus tupakankulutukseen 1970-luvulla. (Finn.)

Suom. Laeaekaeril. 33(9):693-702, Mar. 20, 1978.

Rimpelae, M.

Kaesitykset tupakoinnin vahingollisuudesta ja tupakointi tupakkalain voimaantulon jaelkeen. (Finn.)

Suom. Laeaekaeril. 33(36):2866-2872, Dec. 20, 1978.

Rimpelae, M.

Tuloksia vuoden 1977 terveyskyselystae: Nuorten terveystavat. (Finn.)

Suom. Laeaekaeril. 10(4):849-855, 1979.

Rimsten, A., et al.

Carcinoembryonic antigen in serum of unselected breast-cancer patients and of non-hospitalized controls.

Br. J. Cancer. 39(2):109-115, Feb. 1979.

Rincon, E., et al.

Medicon del volumen de cierre en sujetos fumadores. (Span.)

Invest. Clin. (Venez) 19(2): 68-75, 1978.

Rinkus, S. J. and Legator, M. S.

Chemical characterization of 465 known or suspected carcinogens and their correlation with mutagenic activity in the Salmonella typhimurium system.

Cancer Res. 39(9):3289-3318, Sept. 1979.

Rissanen, A. M.

Familial occurrence of coronary heart disease: Effect of age at diagnosis.

Am. J. Cardiol. 44(1):60-66, July 1979.

Rissanen, V., et al.

Prehospital sudden death from ischaemic heart disease: A postmortem study.

Br. Heart J. 40(9):1025-1033, Sept. 1978.

Ritts, Jr., R. E.

Mutagenesis versus carcinogenesis of plastic implants.

J. Bone Joint Surg. 61-A(8):1201-1202, Dec. 1979.

Rivedal, E. and Sanner, T.

Synergistic effect on morphological transformation of hamster embryo cells. by nickel sulphate and benz[a]pyrene.

Cancer Lett. 8(3):203-208, Jan. 1980.

Robbins, L. C.

Prospective medicine.

Contin. Educ. Fam. Physician 8(2):24-35, Feb. 1978.

Roberts, B. W. and Forester, W. E.

Group relaxation - acute and chronic effects on essential hypertension.

Cardiovasc. Med. 4(5):575-580, May 1979.

Roberts, D. and Cole, P.

Effect of tobacco and nicotine on growth of Haemophilus influenzae in vitro.

J. Clin. Pathol. 32(7):728-731, July 1979.

Roberts, R. K., et al.

Drug prescribing in hepatobiliary disease.

Drugs 17(3):198-212, Mar. 1979.

Robertson, F. W. and Cumming, A. M.

Genetic and environmental variation in serum lipoproteins in relation to coronary heart disease.

J. Med. Genet. 16(2):85-100, Apr. 1979.

Robertson, L. W., et al.

Induction of both cytochromes P-450 and P-448 by 2'3,4,4',5-pentabrombiphenyl a component of firemaster.

Biochem. Biophys. Res. Commun. 92(1):175-182, Jan. 15, 1980.

Robillard, D.

L'ICM veut se doter dun service de rehabilitation cardiague. (Fr.)

Can. Med. Assoc. J. 121(2):228-230 July 21, 1979.

Robins, P. and Cairns, J.

Quantitation of the adaptive response to alkylating agents.

Nature 280(5717):74-76, July 5, 1979.

Robinson, J. S.

Growth of the fetus.

Br. Med. Bull. 35(2):137-144, June 1979.

Robitaille, N.-M., et al.

Prevalence des facteurs de risque de la maladie coronarienne dans la region de Quebec. (Fr.)

Clin. Invest. Med. 2(1):13-16, 1979.

Robkin, M. A. and Cockroft, D. L.

The effect of carbon monoxide on glucose metabolism and growth of rat embryos.

Teratology 18(3):337-342, Dec. 1978.

Robles, R., et al.

Drug use among public and private secondary school students in Puerto Rico.

Int. J. Addict. 14(2):243-258, 1979.

Roboz, J.

Mass spectrometry in cancer research.

Adv. Cancer Res. 27:201-267, 1978.

Rocci, R., et al.

Thallium-201 myocardial imaging in young asymptomtic subjects with "ischaemic" changes in exercise electrocardiogram.

Acta Cardiol. (Brux.) 34(4):217-232, 1979.

Rodgers, R. J.

Effects of nicotine, mecamylamine, and hexamethonium on shock-induced fighting, pain reactivity, and locomotor behaviour in rats.

Psychopharmacology 66(1):93-99, Nov. 1979.

Rodgers, R. L., et al.

Comparison of the cardiostimulatory effects of acetylcholine and nicotine on the working guinea-pig heart.

Naunyn-Schmiedebergs Arch. Pharmacol. 310(2):97-101, Dec. 1979.

Rodriguez, J. R., et al.

Neutrophil lysosomal elastase activity in normal subjects and in patients with chronic obstructive pulmonary disease.

Am. Rev. Respir. Dis. 119(3):409-417, Mar. 1979.

Rogan, E. G., et al.

Horseradish peroxidase/hydrogen peroxide-catalyzed binding of aromatic hydrocarbons to DNA.

J. Biol. Chem. 254(15):7055-7059, Aug. 10, 1979.

Rogan, E., et al.

Binding of benzo[a]pyrene at the 1,3,6 postitions to nucleic acids in vivo on mouse skin and in vitro with rat liver microsomes and nuclei.

Chem. Biol. Interact. 22(1):35-51, July 1978.

Rogot, E.

Cardiorespiratory disease mortality among British and Norwegian migrants to the United States.

Am. J. Epidemiol. 108(3):181-191, Sept. 1978.

Rogot, E.

Smoking and life expectancy among U.S. Veterans.

Am. J. Public Health 68(10):1023-1025, Oct. 1978.

Romanski, B., et al.

The immunologic response to tobacco antigens in smokers: II. Specific precipitins against tobacco antigens in the serum of smokers suffering from coronary heart disease.

Allergol. Immunopathol. (Madr.) 6(5):383-390, Sept.-Oct. 1978.

Romanski, B., et al.

The immunologic response to tobacco antigens in smokers: III. Type III hypersensitivity skin reactions and specific serum precipitins to four different tobacco extracts in patients suffering from coronary artery disease.

Allergol. Immunopathol. (Madr.) 7(3): 187-196, May-June 1979.

Romero Romero, J. M., et al.

Contenido de cadmio en el tabaco y su contribucion a la acumulacion de este metal en el organismo humano. (Span.)

Rev. Sanid. Hig. Publica (Madr.) 52(9-10):1275-1282, Sept.-Oct. 1978.

Rooke, G. B., et al.

Carcinoma of the lung in Lancashire coalminers.

Thorax 34(2):229-233, Apr. 1979.

Roscoe, J. P.

In-vivo-in vitro analysis of ethylnitrosourea-induced brain carcinogenesis in the rat.

Br. Med. Bull. 36(1):33-38, Jan. 1980.

Rose, C. L. and Cohen, M. L.

The Marathon: Physiological, Medical, Epidemiological, and Psychological Studies. Relative importance of physical activity for longevity.

Ann. NY Acad. Sci. 301:671-702, 1977.

Rose, D. P. and Pruitt, B.

Modification of the effect of a gonadoliberin analog on 7,12-dimethylbenz(a)anthracene-induced rat mammary tumors by hormone replacement.

Cancer Res. 39(10):3968-3970, Oct. 1979.

Rose, D. P., et al.

Influence of dosage schedule on the biological characteristics of N-nitrosomethylurea-induced rat mammary tumors.

Cancer Res. 40(2):235-239, Feb. 1980.

Rose, F. L.

Aquatic Pollutants and Biologic Effects with Emphasis on Neoplasia. Tissue lesions of tiger salamanders (Ambystoma tigrinum): Relationship to sewage effluents.

Ann. NY Acad. Sci. 298:270-279, Sept. 29, 1977.

Rose, G., et al.

Epidemiologic methods in diabetic macrovascular disease.

Diabetes Care 2(2):91-97, Mar.-Apr. 1979.

Rose, J. Q., et al.

Phenytoin disposition in smokers and nonsmokers.

Int. J. Clin. Pharmacol. Biopharm. 16(11):547-550, Nov. 1978.

Rosen, C. and Ashley, M. J.

Smoking and the health professional: Recognition and performance of roles.

Can. J. Public Health 69(5):399-406, Sept.-Oct. 1978.

Rosenbaum, J. F., et al.

Psychosis and water intoxication.

J. Clin. Psychiatry 40(7):287-291, July 1979.

Rosenbaum, M. and Argon, S.

Locus of control and success in self-initiated attempts to stop smoking.

J. Clin. Psychol. 35(4):870-872, Oct. 1979.

Rosenberg, L., et al.

Oral contraceptive use in relation to nonfatal myocardial infarction.

Am. J. Epidemiol. 111(1):59-66, Jan. 1980.

Rosenfield, A.

Oral and intrauterine contraception: A 1978 risk assessment.

Am. J. Obstet. Gynecol. 132(1):92-106, Sept. 1, 1978.

Rosenkranz, H. S. and Poirier, L. A.

Evaluation of the mutagenicity and DNA-modifying activity of carcinogens and noncarcinogens in microbial systems.

JNCI 62(4):873-892, Apr. 1979.

Rosenman, K. D.

Cardiovascular disease and environmental exposure.

Br. J. Ind. Med. 36(2): 85-97, May 1979.

Ross, J. L. and Shenkman, L.

Diabetes insipidus.

Compr. Ther. 5(4):30-35, Apr. 1979.

Rosser, W. W.

Screening in family medicine: The current situation.

J. Fam. Pract. 6(3):503-509, Mar. 1978.

Rossi, L., et al.

Induction of tumors by direct injection of N-ethyl-N-nitrosourea into the amniotic space of the mouse fetus.

JNCI 63(4):987-989, Oct. 1979.

Rossiter, C. E. and Harries, P. G.

UK Naval Dockyards asbestosis study: Survey of the sample population aged 50-59 years.

Br. J. Ind. Med. 36(4):281-291, Nov. 1979.

Rostad, H. and Hall, K. V.

In situ vene-bypass: Senresultater. (Norw. Engl. Summary)

Tidsskr. Nor Laegeforen. 99(8):410-412; 434, Mar. 20, 1979.

Rostenberg, I., et al.

Exceso de cadenas ligeras libres de tipo lambda en el suero de fumadores sanos. (Span.)

Rev. Invest. Clin. 30(3):273-275, July-Sept. 1978.

Rostenberg, I., et al.

Serum concentration of alfa-2 HS glycoprotein, prealbumin, beta-lipoprotein, alfa-1-antitripsin and IgG in healthy smokers.

Rev. Invest. Clin. 30(4):367-368, Oct.-Dec. 1978.

Rostenberg, I., et al.

Gc globulin and prealbumin serum levels in patients with cancer and benign inflammatory diseases and in asymptomatic smokers.

JNCI 62(2):299-300, Feb. 1979.

Rostenberg, I., et al.

Congreso Nacional de Genetica Humana: Altered carbohydrates of the IgG in asymptomatic smokers. (Span.) (Abstr.)

Rev. Invest. Clin. 31(1): 106-107, Jan.-Mar. 1979.

Roszinsky-Koecher, G., et al.

Mutagenicity of polycyclic hydrocarbons: V. Induction of sister-chromatid exchanges in vivo.

Mutat. Res. 66(1):65-67, Jan. 1979.

Roszinsky-Koecher, G. and Roehrborn, G.

Increase in genetic acitivity of the polycyclic hydrocarbon benzo[a]pyrene by inhibition of the epoxide hydrase in an activation system in vitro.

Mutat. Res. 66(2):199-203, Feb. 1979.

Roth, J. and Binder, M.

Cellular responses to surface binding and internalization of concanavalin A: An electron microscopic investigation on the problem of membrane cycling.

Exp. Pathol. (Jena) 16(1-6):43-59, 1978.

Rothstein, R. J.

Emergency management of poisoning and overdose.

Compr. Ther. 5(1):7-14, Jan. 1979.

Cathartics are useful in treatment of poisoning. Sodium sulfate, Fleet's phosphosoda or epsom salts can be given orally.

Routledge, P. A. and Shand, D. G.

Clinical pharmacokinetics of propranolol.

Clin. Pharmacokinet. 4(2):73-90, Mar.-Apr. 1979.

Rowe, B. P., et al.

Blockade of pressor responses to angiotensins I and II and noradrenaline using phentolamine, propranolol and hexamthonium in conscious rabbits.

Eur. J. Physiol. 382(3):269-274, Nov. 1979.

Rozenbaum, H.

Precautions a observer avant de prescrire un contraceptif oral. (Fr.)

Concours Med. 100(35):5519-5523, Sept. 30, 1978.

Rozhkova, E. K., et al.

Pharmacological characteristics of cholinoreception in somatic muscles of the nematode, Ascaris suum.

Gen. Pharmacol. 11(1):141-146, 1980.

Rubino, G. F., et al.

Mortality of chrysotile asbestos workers at the Balangero Mine, Northern Italy.

Br. J. Ind. Med. 36(3):187-194, Aug. 1979.

Rubio, C. A. and Biberfield, P.

The basement membrane in experimentally induced atypias and carcinoma of the uterine cervix in mice: An immunofluorescence study.

Virchows Arch. [Pathol Anat.] 38(2):205-209, Feb. 9, 1979.

Rubio, C. A., et al.

Kinetics of cell replication of the uterine cervix. III. Delayed migration in atypical epithelia of mice.

JNCI 64(1):151-156, Jan. 1980.

Ruchirawat, M., et al.

Effects of thiamine deficiency on the metabolism and acute toxicity of dimethylnitrosamine in the rat.

Biochem. Pharmacol. 27(13):1783-1786, 1978.

Rudali, G.

Inhibition of mammary carcinogenesis of dimethylbenzanthracene treated rats with a brominated triphenylethylene.

Biomedicine [Express] 31(5):142-146, Sept. 1979.

Ruddell, W. S. J., et al.

Gastric cancer in patients who have taken cimetidine. (Letter to the Editor.)

Lancet 1(8128):1234-1236, June 9, 1979.

Rudolf, M., et al.

Changes in arterial blood gases during and after a period of oxygen breathing in patients with chronic hypercapnic respiratory failure and in patients with asthma.

Clin. Sci. 57(5):389-396, Nov. 1979.

Ruediger, H. W., et al.

Metabolism and formation of DNA adducts of benzo(a)pyrene in human diploid fibroblasts.

Cancer Res. 39(3):1083-1088, Mar. 1979.

Ruff, W. L., et al.

Carcinoembryonic antigen in a black hospital population.

J. Natl. J. Med. 71(10):971-976, Oct. 1979.

Runge, R., et al.

Pancreatic ductulitis in Syrian golden hamsters bearing homologous transplantable pancreatic adenocarcinomas.

Cancer Lett. 5(4):225-229, Oct. 1978.

Rupp, M., et al.

Prognosi a breve e lungo termine dell'arresto circolatorio nell'infarto miocardico acuto. (Ital.)

Minerva Med. 69(27):1839-1845, May 31, 1978.

Russell, M. A. H., et al.

Effect of general practitioners' advice against smoking.

Br. Med. J. 2(6184):231-235, July 28, 1979.

Russell, M. A. H., et al.

Smokers' response to shortened cigarettes: Dose reduction without dilution of tobacco smoke.

Clin. Pharmacol. Ther. 27(2):210-218, Feb. 1980.

Russell, W.

Tougher curbs on smoking.

Br. Med. J. 208(6208):197, Jan. 19, 1980.

Russo, D. M. and Kaplan, H. L.

Effects of carbon monoxide on two behavioral measures in the rat.

Proc. West. Pharmacol. Soc. 21:419-425, 1978.

Russo, I. H. and Russo, J.

Devekionebtak stage of the rat mammary gland as determinant of its susceptibility to 7,12-dimethylbenz[a]anthracene.

JNCI 61(6):1439-1449, Dec. 1978.

Russo, J. and Russo, I. H.

DNA labelling index and structure of the rat mammary gland as determinants of its susceptibility to carcinogenesis.

JNCI 61(6):1451-1459, Dec. 1978.

Russo, J., et al.

Susceptibility of the mammary gland to carcinogenesis: I. Differentiation of the mammary gland as determination of tumor incidence and type of lesions.

Am. J. Pathol. 96(3):721-736, Sept. 1979.

Rutishauser, I. H. E., et al.

Long-term vitamin status and dietary intake of healthy elederly subjects: 1. Riboflavin.

Br. J. Nutr. 42(1):33-42, July 1979.

Rutstein, D. D., et al.

Mesure de la qualite des soins medicaux: Une methode clinique. (Fr.)

Concours Med. 100(42):6921-6939, Nov. 18, 1978.

Ruzicka, T., et al.

Effects of intravenous and intracutaneous bacillus Calmette-Guerin application on the drug metabolizing system of the liver.

Dermatologica 160(2):135-141, 1980.

Ryan, L. J. and Sharpless, S. K.

Genetically determined spontaneous and pentylenetetrazol-induced brief spindle episodes in mice.

Exp. Neurol. 66(3):493-508, Dec. 1979.

Sabadie, N., et al.

Comparison of the hydroxylation of benzo(a)pyrene with the metabolism of vinyl chloride, N-nitrosomorpholine, and N-nitroso-N'-methylpiperazine to mutagens by human and rat liver microsomal fractions.

Cancer Res. 40(1):119-126, Jan. 1980.

Sachs, L.

The differentiation of myeloid leukaemia cells: New possibilities for therapy.

Br. J. Haematol. 40(4):509-517, Dec. 1978.

Sackner, M. A., et al.

Effect of adrenergic agonists on tracheal mucous velocity.

Bull. Eur. Physiopathol. Respir. 15(3):505-511, 1979.

Sadeghi, A., et al.

Opium: A potential urinary bladder carcinogen in man.

Cancer 43(6):2344-2347, June 1979.

Saffran, W. A. and Gibson, Q. H.

The effect of temperature on carbon monoxide binding to a root effect hemoglobin.

J. Biol. Chem. 254(5):1666-1670, Mar. 10, 1979.

Sahley, T. L. and Bernston, G. G.

Antinociceptive effects of central and systemic administrations of nicotine in the rat.

Psychopharmacology (Berlin) 65(3):279-283, Nov. 1979.

Saine, S. E., et al.

Drug metabolism in the Novikoff hepatoma: Evidence for a mixed function oxidase system and partial purigication of cytochrome P-450 reductase.

Biochem. Biophys. Acta 526(2):345-358, Oct. 12, 1978.

Sakamoto, S., et al.

The behavior of 7,12-dimethylbenz(a)-anthracene (DMBA)-induced mammary tumours in rats during pregnancy and lactation and hormone levels in the pituitary and plasma. (Jpn.)

Folia Endocrinol. Jpn. 55(3):210-218, Mar. 20, 1979.

Sakuma, K., et al.

Asymptomatic Hyperglycemia and Coronary Heart Disease: Report on hyperglycemia in middle-aged male Japanese national railways workers.

J. Chronic Dis. 32(11/12):779-786, 1979.

Sakurai, M.

Influence of the skin temperature on the axon reflex pilomotion produced by nicotine in human skin.

Tohoku J. Exp. Med. 128(1):1-12, May 1979.

Salaman, J. R. and Miller, J. J.

Proceedings of the International Congress of the Transplantation Society: Nonspecific chemical immunosuppression.

Transplant. Proc. 11(1):845-850, Mar. 1979.

Salariya, E. M., et al.

Duration of breast-feeding after early initiation and frequent feeding.

Lancet 2(8100):1141-1143, Nov. 25, 1978.

Salo, M. K., et al.

Plasma lipids and lipoproteins in Down's syndrome.

Scand. J. Clin. Lab. Invest. 39(5): 485-490, Sept. 1979.

Salorinne, Y., et al.

Scandinavian Symposium on Chronic Obstructive Airways Disease: Ipratropium bromide and fenoterol in pulmonary tuberculosis.

Scand. J. Respir. Dis. Suppl. 103:183-185, 1979.

Saltiel, M. J.-C.

Les effets nocifs du tabac. (Fr.)

J. Med. Chir. Prat. 150(5):208-213, Mar. 1979.

Samet, J. M.

A historical and epidemiologic perspective on respiratory symptoms questionnaires.

Am. J. Epidemiol. 108(6):435-446, Dec. 1978.

Samuels, M. S., et al.

Overdose patterns: A five year study at Charity Hospital of Louisiana in New Orleans.

J. La. State Med. Soc. 131(3): 74-78, Mar. 1979.

Sanger, D. J.

Effects of d-amphetamine on temporal and spatial discrimination in rats.

Psychopharmacology 58(2):185-188, July 6, 1978.

Saniie, J., et al.

Real-time moment analysis of pulmonary nitrogen washout.

J. Appl. Physiol. 46(6):1184-1190, June 1979.

Saracci, R.

Aspects socio-economiques du cancer du poumon. (Fr.)

Schweiz. Med. Wochenschr. 109(22):820-824, June 2, 1979.

Sarantos-Laska, C., et al.

Facilitatory effect of nicotine on adrenergic neuroeffector transmission in the isolated ear artery of the rabbit.

J. Pharm. Pharmacol. 32(2):92-96, Feb. 1980.

Saravolatz, L. D., et al.

International Symposium on Legionnaires' Disease: The compromised host and Legionnaires' disease.

Ann. Intern. Med. 90(4):533-537, Apr. 1979.

Saric, M., et al.

Bronchoconstriction in potroom workers.

Br. J. Ind. Med. 36(3):211-215, Aug. 1979.

Sarles, H. and Crousillat, B.

Frequence des arteriopathies dans les pancreatites chroniques. (Fr.)

Gastroenterol. Clin. Biol. 2(10): 791-796, Oct. 1978.

Sarles, H., et al.

A multicenter inquiry into the etiology of pancreatic diseases.

Digestion 19(2):110-125, 1979.

Sarthy, P. V. and Lam, D. M. K.

The uptake and release of [3H]dopamine in the goldfish retina.

J. Neurochem. 32(4):1269-1277, Apr. 1979.

Sassa, S., et al.

Heme biosynthesis and drug metabolism in mice with hereditary hemolytic anemia: Heme oxygenase induction as an adaptive response for maintaining cytochrome P-450 in chronic hemolysis.

J. Biol. Chem. 254(3):729-735, Feb. 10, 1979.

Sastry, B. V. R. and Sadavongvivad, C.

Cholinergic systems in non-nervous tissues.

Pharmacol. Rev. 30(1):65-132, Mar. 1978.

Satake, T. and Arai, T.

Annual Meeting Symposium on Smoking and Cardiopulmonary Function: Effects of smoking on respiratory functions, especially with particular reference to normal Vmax values. (Jpn.)

Jpn. J. Thorac. Dis. 15(9):611-613, Sept. 1977.

Sato, S., et al.

Reduction in mutagenicity of cigarette smoke condensate by added sugars.

Mutat. Res. 60(2):155-161, Apr. 1979.

Sawicki, C. A. and Gibson, Q. H.

Biophysical Discussions. Fast Biochemical Reactions in Solutions, Membranes, and Cells: The relations between carbon monoxide binding and the conformational change of hemoglobin.

Biophys. J. 24(1):21-33, Oct. 1978.

Sawicki, C. A. and Gibson, Q. H.

A photochemical method for rapid and precise determination of carbon monoxide levels in blood.

Anal. Biochem. 94(2):440-449, Apr. 15, 1979.

Saxholm, H. J. K., et al.

Carcinogenesis testing of saccharin. No transformation or increased sister chromatid exchange observed in two mammalian cell system.

Eur. J. Cancer 15(4):509-513, Apr. 1979.

Saxholm, H. J. K.

The oncogenic potential of three different 7,12-dimethylbenz(a)anthracene transformed C3H/10T1/2 cell clones at various passages and the importance of the mode of immunosuppression.

Eur. J. Cancer 15(4):515-526, Apr. 1979.

Scally, M. C., et al.

Choline administration to the rat increases urinary catecholamines.

J. Neural Transm. 43(2):103-112, 1978.

Scarpelli, D. G., et al.

Activation of nitrosamines to mutagens by postmitochondrial fraction of hamster pancreas.

Cancer Res. 40(1):67-74, Jan. 1980.

Schaefer, H.

Rauchen als psychologisches und gesellschaftliches problem. (Ger.)

Bull. Schweiz. Akad. Med. Wiss. 35(1-3):15-23, Mar. 1979.

Schaer, B.

Problemes respiratoires lies a l'anesthesie et a l'acte chirurgical. (Fr.)

Rev. Med. Suisse Romande 99(1):15-18, Jan. 1979.

Schaer, M.

Praevention und ihre Moeglichkeiten: Erfolge der Praevention - Eine schweizerische Bestandesaufnahme. (Ger.)

Soz. Praventivmed. 23(5-6):327-331, Dec. 1978.

Schaer, M.

Das Institut fuer Sozial-und Praeventivmedizin der Universitaet Zuerich. (Ger.)

Soz. Praeventivmed. 24(4):267-268, Aug. 1979.

Schafer, A. I. and Handin, R. I.

The role of platelets in thrombotic and vascular disease.

Prog. Cardiovasc. Dis. 22(1):31-52, July/Aug. 1979.

Schenker, M. B.

Diesel exhaust - An occupational carcinogen?

JOM 22(1):41-46, Jan. 1980.

Scher, C. D., et al.

Platelet-derived growth factor prevents Go growth arrest.

Nature 281(5730):390-392, Oct. 4, 1979.

Scherrer, M., et al.

Entretiens de Physiopathologie Respiratoire: Les echanges gazeux pendant la phase de recuperation de l'effort chez des sujets asthmatiques. (Fr.)

Bull. Eur. Physiopathol. Respir. 15(2):379-383, 1979.

Schettler, G.

Die Aetiologie der Arteriosklerose. (Ger.)

Internist (Berlin) 19(11):611-620, Nov. 1978.

Schettler, G. and Greten, H.

Fettstoffwechselstoerungen in der Intensivmedizin: Klinische Aspekte und Diagnosemoeglichkeiten. (Ger.)

Intensivmedizin 15(3):91-95, May-June 1978.

Schievelbein, H.

Wissenschaft nicht mehr gefragt? Gedanken zu einem Antiraucher-Kongress. (Ger.)

MMW 121(34):1058-1059, Aug. 24,1979.

Schievelbein, H.

Workshop on Carbon Monoxide and Cardiovascular Disease: Evaluation of the role of carbon monoxide and nicotine in the pathogenesis of arteriosclerosis and cardiovascular disease.

Prev. Med. 8(3):379-389, May 1979.

Schilling, R. S. F., et al.

Breathing other people's smoke. (Letters to the Editor.)

Br. Med. J. 2(6141):895, Sept. 23, 1978.

Schimz, A. and Hildebrand, E.

Chemosensory responses of Halobacterium halobium.

J. Bacteriol. 140(3):749-753, Dec. 1979.

Schlager, S. I. and Ohanian, S. H.

A role for fatty acid composition of complex cellular lipids in the susceptibility of tumor cells to humoral immune killing.

J. Immunol. 123(1):146-152, July 1979.

Schlatter, J. and Baettig, K.

Differential effects of nicotine and amphetamine on locomotor activity and maze exploration in two rat lines.

Psychopharmacolgy (Berlin) 64(2):155-161, Aug. 8, 1979.

Schlesinger, M., et al.

Hyperlipoproteinemie de type V: 54 observations. (Fr.)

Nouv. Presse Med. 8(11):933-837, Mar. 10, 1979.

Schmaehl, D., et al.

Carcinogenesis of N-nitrosodiethylamine (DENA) in chickens and domestic cats.

Int. J. Cancer 22(5):552-557, Nov. 15, 1978.

Schmassmann, H., et al.

Epoxide hydratase and benzo(a)pyrene monooxygenase activities in liver, kidney and lung after treatment of rats with epoxides of widely varying structures.

Biochem. Pharmacol. 27(18):2237-2245, 1978.

Schmeltz, I., et al.

Comparison of the metabolic profiles of benzo[a]pyrene obtained from primary cell cultures and subcellular fractions derived from normal and methylcholanthrene-induced rat liver.

Cancer Lett. 5(2):81-89, Aug. 1978.

Schmeltz, I., et al.

Formation and determination of ethyl carbamate in tobacco and tobacco smoke.

J. Anal. Toxicol. 2(6):265-268, Nov.-Dec. 1978.

Schmidt. F.

Gesundheitsschaeden durch Rauchen. (Ger.)

Fortsch. Med. 97(10):V-VI, Mar. 15, 1979.

Schmidt, F.

Nikotinaufnahme beim Tabakschnupfen? (Ger.)

Med. Welt 30(7):263, Feb. 16, 1979.

Schmidt, F.

Tabakwarenreklame in der Oeffentlichkeit ist verfassungswidrig. (Ger.)

Fortsch. Med. 97(9):414-417, Mar. 8, 1979.

Schmidt, F.

Zwangsrauchen und Krebs. (Ger.)

Med. Klin. 74(51/52):1967-1973, Dec. 21, 1979.

Schmidt, W.

The Induction of Drug Metabolism: Greetings.

Symp. Med. Hoechst 14:1-2, 1979.

Schmoldt, A., et al.

Effects of inducers and inhibitors of rat liver mono-oxygenases on digitoxin metabolism.

Biochem. Pharmacol. 29(3):405-409, Feb. 1, 1980.

Schneeweiss, F., et al.

Cholinergic stimulants and excess potassium ion increase the fluidity of plasma membranes isolated from adrenal chromaffin cells.

Biochim. Biophys. Acta 555(3):460-471, Aug. 23, 1979.

Schneider, L. and Henrion, R.

Tabac et grossesse. (Fr.)

J. Gynecol. Obstet. Biol. Reprod. (Paris) 8(1):7-12, Jan. 1979.

Schneider, M., et al.

Clinical Application of Carcinoembryonic Antigen Assay: Carcinoembryonic antigen determinations in head and neck cancer.

Int. Congr. Ser. No. 439:384-388, 1978.

Schoenberg, B. S.

Neurological Epidemiology: Principles and Clinical Applications. Analytic, experimental, and theoretical epidemiology.

Adv. NuFob. 19:43-54, 1978.

Schoental, R., et al.

Cardiovascular lesions and various tumors found in rats given T-2 toxin, a trichothecene metabolite of Fusarium.

Cancer Res. 39(6, Part 1):2179-2189, June 1979.

Schottenfeld, D.

Proceedings of the American Cancer Society and National Cancer Institute National Conference on Nutrition in Cancer: Alcohol as a co-factor in the etiology of cancer.

Cancer 43(5, Suppl.):1962-1966, May 1979.

Schreiber, H., et al.

Bronchial metaplasia as a benign or premalignant lesion: I. Cytologic and ultrastructural discrimination between acute carcinogen effects and toxin-induced changes.

Acta Cytol. (Baltimore) 23(6):496-503, Nov.-Dec. 1979.

Schroll, M. and Hagerup, L.

Asymptomatic Hyperglycemia and Coronary Heart Disease: Relationship of fasting blood glucose to prevalence of ECG abnormalities and 10 yr. risk of mortality from cardiovascular diseases in men born in 1914: From the Glostrup Population Studies.

J. Chronic Dis. 32(11/12):699-707, 1979.

Schuder, S., et al.

Spectrophotometric determination of myoglobulin in cardiac and skeletal muscle: Separation from hemoglobin by subunit-exchange chromatography.

Anal. Biochem. 92(2):473-481, Jan. 15, 1979.

Schuettmann, W.

Die kombinierte Wirkung von ionisierender Strahlung und Rauchen bei der Verursachung des Lungenkrebses. (Ger.)

Z. Erkr. Atmungsorgane 150(3):243-249, 1978.

Schulte, B. P. M., et al.

Cerebral Vascular Disease 2: A retrospective and follow-up study of carotid endarterectomy in the treatment of ischemic brain disease.

I. C. S. No. 449:301-312, 1979.

Schumann, C. B. and Colon, V. F.

Sputum cytology.

Am. Fam. Physician 19(4):81-84, Apr. 1979.

Schwalb, H. and Strobl, G.

Sport und kardiale Risikofaktoren im mittleren Lebensalter. (Ger.)

Med. Klin. 73(35):1203-1208, Sept. 1, 1978.

Schwartz, A. G.

Inhibition of spontaneous breast cancer formation in female C3H (Avy/a) mice by long-term treatment with dehydroepiandrosterone.

Cancer Res. 39(3):1129-1132, Mar. 1979.

Schwartz, A. G. and Moore, C. J.

Inverse correlation between species life span and capacity of cultured fibroblasts to metabolize polycyclic hydrocarbon carcinogens.

Fed. Proc. 38(6):1989-1992, May 1979.

Schwartz, J. L.

Review and evaluation of methods of smoking cessation, 1969-77: Summary of a monograph.

Public Health Rep. 94(6):558-563, Nov.-Dec. 1979.

Schwartz, S. L.

Smoking and health.

Georgetown Med. Bull. 32(1):14-20, Aug. 1978.

Schwarz, M., et al.

DNA damage induced in vivo evaluated with a non-radioactive alakaline elution technique.

Cancer Lett. 6(4-5):221-226, Apr. 1979.

Schweinsberg, F., et al.

Metabolism of isomeric N-methyl-N-nitroso-(Methylphenyl)-methylamines.

Cancer Lett. 8(2):125-132, Dec. 1979.

Schwerd, W. and Schulz, E.

Carboxyhaemoglobin and methaemoglobin findings in burnt bodies.

Forensic Sci. 12(3):233-235, Nov.-Dec. 1978.

Schwetz, B. A., et al.

Teratogenic potential of inhaled carbon monoxide in mice and rabbits.

Teratology 19(3):385-391, June 1979.

Sclesi, R., et al.

Bacillus of Calmette and Guerin and 7,12-dimethylbenz(alpha)-anthracene carcinogenesis in mice.

Tumori 64(4):353-360, Aug. 31, 1978.

Scott, A.-M., et al.

Synthesis of DNA and lecithin in tissue culture and oestrogen receptor activity in rat mammary tumours dependent on and independent of the ovary.

J. Endocrinol. 81(2):183-198, May 1979.

Scott, C. C., et al.

Metabolism of ether-linked glycerolipids in cultures of normal and neoplastic rat respiratory tract epithelium.

Cancer Res. 39(1):207-214, Jan. 1979.

Scott, J. and Poffenbarger, P. L.

Pharmacogenetics of tolbutamide metabolism in humans.

Diabetes 28(1):41-51, Jan. 1979.

Scott, P. P.

Food additives and contaminants.

Practitioner 222(1331):648-655, May 1979.

Scully, R. E., (Editor)

Normal reference laboratory values.

N. Engl. J. Med. 302(1):37-48, Jan. 3, 1980.

Seagren, S. L.

A detailed guide to managing the patient with lung cancer.

Med. Times 107(5):31-38, May 1979.

Sedlak, J., et al.

Prevention, diagnosis and treatment of carbon monoxide poisoning in an East-Slovakian iron works.

Resuscitation 6(3):155-161, 1978.

Seffrin, J. R., et al.

A state-wide survey of hospital policy and practice concerning cigarette sales.

Am. Rev. Respir. Dis. 118(6):1105-1107, Dec. 1978.

Seftel, H. C.

The first published chemical analyses of smoke from South African cigarettes.

S. Afr. Med. J. 55(19): 743-748, May 5, 1979.

Seif, S. M. and Robinson, A. G.

Localization and release of neurophysins.

Ann. Rev. Physiol. 40:345-376, 1978.

Seitz, H. K., et al.

Effect of chronic ethanol ingestion on intestinal metabolism and mutagenicity of benzo(alpha)pyrene.

Biochem. Biophys. Res. Commun. 85(3): 1061-1066, Dec. 14, 1978.

Seixas, F. A.

Drug/alcohol interactions: Avert potential dangers.

Geriatrics 34(10):89-102, Oct. 1979.

Sekine, K., et al.

The prediction equations and the normal limits of the parameters of MEFV curve using a direct writing flow-volume curve recorder.(Jpn.)

Jpn. J. Thorac. Dis. 16(6):428-434, June 1978.

Sekiya, S., et al.

Effect on ovariectomy, adrenalectomy, and hypophysectomy on carcinogenesis of the endometrium by 7,12-dimethylbenz[a]anthracene in rats.

Gynecol. Oncol. 7(3):281-287, June 1979.

Sekiya, S., et al.

In vivo and in vitro studies of experimental ovarian adenocarcinoma in rats.

Cancer Res. 39(3):1108-1112, Mar. 1979.

Seliger, V., et al.

Activity pattern, smoking habits, and somatometric variables of the Czechoslovakian population.

Eur. J. Appl. Physiol. 39(3):165-171, Sept. 15, 1978.

Sellars, S. L.

Symposium on Malignant Disease of the Oral Cavity and Related Structures: Epidemiology of oral cancer.

Otolaryngol. Clin. North Am. 12(1): 45-55, Feb. 1979.

Selmonosky, C. A. and Byrd, R.

Pulmonary function tests in a community hospital.

South. Med. J. 72(8):946-949, Aug. 1979.

Seltzer, C. C.

The absence of excess coronary heart disease among the elderly in the continuation of cigarette smoking: A reply.

Am. J. Med. Sci. 276(2):185-187, Sept.-Oct. 1978.

Selvester, R., et al.

The Marathon: Physiological, Medical, Epidemiological, and Psychological Studies. Effects of exercise training on progression of documented coronary arteriosclerosis in men.

Ann. NY Acad. Sci. 301:495-508, 1977.

Semple, P. d'A

Alpha-1-antitrypsin deficiency and chest disease: A clinical and physiological study.

Scott. Med. J. 23(4):281-285, Oct. 1978.

Senft, D., et al.

Lipidsenkung bei gleichzeitig niedriger Substanzbelastung: Erfahrungen aus einer Gemeinschaftspraxis. (Ger.)

Med. Welt 29(38):1499-1502, Sept. 22, 1978.

Senties, R., et al.

Informacion sobre tabaquismo a la ninez: Report preliminar. (Span.)

Neumol. Cir. Torax 39(4):265-277, June 17, 1978.

Seppaelaeinen, A. M.

Tyoeympaeristoen neurotoksiset kemialliset tekijaet. (Finn.)

Duodecim 94(14-15):915-927, 1978.

Serebriakova, I. K.

Significance of some "risk factors" in development of myocardial infarction. (Russ.)

Zh. Eksp. Klin. Med.18(6):65-68, 1978.

Sershen, H. and Lajtha, A.

The effect of nicotine on the metabolism of brain proteins.

Neuropharmacology 18(10):763-766, Oct. 1979.

Sershen, H. and Lajtha, A.

Cerebral uptake of nicotine and of amino acids.

J. Neurosci. Res. 4(2):85-91, 1979.

Seshia, S. S., et al.

Coma following cardiorespiratory arrest in childhood.

Dev. Med. Child Neurol. 21(2):143-153, Apr. 1979.

Sessa, T., et al.

Influence de l'habitude de fumer chez des ouvriers exposes a la pollution du milieu ambiant. (Fr.)

Bronchopneumologie 28(3):195-204, May-June 1978.

Setchell, B. P. and Main, S. J.

Drugs and the blood-testis barrier.

Environ. Health Perspect. 24:61-64, June 1978.

Sevitt, S.

A review of the complications of burns, their origin and importance for illness and death.

J. Trauma 19(5):358-369, May 1979.

Shafie, S. M., et al.

Cyclic adenosine 3':5'-monophosphate and protein kinase activity in insulin-dependent and -independent mammary tumors.

Cancer Res. 39(7, Part 1):2501-2504, July 1979.

Shamberger, R. J., et al.

Antioxidants reduce the mutagenic effect of malonaldehyde and beta-propiolactone. Part IX, antioxidants and cancer.

Mutat. Res. 66(4):349-355, Apr. 1979.

Shapiro, A. P., et al.

Five-year findings of the Hypertension Detection and Follow-up Program: II. Mortality by race-sex and age.

JAMA 242(23):2572-2577, Dec. 7, 1979.

Shapiro, A. P., et al.

Five-year findings of the Hypertension Detection and Follow-up Program: 1. Reduction in mortality of persons with high blood pressure, including mild hypertension.

JAMA 242(23):2562-2571, Dec. 7, 1979.

Shapiro, S., et al.

Oral-contraceptive use in relation to myocardial infarction.

Lancet 1(8119):743-747, Apr. 7, 1979.

Shapiro, S., et al.

Oral-contraceptive use in relation to myocardial infarction.

Obstet. Gynecol. Surv. 34(9):691-693, Sept. 1979.

Sharpe, I. K. and Tomashefski, J. F.

The physician's role in the evaluation of disability due to pulmonary disease.

Clin. Notes Respir. Dis. 17(4):3-12, Spring 1979.

Sharratt, M. T. and Cerny, F. J.

Pulmonary function and health status of children in two cities of different air quality: A pilot study.

Arch. Environ. Health 34(2):114-119, Mar.-Apr. 1979.

Shatton, J. B., et al.

Creatine kinase activity and isozyme composition in normal tissues and neoplasms of rats and mice.

Cancer Res. 39(2, Part 1):492-501, Feb. 1979.

Shaw, C. R. and Leal, N.

Proceedings of a Conference on the Relationship between Environmental Chemicals and Cancer: How do we know what causes cancer.

Tex. Rep. Biol. Med. 37:21-25, 1978.

Shaw, H. M., et al.

Effect of smoking on the recurrence of malignant melanoma.

Med. J. Aust. 1(6):208-209, Mar. 24, 1979.

Shearman, G. and Lal, H.

Discriminative stimulus properties of pentylenetetrazol and bemegride: Some generalization and antagonism tests.

Psychopharmacology (Berlin) 64(3):315-319, Sept. 1979.

Sheehan, A. J. and Shaw, H. J.

Total laryngectomy for squamous carcinoma of the glottis.

J. Laryngol. Otol. 93(5):461-475, May 1979.

Shehata, W.

Carcinoma of the oesophagus.

IMJ 155(4):215-217, Apr. 1979.

Shelley, E., et al.

Farmer's lung: A study in North-West Ireland.

Ir. Med. J. 72(5):261-264, June 30, 1979.

Shen, A. L., et al.

Inhibition of benzo(a)pyrene and benzo(a)pyrene 7,8-dihydrodiol metabolism by benzo(a)pyrene quinones.

Cancer Res. 39(10):4123-4129, Oct. 1979.

Shepard, R. J. and Labarre, R.

Attitudes of the public towards cigarette smoking in public places.

Can. J. Public Health 69(4):302-310, July-Aug. 1978.

Shepard, R. J., et al.

Effects of cigarette smoking on intraocular pressure and vision.

Br. J. Ophthalmol. 62(10):682-687, Oct. 1978.

Shephard, R. J.

Recurrence of myocardial infarction in an exercising population.

Br. Heart J. 42(2):133-138, Aug. 1979.

Shephard, R. J., et al.

Effect of cigarette smoke on the eyes and airway.

Int. Arch. Occup. Environ. Health 43(2):135-144, Apr. 20, 1979.

Sheps, D. S., et al.

Resting peripheral blood lactate elevation in survivors of prehospital cardiac arrest: Correlation with hemodynamic, electrophysiologic and oxyhemoglobin dissociation indexes.

Am. J. Cardiol. 44(7):1276-1282, Dec. 1979.

Sherwin, R. P., et al.

Silicate pneumoconiosis of farm workers.

Lab. Invest. 40(5):576-582, May 1979.

Sherwood Burge, P., et al.

Occupational asthma in an electronics factory.

Thorax 34(1):13-18, Feb. 1979.

Sheveleva, G. A. and Lukiyanova, L. V.

On the effect of 3,4-benzpyrene on the development of the fetus applied at different periods of gestation. (Russ.)

Gig. Tr. Prof. Zabol. No. 7:54, July 1978.

Shiau, Y.-Y. and Kwan, H.-W.

Submucous fibrosis in Taiwan.

Oral Surg. 47(5):453-457, May 1979.

Shim, C., et al.

Response to corticosteroids in chronic bronchitis.

J. Allergy Clin. Immunol. 62(6):363-367, Dec. 1978.

Shimada, T. And Sato, R.

Inhibition of mono-oxygenase activities by 1,1,1-trichloropropene 2,3-oxide, an inhibitor of epoxide hydrase, in rat liver microsomes.

Biochem. Pharmacol. 28(11): 1771-1781, June 1, 1979.

Shimizu, H., et al.

Diphenylhydantoin as an inducer for mutation test. (Jpn.)

Jpn. J. Ind. Health 19(4):202-203, July 1977.

Shimkin, M. B.

In the middle: 1954-63 - Historical note.

JNCI 62(5):1295-1317, May 1979.

Shinozuka, H., et al.

Effects of a choline-devoid diet on the emergence of gamma-glutamyltrans-peptidase-positive foci and the liver of carcinogen-treated rats.

Cancer Res. 39(7, Part 1):2515-2521, July 1979.

Shiraishi, Y. and Sandberg, A. A.

Effects of various chemical agents on sister chromatid exchanges, chromosome aberrations, and DNA repair in normal and abnormal human lymphoid cell lines.

JNCI 62(1):27-35, Jan. 1979.

Shor, R. E. and Williams, D. C.

A brief survey of beliefs about the effects of tobaccco smoke pollution on intellectual performance in college classrooms.

Psychol. Rep. 43(3, Part 2):1047-1050, Dec. 1978.

Shore, R. E., et al.

A case-control study of hair dye use and breast cancer.

JNCI 62(2):277-283, Feb. 1979.

Shoyab, M.

Dose-dependent preferential binding of polycyclic aromatic hydrocarbons to reiterated DNA of murine skin cells in culture.

Proc. Natl. Acad. Sci. USA 75(12):5841-5845, Dec. 1978.

Shoyab, M.

Caffeine inhibits the binding of dimethylbenz(a)anthracene to murine epidermal cells DNA in culture.

Arch. Biochem. Biophys. 196(1):307-310, Aug. 1979.

Shoyab, M.

Binding of polycyclic aromatic hydrocarbons to DNA of cells in culture: A rapid method for its analysis using hydroxylapatite column chromatography.

Chem. Biol. Interact. 25(1):71-85, Apr. 1979.

Shu, H. P. and Nichols, A. V.

Benzo(a)pyrene uptake by human plasma lipoproteins in vitro.

Cancer Res. 39(4):1224-1230, Apr. 1979.

Shubik, P.

Proceedings of the American Cancer Society and National Cancer Institute National Conference on Nutrition in Cancer: Food additives (natural and synthetic).

Cancer 43(5, Suppl.):1982-1986, May 1979.

Shuler, C. F. and Latt, S. A.

Sister chromatid exchange induction resulting from systemic, topical, and systemic-topical presentations of carcinogens.

Cancer Res. 39(7, Part 1):2510-2514, July 1979.

Sidransky, H. and Verney, E.

Effect of inhibitory and stimulator agents on protein synthesis in hepatomas and host livers of rats.

JNCI 63(1):81-87, July 1979.

Sieber, M. and Angst, J.

Risikofaktoren fuer starkes Zigaretten-rauchen bei jungen Maennern: Eine Langsschnittuntersuchung. (Ger.)

Schweiz. Med. Wochenschr. 109(4):115-122, Jan. 27, 1979.

Siemann, D. W., et al.

Smoking: The influence of carboxy-hemoglobin (HbCO) on tumor oxygenation and response to radiation.

Int. J. Radiat. Oncol. Biol. Phys. 4(7-8):657-662, July-Aug. 1978.

Sifontes, J. E.

Los effectos del cigarrillo. (Span.)

Bol. Asoc. Med. P.R. 71(5):169-173, May 1979.

Sigurdsson, G.

Aedakoelkun og ahaettuthaettir: Yfirlitsgrein. (Icelandic)

Laeknabladid 64(2):65-82, Apr. 1978.

Silbert, N. E. and Dudani, N.

Epidemiology of respiratory allergic disorders in a geriatric age group.

Ann. Allergy 43(1):26-31, July 1979.

Sillett, R. W., et al.

Deception among smokers.

Br. Med. J. 2(6146):1185-1186, Oct. 28, 1978.

Silvestre, A., et al.

Abnormal electrocardiographic responses to exercise patients referred for noninvasive evaluation of occlusive peripheral arterial disease.

Am. J. Cardiol. 43(4):713-716, Apr. 1979.

Simberg, N. and Uotila, P.

Stimulatory effect of cigarette smoke on the metabolism and covalent binding of benzo(a)pyrene in the trachea of the rat.

Int. J. Cancer 22(1):28-31, July 15, 1978.

Simmon, V. F.

In vitro assays for recombinogenic activity of chemical carcinogens and related compounds with Saccharomyces cerevisiae D3.

JNCI 62(4):901-909, Apr. 1979.

Simmon, V. F.

In vitro mutagenicity assays of chemical carcinogens and related compounds with Salmonella typhimurium.

JNCI 62(4):893-899, Apr. 1979.

Simmon, V. F., et al.

Mutagenic activity of chemical carcinogens and related compounds in the intraperitoneal host-mediated assay.

JNCI 62(4):911-918, Apr. 1979.

Simons, L. A. and Jones, A. S.

Coronary risk factor screening and long-term follow up: Year 1 of the Sydney Coronary Heart Disease Prevention Programme.

Med. J. Aust. 2(10):455-458, Nov. 4, 1978.

Simons, P. J., et al.

Squamous lesions in lungs of rats exposed to tobacco-smoke-condensate fractions by repeated intratracheal instillation.

Br. J. Cancer 37(6):965-973, June 1978.

Sims, P.

The metabolic activation of chemical carcinogens.

Br. Med. Bull. 36(1):11-18, Jan. 1980.

Sinclair, G. E.

Diagnosing hiatus hermia.

Can. Fam. Physician 24:1015-1017, Oct. 1978.

Sindelar, R. D., et al.

N-Demethylation of nicotine and reduction of nicotine-1'-N-oxide by Microsporum gypseum.

Appl. Environ. Microbiol. 38(5):836-839, Nov. 1979.

Sine, S. and Taylor, P.

Functional consequences of agonist-mediated state transitions in the cholinergic recpetor: Studies in cultured muscle cells.

J. Biol. Chem. 254(9):3315-3325, May 10, 1979.

Singer, B.

N-nitroso alkylating agents: Formation and persistence of alkyl derivatives in mammalian nucleic acids as contributing factors in carcinogenesis.

JNCI 62(6):1329-1339, June 1979.

Singer, G., et al.

Schedule induced self injections of nicotine with recovered body weight.

Pharmacol. Biochem. Behav. 9(3):387-389, Sept. 1978.

Sipahi, N.

Gastrointestinal kanalin malign tumorlerinde karsinoembriyonik antijenin (CEA) tani degeri. (Turk.)

Tip. Farm. Mecm. 30(Suppl. 112):3-23, 1977.

Sirica, A. E., et al.

Definition of stages during hepatocarcinogenesis in the rat: Potential application to the evaluation of initiating and promoting agents in the environment.

J. Environ. Pathol. Toxicol. 2(1):21-28, Sept.-Oct. 1978.

Sirtori, C., et al.

Mutagenic substances as possible senility factors.

Pharmacol. Res. Commun. 10(9):809-812, Oct. 1978.

Sithichoke, N. and Marotta, S. F.

Cholinergic influences on hypothalamic-pituitary-adrenocortical activity of stressed rats: An approach utilizing agonists and antagonists.

Acta Endocrinol. (Kbh.) 89(4):726-736, Dec. 1978.

Sivarajah, K., et al.

Metabolism of benzo(a)pyrene to reactive intermediate(s) via prostaglandin biosynthesis.

Life Sci. 23(26):2571-2578, Dec. 25, 1978.

Sjoeberg, L. and Johnson, T.

Trying to give up smoking: A study of volitional breakdowns.

Addict. Behav. 3(3-4):149-164, 1978.

Skaare, J. U. and Nafstad, I.

Interaction of vitamin E and selenium with the hepatotoxic agent dimethylnitrosamine.

Acta Pharmacol. Toxicol. (Kbh.) 43(2):119-128, Aug. 1978.

Skopek, T. R., et al.

Mutation of human cells by kerosene soot.

JNCI 63(2):309-312, Aug. 1979.

Sladek, C. D. and Joynt, R. J.

Angiotensin stimulation of vasopressin release from the rat hypothalamo-neurohypophyseal system in organ culture.

Endocrinology 104(1):148-153, Jan. 1979.

Sladek, C. D. and Joynt, R. J.

Characterization of cholinergic control of vasopressin release by the organ-cultured rat hypothalamo-neurohypophyseal system.

Endocrinology 104(3):659-663, Mar. 1979.

Sladek, C. D. and Joynt, R. J.

Role of angiotensin in the osmotic control of vasopressin release by the organ-cultured rat hypothalamo-neurohypophyseal system.

Endocrinology 106(1):173-178, Jan. 1980.

Slaga, T. J.

Carcinogenesis study of benzo[e]pyrene in mice.

Tox Tips No. 32:11-12, Jan. 1979.

Slaga, T. J.

Carcinogenesis study of dibenz[a,h]-anthracene in mice.

Tox Tips No. 32:15-16, Jan. 1979.

Slaga, T. J., et al.

The effects of weak or non-carcinogenic polycyclic hydrocarbons on 7, 12-dimethylbenz[a]anthracene and benzo[a]pyrene skin tumor-initiation.

Cancer Lett. 7(1):51-59, June 1979.

Slaga, T. J., et al.

In vitro transformation of epidermal cells from newborn mice.

Cancer Res. 38(8):2246-2252, Aug. 1978.

Slaga, T. J., et al.

Lack of involvement of 6-hydroxymethylation in benzo[a]pyrene skin tumor initiation in mice.

JNCI 61(2):451-455, Aug. 1978.

Slaga, T. J., et al.

Marked differences in the skin tumor-initiating activities of the optical enantiomers of the diastereomeric benzo(a)-pyrene 7,8-diol-9,10-epoxides.

Cancer Res. 39(1):67-71, Jan. 1979.

Slaga, T. J., et al.

Potent tumor-initiating activity of the 3,4-dihydrodiol of 7,12-dimethyl-benz(a)anthracene in mouse skin.

Cancer Res. 39(6, Part 1):1934-1936, June 1979.

Slaga, T. J., et al.

The importance of the 'Bay Region' diol-epoxide in 7,12-dimethylbenz[a]anthracene skin tumor initiation and mutagenesis.

Cancer Lett. 6(4-5):213-220, Apr. 1979.

Slagle, D. J.

Tobacco.

J. Tenn. Med. Assoc. 72(2):127;129, Feb. 1979.

Sliwinski, S.

Niektore uwagi dotyczace szkodliwego wplywu dymu nikotynowego na narzad oddechowy. (Pol).

Wiad. Lek. 32(7):479-481, Apr. 1, 1979.

Smaldone, G. C., et al.

Effect of flow-limiting segments and cough on particle deposition and mucociliary clearance in the lung.

Am. Rev. Respir. Dis. 120(4):747-758, Oct. 1979.

Small, W. P. and Tucker, L.

The smoking habits of hospital nurses.

Nurs. Times 74(46):1878-1879, Nov. 16, 1978.

Smidt, U.

Problems and results in the simultaneous assessment of the role of smoking and occupational dust exposure for chronic bronchitis and pulmonary emphysema.

Bronchopneumologie 28(3):177-185, May-June 1978.

Smith, B. R. and Bend, J. R.

Metabolism and excretion of benzo(a)pyrene 4,5-oxide by the isolated perfused rat liver.

Cancer Res. 39(6, Part 1):2051-2056, June 1979.

Smith, B. R. and Bend, J. R.

Metabolism and toxicity of benzo(a)-pyrene-4,5-oxide in the isolated perfused rat liver.

Toxicol. Appl. Pharmacol. 49(2): 313-321, June 30, 1979.

Smith, B. R., et al.

Characterization of pulmonary arene oxide biotransformation using the perfused rabbit lung.

Cancer Res. 40(1):101-106, Jan. 1980.

Smith, E. M.

Epidemiology of oral and pharyngeal cancers in the United States: Review of recent literature.

JNCI 63(5):1189-1198, Nov. 1979.

Smith, E. R.

Epidemiology of gastrointestinal disorders.

Can. Fam. Physician 24:1007-1010, Oct. 1978.

Smith, G. H., et al.

Chemical carcinogenesis in C3H/StWi mice, a worthwhile experimental model for breast cancer.

Cancer Res. 38(12):4504-4509, Dec. 1978.

Smith, G. H., et al.

Chemical carcinogenesis in C3H/StWi mice, a worthwhile experimental model for breast cancer.

Cancer Res. 38(12):4504-4509, Dec. 1978.

Smith, G. J., et al.

Increased sensitivity for detection of carcinogen-induced DNA repair with the chain terminator dideoxythymidine.

Biochem. Biophys. Res. Commun. 83(4):1538-1544, Aug. 29, 1978.

Smith, I. A., et al.

Relationships between carcinogenicity and theoretical reactivity indices in polycyclic aromatic hydrocarbons.

Cancer Res. 38(9):2968-2977, Sept. 1978.

Smith, R. J., (Chairman) et al.

Smoking and health: Council on scientific affairs.

JAMA 243(8):779-781, Feb. 22/29. 1980.

Smith, S. A., et al.

Inhibition of hepatic gluconeogenesis by tryptophan metabolites in rats and guinea pigs.

Biochem. Pharmacol. 28(14):2145-2148, July 15, 1979.

Smith, S. E., et al.

Pupillary signs in diabetic autonomic neuropathy.

Br. Med. J. 2(6142):924-927, Sept. 30, 1978.

Smulevich, V. B., et al.

Epidemiology of malignant tumors in occupational groups: Methods and peculiarities of study.

JOM 21(1):11-14, Jan. 1979.

Snider, G. L. and Proppe, K. H.

Pulmonary infiltrates in a 42-year-old man.

N. Engl. J. Med. 299(12):644-650, Sept. 21, 1978.

Snyder, S. H.

Receptors, neurotransmitters and drug responses.

N. Engl. Med. J. 300(9):465-472, Mar. 1, 1979.

Soares de Moura, R., et al.

Effect of strophantin on the isolated guinea-pig ileum.

Arch. Int. Pharmacodyn. Ther. 239(1):45-51, May 1979.

Soffer, A.

You've regressed a long way, baby. (Editorial)

Arch. Intern. Med. 138(12):1779, Dec. 1978.

Sohji, Y., et al.

Pharmacological studies of loperamide, an anti-diarrheal agent. III. Interaction between loperamide and various agonists in the guinea pig intestine. (Jpn.)

Folia Pharmacol. Jpn. 74(2):213-223, Mar. 1978.

Sokolowski, J. W. and Harrer, W. V.

Desquamative interstitial pneumonia associated with normal chest film.

Postgrad. Med. 66(2):135-136, Aug. 1979.

Solbakken, J. E., et al.

Urinary and biliary metabolites of phenanthrene in the coalfish (Pollachius virens).

Acta Pharmacol. Toxicol. (Copenh.) 46(2):127-132, Feb. 1980.

Soldatos, C. R., et al.

Cigarette smoking associated with sleep difficulty.

Science 207(4430):551-553, Feb. 1, 1980.

Sole, M. J., et al.

The extraction of circulating catecholamines by the lungs in normal man and in patients with pulmonary hypertension.

Circulation 60(1):160-163, July 1979.

Solomon, A., et al.

Brochogenic carcinoma with coexisting active pulmonary tuberculosis in urban blacks.

S. Afr. Med. J. 55(24):979-981, June 9, 1979.

Somogyi, E., et al.

Ultrastructural examination of blood dialysate effects in experimental carbon monoxide poisoning of the heart muscle.

Arzneim. Forsch. 28(11):2070-2075, 1978.

Son, O. S., et al.

2-Acetylaminofluorene metabolism in rat liver microsomes: Formation of 9-hydroxy-2-acetylaminofluorene and effect of hepatic enzyme modifiers.

Toxicol. Appl. Pharmacol. 51(2): 367-377, Nov. 1979.

Sonnenberg, A., et al.

Rezidivprophylaxe des Ulcus duodeni mit Cimetidin. (Ger.)

Dtsch. Med. Wochenschr. 104(20):725-730, May 18, 1979.

Soorae, A. and Gibbons, J. R. P.

Primary oat cell carcinoma of the trachea.

Thorax 34(1):130-131, Feb. 1979.

Spector, S. L.

Use of provocation techniques for the evaluation of drug efficacy.

J. Allergy Clin. Immunol. 64(6, Part 2): 677-684, Dec. 1979.

Speizer, F. E., et al.

Respiratory disease rates and pulmonary function in children associated with NO2 exposure.

Am. Rev. Respir. Dis. 121(1):3-10, Jan. 1980.

Spicer, J., et al.

Distributions and interrelations of coronary risk factors in community sample of Auckland men.

Aust. NZ J. Med. 9(2):158-169, Apr. 1979.

Spiegelhalder, B., et al.

Contamination of beer with trace quantities of n-nitrosodimethylamine.

Food Cosmet. Toxicol. 17(1):29-31, Feb. 1979.

Spiliopoulos, A., et al.

Les carcinomes bronchiques au stade occulte: A propos de 3 observations. (Fr.)

Med. Hyg. 36(1292):2349-2353, June 21, 1978.

Spira, A. and Lazar, P.

Spontaneous abortions in sibship of children with congenital malformation or malignant disease.

Eur. J. Obstet. Gynecol. Reprod. Biol. 9(2):89-95, Apr. 2, 1979.

Spitzer, S. A., et al.

The effect of thymic humoral factor (THF) in sarcoidosis: Report of a case.

Ann. Allergy 43(3):193-196, Sept. 1979.

Spohr, U., et al.

Evaluation of smoking-induced effects on sympathetic, hemodynamic and metabolic variables with respect to plasma nicotine and COHb levels.

Atherosclerosis 33(3):271-283, July 1979.

Spooner, C. M.

Asbestos in schools - A public health problem.

N. Engl. J. Med. 301(14):782-784, Oct. 4, 1979.

St. Onge, L. M., et al.

Improved determination of phenobarbital, primidone, and phenytoin by use of a preparative instrument for extraction, followed by gas chromatography.

Clin. Chem. 25(8):1373-1376, Aug. 1979.

Staahle, I. and Tibbling, L.

Tobaksallergi hos patienter med asthma bronchiale. (Swed.)

Lakartidningen 75(17):1711-1713, Apr. 26, 1978.

Stableforth, D. E.

Lung function in alpha-1-antitrypsin deficient sisters.

Br. J. Dis. Chest 72(2):125-130, Apr. 1978.

Stadnicki, S. S., et al.

DNA single strand breaks caused by 2,2',5,5'-tetrachlorobiphenyl and its metabolites.

Res. Commun. Chem. Pathol. Pharmacol. 24(2):313-327, May 1979.

Stamler, J.

Mild Hypertension: To Treat or Not to Treat. Hypertension, blood lipids, and cigarette smoking as co-risk factors for coronary heart disease: Discussion.

Ann. NY Acad. Sci. 304:140-143, 1978.

Stamler, J.

Research related to risk factors.

Circulation 60(7):1575-1587, Dec. 1979.

Stamler, R. and Stamler, J.

Asymptomatic Hyperglycemia and Coronary Heart Disease: A series of papers by the international collaborative group, based on studies in fifteen populations.

J. Chronic Dis. 32(11/12):683-691, 1979.

Stamler, R., et al.

Asymptomatic Hyperglycemia and Coronary Heart Disease: Asymptomatic hyperglycemia and coronary heart disease in middle-aged men in two employed populations in Chicago.

J. Chronic Dis. 32(11/12):805-815, 1979.

Stamler, R., et al.

Asymptomatic Hyperglycemia and Coronary Heart Disease: Relationship of glucose tolerance to prevalence of ECG abnormalities and to 5-year mortality from cardiovascular disease: Findings of the chicago heart association detection project in industry.

J. Chronic Dis. 32(11/12):817-828, 1979.

Stanhope, J. M.

Social patterns of adolescent cigarette smoking in a rural community.

N.Z. Med. J. 87(612):343-348, May 24, 1978.

Stanhope, J. M., et al.

Asthma and wheeze in New Zealand adolescents.

NZ Med. J. 90(645):279-282, Oct. 10, 1979.

Stanton, M. F., et al.

Coffee and cola beverage consumption as heart disease risk factors in men.

Experientia 34(9):1182-1183, Sept. 15, 1978.

Stanulovic, D. (Moderator), et al.

Pusenje i zdravlje (usmerena diskusija). (Ser.)

Med. Pregl. 31(9-10):389-402, 1978.

Starke, K. and Weitzell, R.

Is histamine involved in the sympathomimetic effect of nicotine?

Naunyn Schmiedebergs Arch. Pharmacol. 304(3):237-248, Oct. 16, 1978.

Staugaard, F.

Foersoek med haelsoundervisning baserad paa riktad haelsokontroll. (Swed.)

Nord. Med. 93(11-12):287-288, Dec. 1978.

Steele, V. E., et al.

Transformation of rat tracheal epithelial cells by benzo[a]pyrene and its metabolites.

Cancer Lett. 8(4):291-298, Feb. 1980.

Stefanis, C.

The International Challenge of Drug Abuse: Biological aspects of cannabis use.

Natl. Inst. Drug Abuse Res. Monogr. Ser. 19:149-178, 1978.

Stegeman, J. J. and Binder, R. L.

High benzo[a]pyrene hydroxylase activity in the marine fish Stenotomus versicolor.

Biochem. Pharmacol. 28(10): 1686-1688, May 15, 1979.

Stegeman, J. J., et al.

Hepatic and extrahepatic microsomal electron transport components and mixed-function oxygenases in the marine fish Stenotomus versicolor.

Biochem. Pharmacol. 28(23):3431-3439, Dec. 1, 1979.

Stein, Z., et al.

Prenatal nutrition and birth weight: Experiments and quasi-experiments in the past decade.

J. Reprod. Med. 21(5):287-297, Nov. 1978.

Steinbrueck, P.

Informationen zum Problem Rauchen und Gesundheit. (Ger.)

Z. Erkr. Atmungsorgane 150(2):206-209, 1978.

Steiner, M. R., et al.

Differential response to cultured mouse mammary cells of varying tumorigenicity of cytochalasin B.

Cancer Res. 38(9):2719-2721, Sept. 1978.

Steinmetz, J., et al.

Factors affecting the concentration of triacylglycerols (triglycerides) in plasma: Reference values for adults.

Clin. Chem. 25(6):924-932, June 1979.

Steinmetz, J., et al.

Personal and familial factors in cholesterolemia: Criteria for selection of a reference population.

Clin. Chem. 26(2):219-226, Feb. 1980.

Stellman, J. M.

The effects of toxic agents on reproduction.

Occup. Health Saf. 48(3):36-43, Apr. 1979.

Stembaeck, F.

Life history and histopathology of ultraviolet light-induced skin tumors.

Natl. Cancer Inst. Mongr. 50:57-70, Dec. 1978.

Stembaeck, F.

Skin carcinogenesis as a model system: Observations on species, strain and tissue sensitivity to 7,12-dimethylbenz(a)anthracene with or without promotion from croton oil.

Acta Pharmacol. Toxicol. (Copenh.) 46(2):89-97, Feb. 1980.

Stenbeck, F. and Rowland, J.

Role of talc and benzo(a)pyrene in respiratory tumor formation: An experimental study.

Scand. J. Respir. Dis. 59(3):130-140, June 1978.

Stenhouse, N. S., et al.

Asymptomatic Hyperglycemia and Coronary Heart Disease. Busselton population study: Risk associated with asymptomatic hyperglycemia.

J. Chronic Dis. 32(11/12):693-698, 1979.

Stephan, E.

Kombination Schirmbild - Blutdruckmessung: Erfahrungen und Ergebnisse im Kanton Bern. (Ger.)

Schweiz. Med. Wochenschr. 109(7):234-243, Feb. 17, 1979.

Stepney, R.

The Indians revenge or drunk without drinking.

Practitioner 224(1339):109-111, Jan. 1980.

Sterling, T. D. and Weinkam, J. J.

Smoking patterns by occupation, industry, sex, and race.

Arch. Environ. Health 33(6):313-317, Nov.-Dec. 1978.

Stern, M. P.

The recent decline in ischemic heart disease mortality.

Ann. Intern. Med. 91(4):630-640, Oct. 1979.

Stevens, J. L. and Anders, M. W.

Metabolism of haloforms to carbon monoxide-III: Studies on the mechanism of the reaction.

Biochem. Pharmacol. 28(21):389-3194, Nov. 1, 1979.

Stevens, M. H.

Synergistic effect of alcohol on epidermoid carcinogenesis in the larynx.

Otolaryngol. Head Neck Surg. 87(6): 751-756, Nov.-Dec. 1979.

Stevens, R. G. and Moolgavkar, S. H.

Estimation of relative risk from vital data: Smoking and cancers of the lung and bladder.

JNCI 63(6):1351-1357, Dec. 1979.

Stevens, R. H., et al.

Cyclic nucleotide concentrations in 7,12-dimethylbenz[a]antracene-induced pancreatic cancer in rats.

JNCI 61(5):1281-1284, Nov. 1978.

Stevenson, D. K., et al.

Effect of erythrocyte destruction on the pulmonary excretion rate of carbon monoxide in adult male Wistar rats.

J. Lab. Clin. Med. 94(4):649-654, Oct. 1979.

Stewart, B. W.

Comparing carcinogens.

Cancer Forum 16:183-185, Mar. 1979.

Stewart, B. W. and Brian, M. J.

Evidence of carcinogen-induced replication of partially-repaired DNA in target cells during nitrosamine carcinogenesis.

Eur. J. Cancer 15(2):251-256, Feb. 1979.

Stier, A., et al.

The Induction of Drug Metabolism: The integrated system of drug metabolism and its perturbation on induction.

Symp. Med. Hoechst 14:225-241, 1979.

Stirling, G. A., et al.

Study of one thousand consecutive malignant neoplasms in Saudis 1975-1977.

Saudi Med. J. 1(2):89-94, Oct. 1979.

Stockley, R. A.

Alpha1-antitrypsin phenotypes in cor pulmonale due to chronic obstructive airways disease.

Q. J. Med. 48(191):419-428, July 1979.

Stohs, S. J., et al.

Benzo[a]pyrene metabolism by hepatic and extrahepatic tissues in streptozotocin-diabetic rats.

Drug Metab. Dispos. 7(1):49-51, Jan.-Feb. 1979.

Stonesifer, L. D., et al.

Thrombotic thrombocytopenic purpura in carbon monoxide poisoning. Report of a case.

Arch. Intern. Med. 140(1):104-105, Jan. 1980.

Stora, C.

Comparative study of the cellular localization of three polycyclic hydrocarbons differing in their carcinogenicity.

Oncology 37(1):23-26, 1980.

Storch, G., et al.

International Symposium on Legionnaires' Disease. Sporadic community-acquired Legionnaires' disease in the United States: A case-control study.

Ann. Intern. Med. 90(4):596-600, Apr. 1979.

Storstein L. and Jervell, J.

Response to bicycle exercise testing in long-standing juvenile diabetes.

Acta Med. Scand. 205(3):227-230, 1979.

Strahilevitz, M., et al.

Air pollutants and the admission rate of psychiatric patients.

Am. J. Psychiatry 136(2):205-207, Feb. 1979.

Stransky, M.

Motiviert Herzinfarkt zu Aenderung ungesunder Gewohnheiten? (Ger.)

Soz. Praeventivmed. 24(4):270, Aug. 1979.

Strasser, A.L.

Smoking in the workplace: Should it be prohibited?

Occup. Health Saf. 48(1):9-10, Jan.-Feb. 1979.

Streja, D. and Mymin, D.

Moderate exercise and high-density lipoprotein-cholesterol.

JAMA 242(20):2190-2192, Nov. 16, 1979.

Strick, R.

DNCB - Useful new compound.

West. J. Med. 130(2):162-163, Feb. 1979.

Strobel, H. W., et al.

The drug metabolism systems of liver and liver tumors: A comparison of activities and characteristics.

Mol. Cell. Biochem. 22(2-3):79-91, Dec. 22, 1978.

Strohl, K. P., et al.

Carbon monoxide poisoning in fire victims: A reappraisal of prognosis.

J. Trauma 20:(1):78-80, Jan. 1980.

Strong, J. P., et al.

The Thrombotic Process in Atherogenesis: The geographic pathology and topography of atherosclerosis and risk factors for atherosclerotic lesions.

Adv. Exp. Med. Biol. 104:11-31, 1978.

Struck, C.-J. and Glossmann, H.

Soluble bovine adrenal cortex guanylate cyclase: Effect of sodium nitroprusside, nitrosamines, and hydrophobic ligands on activity, substrate specificity and cation requirements.

Naunyn Schmiedebergs Arch. Pharmacol. 304(1):51-61, Aug. 24, 1978.

Stumpf, R., et al.

Formation and loss of alkylated purines from DNA of hamster liver after administration of dimethylnitrosamine.

Cancer Res. 39(1):50-54, Jan. 1979.

Stupfel, M., et al.

Workshop on Carbon Monoxide and Cardiovascular Disease: Animal models and acute and long-term carbon monoxide intoxication.

Prev. Med. 8(3):333-343, May 1979.

Sturm, A.

Kontraindikationen stationaerer Heilbehandlung bei koronarer Herzkrankheit und arterieller Hypertonie. (Ger.)

Dtsch. Med. Wochenschr. 103(45):1761-1765, Nov. 10, 1978.

Styka, P. E. and Penney, D. G.

Regression of carbon monoxide-induced cardiomegaly.

Am. J. Physiol. 235(5):H516-H522, Nov. 1978.

Subash Babu, D., et al.

Some epidemiological factors related to smoking among secondary school children of Delhi urban area.

Int. J. Epidemiol. 7(2):183-184, June 1978.

Sudan, B. J. L. and Sterboul, J.

Sensibilisation tabagique. Le tabac: Un allergene, la nicotine; un haptene. Diagnostic par le test de degranulation des basophiles. (Letter to the Editor.) (Fr.)

Nouv. Presse Med. 8(43):3563, Nov. 5, 1979.

Suh, S. K.

Treatment of angina pectoris (review). (Korean)

Korean J. Intern. Med. 20(12):1048-1059, Dec. 1977.

Summer, K.-H., et al.

1-Chloro-2,4-dintrobenzene depletes glutathione in rat skin an is mutagenic in Salmonella typhimurium.

Mutat. Res. 77(1):91-93, Jan. 1980.

Summerhayes, I. C. and Franks, L. M.

Effects of donor age on neoplastic transformation of adult mouse bladder epithelium in vitro.

JNCI 62(4):1017-1023, Apr. 1979.

Sutinen, S., et al.

Prevalence, severity, and types of pulmonary emphysema in a population of deaths in a Finnish city: Correlation with age, sex and smoking.

Scand. J. Respir. Dis. 59(2):101-115, Apr. 1978.

Sutorius, D. J., et al.

Vascular complications as a result of intra-aortic balloon pumping.

Am. Surg. 45(8):512-516, Aug. 1979.

Sutton, S. R., et al.

Adjustment of smokers to dilution of tobacco smoke by ventilated cigarette holders.

Clin. Pharmacol. Ther. 24(4):395-405, Oct. 1978.

Suzuki, E. and Okada, M.

Synthesis of N-nitrosamino aldehydes, metabolic intermediates possibly involved in the induction of tumors in rats by N-butyl-N-(omega-hydroxy-alkyl)nitrosamines.

Chem. Pharm. Bull. 27(2):541-544, Feb. 1979.

Suzuki, M.

Purification and properties of cyto-chrome P-450 from liver microsomes of rat treated with phenobarbital or 3,4-benzpyrene.

Kumamoto Med. J. 31(2):35-47, June 30, 1978.

Suzuki, S.

Annual Meeting Symposium on Smoking and Cardiopulmonary Function: Smoking and mechanical response of the respiratory system. (Jpn.)

Jpn. J. Thorac. Dis. 15(9):565-671, Sept. 1977.

Svaerdsudd, K., et al.

Hypertensive eye ground changes: Prevalence, relation to blood pressure and prognostic importance. The study of men born in 1913.

Acta Med. Scand. 204(3):159-167, 1978.

Swann, P. G.

Smoking or health - A report of the Royal College of Physicians: Review of the publication.

Med. Bull. Exxon Corp. Affil. Co. 38(1):40-65, Spring 1978.

Sylvester, J. T., et al.

Hypoxic and CO hypoxia in dogs: Hemodynamics, carotid reflexes, and catecholamines.

Am. J. Physiol. 236(1):H22-H28, Jan. 1979.

Szklo, M., et al.

Additional data favoring use of anti-coagulant therapy in myocardial infarction: A population-based study.

JAMA 242(12):1261-1264, Sept. 1979.

Szuets, T., et al.

Long-term fate of [14C]nicotine in the mouse: Retention in the bronchi, melanin-containing tissues and urinary bladder wall.

Toxicology 10(3):207-220, July 1978.

Szymanowicz, A., et al.

De la diffulte de selectionner un echantillon de reference. (Letter to the Editor.)

Ann. Biol. Clin. (Paris) 37(2):113-116, 1979.

Tabry, I. F., et al.

American Heart Association Monograph No. 59. Cardiovascular Surgery 1977: Effect of surgery on ventricular tachyarrhythmias associated with coronary arterial occlusive disease.

Circulation 58(3, Suppl. 1):I-166-I-170, Sept. 1978.

Tager, I. B., et al.

Effect of parental cigarette smoking on the pulmonary function of children.

Am. J. Epidemiol. 110(1): 15-26, July 1979.

Takahashi, G.

Macroautoradiographic study of the distribution of 14C-dimethylnitrosamine in mice and fetuses.

Bull. Chest Dis. Res. Inst. Kyoto Univ. 11(1-2):81-85, Mar. 1978.

Takahashi, G., et al.

Indentificaiton of benzo(a)pyrene metabolites by gas chromatograph-mass spectrometer.

Cancer Res. 39(5):1814-1818, May 1979.

Takishima, T.

Annual Meeting Symposium on Smoking and Cardiopulmonary Function: Smoking and cardiopulmonary function. (Abstr.) (Jpn.)

Jpn. J. Thorac. Dis. 15(9):551, Sept. 1977.

Takishima, T.

Lung function tests and its clinical application. (Jpn.)

J. Jpn. Soc. Intern. Med. 67(3): 1-15, Mar. 1978.

Takizawa, S. and Hirose, F.

Modification of renal tumorigenesis by gonadal ablation in rats treated with N-butylnitrosourea or dimethylnitrosamine.

Hiroshima J. Med. Sci. 27(4):27-34, Dec. 1978.

Tallarida, G., et al.

Cardiovascular and respiratory chemoreflexes from the hindlimb sensory receptors evoked by intra-arterial injection of bradykinin and other chemical agents in the rabbit.

J. Pharmacol. Exp. Ther. 208(2):319-329, Feb. 1979.

Tamura, M., et al.

Annual Meeting Symposium on Smoking and Cardiopulmonary Function: Effects of cigarette smoke on airway resistance. (Jpn.)

Jpn. J. Thorac. Dis. 15(9):558-564, Sept. 1977.

Taniguchi, T., et al.

Effect of acetylcholine on the norepinephrine-induced positive chronotropy and increase in cyclic nucleotides of isolated rabbit sinoatrial node.

Circ. Res. 45(4):493-504, Oct. 1979.

Taniyama, T. and Holden, H. T.

In vitro induction of T-lymphocyte mediated cytotoxicity by infectious murine type C oncornaviruses.

J. Exp. Med. 150(6):1367-1382, Dec. 1, 1979.

Tanner, A. R., et al.

Efficacy of cimetidine and tri-potassium di-citrato bismuthate (De-Nol) in chronic gastric ulceration: A comparative study.

Med. J. Aust. 1(1):1-2, Jan. 13, 1979.

Tarhan, S., et al.

Anesthetic considerations for aortocoronary bypass graft surgery.

Ann. Thorac. Surg. 27(4):376-389, Apr. 1979.

Tasman-Jones. C.

A background for the management of peptic ulcer disease.

N.Z. Med. J. 87(610):290-292, Apr. 26, 1978.

Tatematsu, M., et al.

Sequential quantitative studies on hyperplastic nodules in the liver of rats treated with carcinogenic chemicals.

Gann 70(1):125-130, Feb. 1979.

Tattersall, S. F., et al.

The use of tests of peripheral lung function for predicting future disability from airflow obstruction in middle-aged smokers.

Am. Rev. Respir. Dis. 118(6):1035-1050, Dec. 1978.

Tattersall, S. F., et al.

Lung distensibility and airway function in intermediate alpha1-antitrypsin deficiency (Pi MZ).

Thorax 34(5):637-646, Oct. 1979.

Tautu, P. and Wagner, G.

Betrachtungen zum Risikoproblem in der Krebsepidemiologie. (Ger.)

Lebensversicherungsmed 31(4):88-93, July 1979.

Tay, L. K., et al.

Binding of 6-hydroxymethylbenzo[a] pyrene and 6-ace-toxymethylbenzo[a] pyrene to DNA.

Chem. Biol. Interact. 25(1):35-44, Apr. 1979.

Taylor, J. K.

The status of chemical analysis in environmental research and control.

Lung 156(2):109-117, May 18, 1979.

Taylor, J. M.

Early botanists and the introduction of drug specifics.

Bull. NY Acad. Med. 55(7):684-699, July-Aug. 1979.

Taylor, T. V., et al.

Leucocyte ascorbate levels and post-operative deep venous thrombosis.

Br. J. Surg. 66(8):583-585, Aug. 1979.

Teel, R. W. and Douglas, W. H. J.

Aryl hydrocarbon hydroxylase activity in type II alveolar lung cells.

Experientia 36(1):107-109, Jan. 15, 1980.

Tepper, J. M., et al.

Relations between nicotine-induced convulsive behavior and blood and brain levels of nicotine as a function of sex and age in two inbred strains of mice.

Pharmacol. Biochem. Behav. 10(3):349-353, Mar. 1979.

Teramo, K.

Perinatal epidemiologi. (Swed.)

Fin. Lakaresallsk. Handl. 122(3):151-157, 1978.

Territo, M. C. and Golde, D. W.

The function of human alveolar macrophages.

J. Reticuloendothel. Soc. 25(1):111-120, Jan. 1979.

Terzaghi, M. and Nettesheim, P.

Dynamics of neoplastic development in carcinogen-exposed tracheal mucosa.

Cancer Res. 39(10):4003-4010, Oct. 1979.

Terzaghi, M., et al.

Repopulation of denuded tracheal grafts with normal, preneoplastic, and neoplastic epithelial cell populations.

Cancer Res. 38(12):4546-4553, Dec. 1978.

Thamavit, W., et al.

Effects of dimethylnitrosamine on induction of cholangiocarcinoma in Opisthorchis viverrini-infected Syrian golden hamsters.

Cancer Res. 38(12):4634-4639, Dec. 1978.

Thamavit, W., et al.

Effects of dimethylnitrosamine on induction of cholangiocarcinoma in opisthorchis viverrini-infected Syrian golden hamsters.

Cancer Res. 38(12):4634-4639, Dec. 1978.

Thanavaro, S., et al.

In-hospital prognosis of patients with first nontransmural and transmural infarctions.

Circulation 61(1):29-33, Jan. 1980.

Thomas, C. B., et al.

Health of physicians in midlife in relation to use of alcohol: A prospective study of a cohort of former medical students.

Johns Hopkins Med. J. 146(1): 1-10, Jan. 1980.

Thomas, H. F., et al.

Aryl-monoalkyl and cyclic triazenes: Direct-acting mutagens.

Mutat. Res. 60(1):25-32, Mar. 1979.

Thomas, P. C., et al.

Heart disease risk factors in Los Angeles County safety personnel.

JOM 21(10):683-687, Oct. 1979.

Thomison, J. B.

Appendix B: Council on Scientific Affairs Report C Smoking and Health.

J. Tenn. Med. Assoc. 72(11):815-818, Nov. 1979.

Thompson, D. R.

Sudden death and cardiac disease.

R. Soc. Health J. 99(2):84-85, Apr. 1979.

Thompson, H. J., et al.

Effect of the duration of retinyl acetate feeding on inhibition of 1-methyl-1-nitrosourea-induced mammary carcinogenesis in the rat.

Cancer Res. 39(10)3977-3980, Oct. 1979.

Thompson, P. D., et al.

Unexpected decrease in plasma high density lipoprotein cholesterol with weight loss.

Am. J. Clin. Nutr. 32(10):2016-2021, Oct. 1979.

Thoren, P.

Role of cardiac vagal C-fibers in cardiovascular control.

Rev. Physiol. Biochem. Pharmacol. 86:1-94, 1979.

Thorgeirsson, S. S. and Wirth, P. J.

NCTR/NCI Symposium on the use of Inbred and Outbred Animals in Toxocological Testing: Genetic aspects of metabolic processing of chemical substances.

J. Toxicol. Environ. Health 5(1):83-87, Jan. 1979.

Thust, R., et al.

No neoplastic alteration of metabolically competent rat liver cells in vitro by chemical carcinogens: 3-methylcholanthrene dimethylnitrosamine and Natulan.

Cancer Biochem. Biophys. 3(1):1-6, 1978.

Tibblin, E., et al.

Haemoglobin concentration and pheripheral blood cell counts in women: The population study of women in Goeteborg 1968-1969.

Scand. J. Haematol. 22(1):5-16, Jan. 1979.

Tien, Y-K., et al.

Variability of the configuration of maximum expiratory flow-volume curves.

J. Appl. Physiol. 46(3):565-570, Mar. 1979.

Tiendrebeogo, H., et al.

Le cytodiagnostic bronchique: Re sultats d'une serie preliminaire de 204 prelevements bronchiques. (Fr.)

Med. Afr. Noire. 26(5):405-411, May 1979.

Tierney, B., et al.

The formation of dihydrodiols by chemical or enzymic oxidation of 3-methylcholanthrene.

Chem. Biol. Interact. 23(1):121-135, Oct. 1978.

Tierney, B., et al.

Microsomal and nuclear metabolism of 3-methylcholanthrene.

Biochem. Pharmacol. 28(17):2607-2610, Sept. 1, 1979.

Tirmarche, M. and Flamant, R.

Epidemiologie du cancer bronchique a travers le monde. (Fr.)

Ther. Umsch. 35(12):979-982, Dec. 1978.

Tisdale, M. J.

The significance of cyclic AMP and cylic GMP in cancer treatment.

Cancer Treat. Rep. 6(1):1-15, Mar. 1979.

Tisi, G. M.

Preoperative evaluation of pulmonary function: Validity, indications, and benefits.

Am. Rev. Respir. Dis. 119(2):293-310, Feb. 1979.

Tobiasch, V.

Die Bedeutung der Ophthalmodynamographie fuer die Praxis. (Ger.)

Mater. Med. Nordmark 30(7-8):204-227, July-Aug. 1978.

Tola, S. and Vaaranen, V.

Ammattitaudit ja muut tyoeperaeiset sairaudet. (Finn.)

Duodecim 94(14-15):937-944, 1978.

Tola, S., et al.

Lung cancer mortality among iron foundry workers.

JOM 21(11):753-760, Nov. 1979.

Tomatis, L.

The predictive value of rodent carcinogenicity tests in the evaluation of human risks.

Annu. Rev. Pharmacol. Toxicol. 19:511-530, 1979.

Tomatis, L. and Shanmugaratnam, K.

Symposium No. 17: Interaction between genetic and environmental factors in human cancer.

UICC Bull. 16(4):29-31, Dec. 1978.

Tompa, A. and Langenbach, R.

Culture of adult rat lung cells: Benzo(a)pyrene metabolism and mutagenesis.

In Vitro 15(8):569-578, Aug. 1979.

Tonelli, Q. J., et al.

Transformation of cultured mouse mammary glands by aromatic amimes and amides and their derivatives.

Cancer Res. 39(5):1784-1792, May 1979.

Tongas, P. N.

Symposium on Behavior Therapy in Psychiatry: The control of smoking.

Psychiatr. Clin. North Am. 1(2):363-376, Aug. 1978.

Topping, D. C., et al.

Pathologic changes induced in respiratory tract mucosa by polycyclic hydrocarbons of differing carcinogenic activity.

Am. J. Pathol. 93(2):311-324, Nov. 1978.

Torjussen, W.

Rhinoscopical findings in nickel workers, with special emphasis on the influence of nickel exposure and smoking habits.

Acta Otolaryngol. (Stockh.) 88(3-4):279-288, Sept.-Oct. 1979.

Torres, I. J., et al.

Transport of model compounds across the peritoneal membrane in the rat.

Pharmacology 17(6):330-340, 1978.

Torrington, M. and Kotze, T. J. W.

A follow-up study of cardiac patients: A preliminary report.

S. Afr. Med. J. 55(25):1037-1042, June 16, 1979.

Toth, B.

1-Acetyl-2-phenylhydrazine carcinogenesis in mice.

Br. J. Cancer 39(5):584-587, May 1979.

Traul, K. A., et al.

A rapid in vitro assay for carcinogenicity of chemical substances in mammalian cells utilizing an attachment-independence endpoint.

Int. J. Cancer 23(2):193-196, Feb. 15, 1979.

Traver, G. A., et al.

Predictors of mortality in chronic obstructive pulmonary disease: A 15-year follow-up study.

Am. Rev. Respir. Dis. 119(6): 895-902, June 1979.

Tredger, J. M. and Chabra, R. S.

Factors affecting the properties of mixed-function oxidases in the liver and small intestine of neonatal rabbits.

Drug Metab. Dispos. 8(1):16-22, Jan./Feb. 1980.

Trembath, P. W. and Boobis, S. W.

Plasma theophylline levels after sustained-release aminophylline.

Clin. Pharmacol. Ther. 26(5):654-659, Nov. 1979.

Trenckmann, H.

Arteriosklerose: Grundlagen der Arteriosklerosetherapie. (Ger.)

Z. Gesamte Inn. Med. 33(17):625-628, Sept. 1, 1978.

Treves, R., et al.

Polyglobulie du fumeur. (Fr.)

Nouv. Presse Med. 7(46):4230, Dec. 23, 1978.

Trewyn, R. W., et al.

Cell transformation by exogenous methylated purines.

Adv. Enzyme Regul. 16:335-345, 1978.

Tripathi, R. K., et al.

Properties and affinity purification of the mixed-type putative acetylcholine receptor from wild and a mutant strain of house flies.

Biochim. Biophys. Acta 586(3):624-631, Sept. 3, 1979.

Tripier, M. F., et al.

Normal and benzo(a)pyrene-transformed fetal mouse brain cells. II. Ultrastructural study.

Acta Neuropathol. (Berl.) 47(3): 205-211, Aug. 1979.

Trzos, R. J., et al.

The evaluation of sixteen carcinogens in the rat using the micronucleus test.

Mutat. Res. 58(1):79-86, Sept. 1978.

Tsibris, J. C. M.

Carcinogen activation by human uterine enzymes.

Ann. Clin. Lab. Sci. 9(3):236-242, May-June 1979.

Tskahashi, G., et al.

Macroautoradiographic assays of 14C-labeled 4-nitroquinoline 1-oxide in adult and fetal mice.

Bull. Chest Dis. Res. Inst. Kyoto Univ. 11(1-2):85-90, Mar. 1978.

Tsuchida, S., et al.

Purification of gamma-glutamyltransferases from rat hepatomas and hyperplastic hepatic nodules, and comparison with the enzyme from rat kidney.

Cancer Res. 39(10):4200-4205, Oct. 1979.

Tsurutani, H., et al.

Annual Meeting Symposium on Smoking and Cardiopulmonary Function: Gas transport. (Jpn.)

Jpn. J. Thorac. Dis. 15(9):572-579, Sept. 1977.

Tsutsui, T., et al.

Morphological transformation, DNA damage, and chromosomal aberrations induced by a direct DNA perturbation of synchronized Syrian hamster embryo cells.

Cancer Res. 39(7, Part 1):2356-2365, July 1979.

Tucci, M., et al.

Rilevazione epidemiologica sulla bronchite cronica in un gruppo di lavoratori ospedalieri. (Ital.)

Rass. Int. Clin. Ter. 58(22):1562-1576, Nov. 30, 1978.

Tucker, A. N. and Tang, T.

Effects of phenobarbital and methylcholanthrene on hepatic mixed-function-oxidase activities in hamsters.

J. Environ. Pathol. Toxicol. 2(3):613-623, Jan.-Feb. 1979.

Tucker, A. N., et al.

Effects of N-nitrosodiethylamine on murine hepatic mixed-function-oxidase activities.

J. Environ. Pathol. Toxicol. 2(2):571-578, Nov.-Dec. 1978.

Tucker, G. T.

Drug metabolism.

Br. J. Anaesth. 51(7):603-618, July 1979.

Tucker, R. M., et al.

Saralasin infusion in renovascular hypertension: Increased response rate in seated patients.

Mayo Clin. Proc. 55(2):99-102, Feb. 1980.

Tuomilehto, J., et al.

Coronary risk factors and socioeconomic status in Eastern Finland.

Prev. Med. 7(4):539-549, Dec. 1978.

Tuomisto, J.

Toksikologian kriisi: Mikae myrkyllisyys on taerkeaeae, mikae ei. (Finn.)

Soum. Laeaekaeril. 33(16):1309-1313, June 1, 1978.

Turkington, R. W.

Diabetes mellitus: New diagnostic criteria.

Compr. Ther. 5(4):9-16, Apr. 1979.

Turner, D. M.

Workshop on Carbon Monoxide and Cardiovascular Disease: Carbon monoxide, tobacco smoking and the pathogenesis of atherosclerosis.

Prev. Med. 8(3):303-309, May 1979.

Turner, D. M., et al.

Atherogenesis in the White Carneau pigeon: Further studies of the role of carbon monoxide and dietary cholesterol.

Atherosclerosis 34(4):407-417, Dec. 1979.

Turpeinen, O.

Effect of cholesterol-lowering diet on mortality from coronary heart disease and other causes.

Circulation 59(1):1-7, Jan. 1979.

Turpin, J. C., et al.

Intoxication oxycarbonee chez le foetus: A propos d'une observation anatomo-clinique. (Fr.)

Rev. Neurol. (Paris) 134(8-9):485-495, Aug.-Sept. 1978.

Tuyns, A. J.

Proceedings of Alcohol and Cancer Workshop: Epidemiology of alcohol and cancer.

Cancer Res. 39(7, Part 2): 2840-2843, July 1979.

Tuyns, A. J.

Association tabac et alcool dans le cancer. (Fr.)

Bull. Schweiz. Akad. Med. Wiss. 35(1-3):151-158, Mar. 1979.

Tweeddale, M. G. and Fodor, J. G.

Symposium. A New Class of Diuretics with Uricosuric Activity: An examination of elevated serum uric acid values in cardiovascular diseases.

Postgrad. Med. Commun. (Spec. Rep.): 9-18, 1979.

Tyndall, R. L., et al.

Effects of carcinogenic and non-carcinogenic chemicals on plasma esterases in BALB/c mice.

Chem. Biol. Interact. 23(2):159-169, Nov. 1978.

Tyrer, H. W., et al.

Cell sorter analysis of carcinogen metabolites in human tissues.

J. Histochem. Cytochem. 27(1):508-511, Jan. 1979.

Uchida, E. and Hirono, I.,

Effect of phenobarbital on induction of liver and lung tumors by dimethylnitrosamine in newborn mice.

Gan 70(5):639-644, Oct. 1979.

Ueda, N.

Studies on immunogenicity of soluble tumor antigen obtained from transplantable tumor cells of guinea pigs. (Jpn.)

Jpn. J. Dermatol. 88(6):399-409, 1978.

Ulus, I. H. and Wurtman, R. J.

Selective response of rat peripheral sympathetic nervous system to various stimuli.

J. Physiol. (Lond.) 293:513-523, 1979.

Umezawa, K., et al.

In vitro transformation of hamster embryo cells by betel tobacco extracts.

Toxicol. Lett. 2(4):243-246, Oct. 1978.

Unnerus, H.-A.

Maternal Plasma Free Oestriol and 24 Hour Urinary Oestriol Excretion in the Assessment of Foetal Outcome.

Acta Endocrinol. (Copenh.) 91(Suppl. 226):1-80, June 1979.

Uotila, P.

The fate of intratracheally instilled 3H-styrene oxide in the isolated perfused rat lungs.

Res. Commun. Chem. Pathol. Pharmacol. 23(3):561-573, Mar. 1979.

Uotila, P. et al.

Quantitative and qualitative changes in the metabolism of benzo(a)pyrene in rat tissues after intragastric administration of TCDD.

Toxicol. Appl. Pharmacol. 46(3):671-683, Dec. 1978.

Urdiales Campos, J. and Sahagun Salcedo, E.

Rentabilidad de la broncofibroscopia en el diagnostico precoz del cancer broncopulmonar. (Span.)

Enferm. Torax 27(105):83-90, 1978.

Urwitz, S.

Foerbaettrad haelsa och oekad livslaengd. (Swed.)

Lakartidningen 76(9):708-709, Feb. 28, 1979.

Usui, H., et al.

Influence of indapamide on isolated rabbit arteries. (Jpn.)

Folia Pharmacol. Jpn. 74(3):389-396, Apr. 1978.

Utell, M. J., et al.

Development of airway reactivity to nitrates in subjects with influenza.

Am. Rev. Respir. Dis. 121(2):233-241, Feb. 1980.

Utidjian, M. D.

Panel Discussion: Role of high risk groups in standard derivation.

Environ. Health Perspect. 29:161-173, Apr. 1979.

Vachalkova, A., et al.

Electrochemical properties of polycyclic compounds studied by the polarographic method in anhydrous systems: VI. The influence of proton-donor on reduction of carcinogenic aromatic hydrocarbons in anhydrons environment.

Neoplasma 25(6):679-684, 1978.

Vaehaekangas, K., et al.

Proceedings of the International Symposium on Microsomes and Drug Oxidations: The disposition of benzo(a)pyrene in isolated perfused rat lung.

Biochem. Pharmacol. Suppl.:453-458, 1977.

Vaehaekangas, K., et al.

The metabolism of benzo(a)pyrene in isolated perfused lungs from variously-treated rats.

Arch. Pharmacol. Toxicol. (Kbh.) 41(2):129-140, Aug. 1977.

Vaehaekangas, K., et al.

The DNA binding of benzo[a]pyrene metabolites catalysed by rat lung microsomes in vitro and in isolated perfused rat lung.

Chem. Biol. Interact. 24(2):167-176, Feb. 1979.

Vaehaekangas, K. and Pelkonen, O.

The effects of harman and norharman on the metabolism of benzo(a)pyrene in isolated perfused rat lung and in rat lung microsomes.

Biochem. Pharmacol. 28(10):1591-1596, May 15, 1979.

Vaehaekangas, K., et al.

Effects of various in vitro-inhibitors of benzo(a)pyrene metabolism in isolated rat lung perfusion.

Acta Pharmacol. Toxicol. (Copenh.) 45(1):1-8, July 1979.

Vaillant, G. E.

Natural history of male psychologic health: Effects of mental health on physical health.

N. Engl. J. Med. 301(23):1249-1254, Dec. 6, 1979.

Vainio-Mattila, J.

Tupakoinnin vaikutus hengitysteiden oireisiin ja toiminataan. (Finn.)

Suom. Laeaekaeril. 34(1-2): 28-29, Jan. 10, 1979.

Vaino, H., et al.

Urinary thioether of employees of a chemical plant.

Br. J. Ind. Med. 35(3):232-234, Aug. 1978.

Valadaud-Barrieu, D. and Izard, C.

Action de la phase gazeuse de fumee de cigarette sur le taux d'echanges des chromatides-soeurs du lymphocyte humain in vitro. (Fr.)

C. R. Acad. Sci. [D] (Paris) 288(10): 899-901, Mar. 12, 1979.

Valdez, R. S., et al.

Evaluation of the echocardiogram as an epidemiologic tool in an asymptomatic population.

Circulation 60(4):921-929, Oct. 1979.

Valentin, H., et al.

Das Passivrauchen am Arbeitsplatz - eine Gesundheitsschaedigung? (Ger.)

Zentralbl. Bakteriol. [Orig. B] 167(5-6):405-434, Dec. 1978.

Valeriote, C., et al.

Ethanol, tobacco and laterality effects on simple and complex motor performance.

J. Stud. Alcohol 40(9):823-830, Sept. 1979.

Van Cantfort, J., et al.

A new assay for glutathione S-transferase using [3H]-benzo(a)pyrene 4,5-oxide as substrate. Inducibility by various chemicals in different rat tissues compared to that of aryl hydrocarbon hydroxylase and epoxide hydratase.

Biochem. Pharmacol. 28(4):455-460, 1979.

Van De Water, J. M., et al.

Limb salvage and selectivity.

Surg. Gynecol. Obstet. 148(3):349-354, Mar. 1979.

Van Dellen, R. G.

Series on pharmacology in practice. 4. Theophylline: Practical application of new knowledge.

Mayo Clin. Proc. 54(11):733-745, Nov. 1979.

Van Der Burgh, C.

Smoking behaviour of white, black, coloured and Indian South Africans: Some statistical data on a major public health hazard.

S. Afr. Med. J. 55(24):975-978, June 9, 1979.

van der Linde, F. and Abelin, Th.

Massnahmen gegen das Rauchen in der Schweiz und ihre Evaluation. (Ger.)

Bull. Schweiz. Akad. Med. Wiss. 35(1-3):123-130, Mar. 1979.

Van der Molen, H. R., et al.

Resultats a long terme du traitement des arteritiques par les injections intra-arterielles selon la technique de Reboul. (Fr.)

Phlebologie 32(1):57-65, Jan.-Mar. 1979.

Van Duuren, B. L., et al.

Effects of structural changes on the tumor-promoting activity of phorbol myristate acetate on mouse skin.

Cancer Res. 39(7, Part 1):2644-2646, July 1979.

van Gent, C. M., et al.

High-density lipoprotein cholesterol, monthly variation and association with cardiovascular risk factors in 1000 forty-year-old Dutch citizens.

Clin. Chim. Acta 88(1):155-162, Aug. 15, 1978.

Vandeputte-Van Messom, G.

Onderzoekingen over de neurotransmissieprocessen in de hypothalamus bij de vrijstelling van antidiuretisch hormoon bij de giet. (Dut.)

Verh. K. Acad. Geneeskd. Belg. 40(5): 372-434, 1978.

Vanegas Barrios, R., et al.

Revision del infarto del miocardio en el hospital Mexico. (Span.)

Acta Med. Costarric. 21(4):333-337, Oct. 1978.

Varnauskas, E., et al.

Coronary-artery bypass surgery in angina pectoris: Survival at two years.

Lancet 1(8122):889-893, Apr. 28, 1979.

Varpela, E.

Vesirokon jaelkeiset keuhkojen milliaariset kalkkitiivistymaet. (Finn.)

Duodecim 94(8):498-503, 1978.

Vaught, J. B., et al.

Comparison of benzo[a]pyrene metabolism by human peripheral blood lymphocytes and monocytes.

Cancer Lett. 5(5):261-268, Nov. 1978.

Vaught, J. B., et al.

Effects of smoking on benzo(a)pyrene metabolism by human placental microsomes.

Cancer Res. 39(8):3177-3183, Aug. 1979.

Vener, A. M., et al.

Drug usage and health characteristics in noninstitional retired persons.

J. Am. Geriatr. Soc. 27(2):83-90, Feb. 1979.

Verhaeghe, R. and Verstraete, M.

Medical treatment in intermittent claudication.

Acta Cardiol. (Brux.) 34(3):153-161, 1979.

Verma, A. K., et al.

Correlation of the inhibition by retinoids of tumor promoter-induced mouse epidermal ornithine decarboxylase activity and of skin tumor promotion.

Cancer Res. 39(2, Part 1):419-425, Feb. 1979.

Veron, G. and Bremond, J.

Habitudes toxicophiliques avant le service militaire. (Fr.)

Med. Armees 6(6):529-533, June-July 1978.

Vertio, H.

Varusmiesten tupakointitottumukset. (Finn.)

Ann. Med. Milit. Fenn. 54(1):10-20, 1979.

Vesell, E. S.

Proceedings of the International Symposium on Microsomes and Drug Oxidations: Effects of disease states on drug disposition in man.

Biochem. Pharmacol. Suppl.:628-645, 1977.

Vesell, E. S.

The antipyrine test in clinical pharmacology: Conceptions and misconceptions.

Clin. Pharmacol. Ther. 26(3):275-286, Sept. 1979.

Vesely D. L., et al.

Two components of laetrile (mandelonitrile and cyanide) stimulate guanylate cyclase activity.

Proc. Soc. Exp. Biol. Med. 161(3): 319-321, July 1979.

Vesely, D. L.

Biochemical evidence of cocarcinogenesis: Tumor promoting agent enhances methylnitrosourea activation of rat guanylate cyclase activity.

Res. Commun. Chem. Pathol. Pharmacol. 24(2):329-338, May 1979.

Vessey, M., et al.

Outcome of pregnancy in women using different methods of contraception.

Br. J. Obstet. Gynaecol. 86(7):548-556, July 1979.

Vestal, R. E.

Drug use in the elderly: A review of problems and special considerations.

Curr. Ther. 19(8):181-206, Aug. 1978.

Vestal, R. E., et al.

Effects of age and cigarette smoking on propranolol disposition.

Clin. Pharmacol. Ther. 26(1):8-15, July 1979.

Vezzoli, F., et al.

Small airways disease: A trial of an easy functional discrimination of preclinical emphysema.

Respiration 37(5):282-290, 1979.

Vig, B. K.

Somatic mosaicism in plants with special reference to somatic crossing over.

Environ. Health Perspect. 27:27-36, Dec. 1978.

Vincent, J. P., et al.

Interaction of phencyclidine ("angel dust") with a specific receptor in rat brain membranes.

Proc. Natl. Acad. Sci. USA 76(9): 4678-468, Sept. 1979.

Viviani, A. and Lutz, W. K.

Modulation of the binding of the carcinogen benzo(a)pyrene to rat liver DNA in vivo by selective induction of microsomal and nuclear aryl hydrocarbon hydroxylase activity.

Cancer Res. 38(12):4640-4644, Dec. 1978.

Viviani, A. and Lutz, W. K.

Modulation of the binding of the carcinogen benzo(a)pyrene to rat liver DNA in vivo by selective induction of microsomal and nuclear aryl hydrocarbon hydroxylase activity.

Cancer Res. 38(12):4640-4644, Dec. 1978.

Vizi, E. S.

Presynaptic modulation of neurochemical transmission.

Prog. Neurobiol. 12(3/4):181-190, 1979.

Vogt, T. M., et al.

Comparison of biochemical and questionnaire estimates of tobacco exposure.

Prev. Med. 8(1):23-33, Jan. 1979.

Vogt, T. M., et al.

Smoking cessation program: Baseline carbon monoxide and serum thiocyanate levels as predictors of outcome.

Am. J. Public Health 69(11):1156-1159, Nov. 1979.

Voll, M. J., et al.

Aquatic Pollutants and Biologic Effects with Emphasis on Neoplasia: Effects of microbial activity on aquatic pollutants.

Ann. NY Acad. Sci. 298:104-110, Sept. 29, 1977.

von der Hardt, H. and Wenner, J.

Schadstoffe in der Luft und Erkrankungen des Respirationstraktes im Kindesalter. (Ger.)

Dtsch. Med. Wochenschr. 103(37): 1419-1422, Sept. 15, 1978.

von Nieding, G. and Wagner, H. M.

Effects of NO2 on chronic bronchitics.

Environ. Health Perspect. 29:137-142, Apr. 1979.

Vore, M. and Soliven, E.

Organic solvent extraction of liver microsomal lipid: Effect on the kinetic parameters of benzo[a]pyrene hydroxylase and benzphetamine N-demethylase activity.

Biochem. Pharmacol. 28(24):3659-3665, Dec. 15, 1979.

Vourakis, C. and Bennett, G.

Angel dust: Not heaven sent.

Am. J. Nurs. 79(4):649-653, Apr. 1979.

Vraney, G. A. and Pokorny, C.

Pulmonary function in patients with gastroesphageal reflux.

Chest 76(6):678-680, Dec. 1979.

Vutuc, C., et al.

Tabakrauchen und Bronchuskarzinom: Relatives Risiko fuer Kreyberg I- und Kreyberg II-Tumoren. (Ger.)

Zentralbl. Bakteriol. [Orig. B] 167(5-6):443--446, Dec. 1978.

Vutuc, Ch. and Kunze, M.

Teer-Exposition bei tabakkonsumierenden weiblichen Bronchuskarzinompatienten und einer Vergleichspopulation. (Ger.)

Prax. Klin. Pneumol. 11(33):1121-1124, Nov. 1979.

Waddell, W. J. and Marlowe, C.

Inhibition by metyrapone of the accumulation of nicotine-14C in bronchial epithelium of mice.

Arch. Int. Pharmacodyn. Ther. 234(2):294-307, Aug. 1978.

Waern, U.

Health and disease at the age of sixty: Findings in a health survey of 60-year-old men in Uppsala and a comparison with men 10 years younger.

Ups. J. Med. Sci. 83(3):153-162, 1978.

Waern, U. and Aaberg, H.

Blood pressure in 60-year old men: Findings in a health survey and some comparisons with 50-year old men in the same community.

Acta Med. Scand. 206(1-2):99-105, 1979.

Wagner, I. U.

Nikotinvergiftung im kindesalter. (Ger.)

Paediatr. Paedol. 14(2):191-195, 1979.

Wagner, J. C. W., et al.

Carcinogenesis and mineral fibres.

Br. Med. Bull. 36(1):53-56, Jan. 1980.

Wagner, K-H. and Wagner-Hering, E.

Blei, Cadmium und polycyclische aromatische Kohlenwasserstoffe im carcinomatoesen Gewebe des Urogenitalsystems. (Ger.)

Naturwissenschaften 66(7):371-372, July 1979.

Waldron, I.

Type A behavior pattern and coronary heart disease in men and women.

Soc. Sci. Med. 12(3B):167-170, July 1978.

Walker, D., et al.

Inhalation toxicity studies on cigarette smoke (VI). 6-Week comparative experiments using modified flue-cured cigarettes: Histopathology of the lung.

Toxicology 10(3):229-240, July 1978.

Walker, D., et al.

Inhalation toxicity studies on cigarettes smoke (VII). 6-Week comparative experiments using modified flue-cured cigarettes: Histopathology of the conducting airways.

Toxicology 10(3):241-259, July 1978.

Walker, E. A., et al.

N-nitrosamines in the diet of experimental animals.

Cancer Lett. 6(3):175-178, Mar. 1979.

Walker, E. A., et al.

Intake of volatile nitrosamines from consumption of alcohols.

JNCI 63(4):947-951, Oct. 1979.

Walker, R. J. and James, V. A.

The action of putative transmitters and related compounds on neurones in the abdominal ganglia of the horse-shoe crab, Limulus polyphemus.

Neuropharmacology 17(9):765-769, Sept. 1978.

Walker, V. and Taylor, W. H.

Cigarette smoking, chronic peptic ulceration, and pepsin 1 secretion.

Gut 20(11):971-976, Nov. 1979.

Wallace, R. B., et al.

Altered plasma lipid and lipoprotein levels associated with oral contraceptives and oestrogen use.

Lancet 2(8134):112-114, July 21, 1979.

Wallace, R. B., et al.

Plasma lipids, lipoproteins, and blood pressure in female adolescents using oral contraceptives.

J. Pediatr. 95(6):1055-1059, Dec. 1979.

Walle, T., et al.

The predictable relationship between plasma levels and dose during chronic propranolol therapy.

Clin. Pharmacol. Ther. 24(6):668-677, Dec. 1978.

Walter, E., et al.

Jahrestagung der Deutschen Arbeitsgemeinschaft fuer Blutgerinnungsforschung: Diurnaler Rhythmus der Thrombocytenaggregation und Einfluss des Zigarettenrauchens. (Abstr.) (Ger.)

Blut 38(1):86, Jan. 1979.

Walter, S.

The immediate airway response to cigarette smoking.

Indian J. Med. Res. 70:819-824, Nov. 1979.

Walter, S., et al.

Changes in the forced expiratory spirogram in young male smokers.

Am. Rev. Respir. Dis. 119(5):717-724, May 1979.

Walters, C. L., et al.

Environmental Aspects of N-Nitroso Compounds. Gastric juice nitrite: Its source and relationship to hydrogen ion concentration.

IARC Sci. Publ. No. 19:279-288, 1978.

Wambach, G. et al.

Therapieresistentes Zungenbrennen als Fruehsymptom eines Kleinzelligen Bronchialkarzinoms. (Ger.)

Med. Welt. 30(26):993-995, June 29, 1979.

Wang, P., et al.

Purification of human liver cytochrome P-450 and comparison to the enzyme isolated from rat liver.

Arch. Biochem. Biophys. 199(1):206-219, Jan. 1980.

Ward, E., et al.

Aryl hydrocarbon hydroxylase in persons with lung or laryngeal cancer.

Int. J. Cancer 22(4):384-389, Oct. 15, 1978.

Ward, J. M., et al.

The mouse liver tumor as an endpoint in carcinogenesis tests.

Toxicol. Appl. Pharmacol. 51(3): 389-397, Dec. 1979.

Ward, S. D., et al.

Determinants of plasma cholesterol in children - A family study.

Am. J. Clin. Nutr. 33(1):63-70, Jan. 1980.

Warner, K. E., et al.

Toward less hazardous cigarettes. (Letter to the Editor and Reply.)

JAMA 241(20):2143-2144, May 18, 1979.

Warr, G. A.

Symposium de Lille: The biology of normal human bronchoalveolar cells. (Abstr.)

Bull. Eur. Physiopathol. Respir. 15(3):23P-24P, 1979.

Warren, J. R., et al.

Properties of hypolipidemic peroxisoma proliferators in the lymphocyte [3H] thymidine and Salmonella mutagenesis assays.

Cancer Res. 40(1):36-41, Jan. 1980.

Warshaw, R., et al.

Health Effects of Halogenated Aromatic Hydrocarbon: Decrease in vital capacity in PCB-exposed workers in a capacitor manufacturing facility.

Ann. NY Acad. Sci. 320:277-283, 1979.

Watanabe, H.

Clinicopathological and experimental study of pancreatic carcinoma. (Jpn.)

J. Showa Med. Assoc. 38(2):187-196, Apr. 1978.

Watanabe, M., et al.

Effect of trichloropropene oxide and benzoflavone on polycyclic hydrocarbon carcinogenesis in C3H/He and DBA/2 mice.

Gann 70(1):83-87, Feb. 1979.

Waters, R., et al.

Postreplication repair of DNA in human fibroblasts after UV irradiation or treatment with metabolites of benzo(a)pyrene.

Chem. Biol. Interact. 20(3):289-297, Mar. 1978.

Watson, C. S., et al.

Characterization and estrogen stimulation of cytoplasmic progesterone receptor in the ovarian-dependent MXT-3590 mammary tumor line.

Cancer Res. 39(10):4098-4104, Oct. 1979.

Watson, D. S.

Health education for hypertensive patients.

Aust. Fam. Physician 315-320, Mar. 1979.

Wattenberg, L. W., et al.

Neoplastic effects of oral administration of (plus/minus)-trans-7,8-dihydroxy-7,8-dihydrobenzo[a]pyrene and their inhibition by butylated hydroxyanisole.

JNCI 62(4):1103-1106, Apr. 1979.

Wattenberg, L. W., et al.

Inhibition of chemical carcinogen-induced neoplasia by coumarins and alpha-angelicalactone.

Cancer Res. 39(5):1651-1654, May 1979.

Wattenberg, L. W. and Sparnins, V. L.

Inhibitory effects of butylated hydroxyanisole on methylazoxymethanol acetate-induced neoplasia of the large intestine and on nicotinamide adenine dinucleotide-dependent alcohol dehydrogenase activity in mice.

JNCI 63(1):219-222, July 1979.

Wayss, K., et al.

Vascular liver tumors induced in Mastomys (Praomys) natalensis by single or twofold administration of dimethylnitrosamine.

JNCI 62(5):1199-1207, May 1979.

Weathersbee, P. S. and Lodge, R.

Alcohol, caffeine and nicotine as factors in pregnancy.

Postgrad. Med. 66(3):165-171, Sept. 1979.

Weaver, A., et al.

Mouthwash and oral cancer: Carcinogen or coincidence?

J. Oral Surg. 37(4):250-253, Apr. 1979.

Weaver, N. K. and Gibson, R. L.

The U.S. oil shale industry: A health perspective.

Am. Ind. Hyg. Assoc. J. 40(6): 460-467, June 1979.

Webb-Johnson, D. C.

Postoperative pulmonary complications.

Compr. Ther. 5(3):38-45, Mar. 1979.

Weber, A., et al.

Passivrauchen: Reizwirkungen des Gesamtrauches und der Gasphase. (Ger.)

Soz. Praeventivmed. 24(4):280-281, Aug. 1979.

Webster, P. M., et al.

Pulmonary function in identical twins: Comparison of nonsmokers and smokers.

Am. Rev. Respir. Dis. 119(2):223-228, Feb. 1979.

Webster, W. S.

Iron deficiency and its role in cadmium-induced fetal growth retardation.

J. Nutr. 109(9):1640-1645, Sept. 1979.

Wechsler, H. and McFadden, M.

Drinking among college students in New England: Extent, social correlates and consequences of alcohol use.

J. Stud. Alcohol 40(11):969-996, Nov. 1979.

Wechsler, H., et al.

Lifestyle, conditions of life, and health care in urban and suburban areas.

Public Health Rep. 94(5):477-482, Sept.-Oct. 1979.

Weeks , D. J.

Do chronic cigarette smokers forget people's names?

Br. Med. J. 2(6205):1627, Dec. 22-29, 1979.

Weeks, C. E., et al.

Inhibition of phorbol ester-induced tumor promotion in mice by vitamin A analog and anti-inflammatory steroid.

JNCI 63(2):401-406, Aug. 1979.

Wehner, A. P., et al.

Inhalation studies with Syrian golden hamsters.

Prog. Exp. Tumor Res. 24:177-198, 1979.

Wehner, F. C., et al.

Mutagenicity of marijuana and Transkei tobacco smoke condensates in the salmonella/microsome assay.

Mutat. Res. 77(2):135-142, Feb. 1980.

Wei, J.-W. and Sulakhe, P. V.

Properties of the muscarinic cholinergic receptors in rat atrium.

Naunyn Schmiedebergs Arch. Pharmacol. 309(3):259-269, Nov. 1979.

Weidmann, P. and Glueck, Z.

Grenzwert-Hypertonie. (Ger.)

Schweiz. Med. Wochenschr. 109(12):417-422, Mar. 24, 1979.

Weiler, E. W. and Zenk, M. H.

Autoradiographic immunoassay (ARIA): A rapid technique for the semiquantitative mass screening of haptens.

Anal. Biochem. 92(1):147-155, Jan. 1, 1979.

Weisburger, J. H.

Proceedings of a Conference on the Relationship between Environmental Chemicals and Cancer. Environmental cancer: On the causes of the main human cancers.

Tex. Rep. Biol. Med. 37:1-18, 1978.

Weiss, W.

Lung cancer due to chemicals.

Compr. Ther. 5(2):18-23, Feb. 1979.

Weiss, W., et al.

Lung cancer in chloromethyl ether workers.

Am. Rev. Respir. Dis. 120(5):1031-1037, Nov. 1979.

Weitzman, R. E. and Kleeman C. R.

The clinical physiology of water metabolism: Part II. Renal mechanisms for urinary concentration: Diabetes insipidus.

West. J. Med. 131(6):486-515, Dec. 1979.

Welch, R. M.

Pharmaceutical Manufacturers Association Foundation Inc. Workshop on Cellular and Molecular Toxicology: Toxicological implications of drug metabolism.

Pharmacol. Rev. 30(4):457-467, Dec. 1978.

Welsch, F.

Release of human chorionic somatomammotrophin from isolated perfused lobules and superfused fragments of term placenta: Spontaneous liberation and the effects of cholinergic drugs, dibutyrylcyclic adenosine monophosphate and calcium.

Res. Commun. Chem. Pathol. Pharmacol. 24(2):211-222, May 1979.

Wenger, N. K. and Felner, J. M.

Management of the patient with myocardial infarction.

DM 25(7):1-68, Apr. 1979.

The use of laxatives such as diocytyl succinate (colace) in cardiac patients is discussed.

Wennmalm, A.

Effects of nicotine on cardiac prostaglandin and platelet thromboxane synthesis.

Br. J. Pharmacol. 64(4):559-563, Dec. 1978.

Wennmalm, A.

Cigarette smoking, prostaglandins and reactive hypermia.

Prostaglandins Med. 3(6):321-326, Dec. 1979.

Werkoe, L.

Blodtryckskomplikationer och roekning. (Swed.)

Lakartidningen 76(14):1254, Apr. 4, 1979.

Werkoe, L.

Prevention of heart attacks: A multifactorial preventive trial in Gothenburg, Sweden.

Ann. Clin. Res. 11(2):71-79, Apr. 1979.

Werringloer, J. and Estabrook, R. W.

The Induction of Drug Metabolism: The characterization of product adducts of liver microsomal cytochrome P-450 and their use as probes for the heterogeneity of cytochrome P-450 as modified by the induction of drug metabolism.

Symp. Med. Hoechst 14:269-307, 1979.

Werringloer, J., et al.

The interaction of divalent copper and the microsomal electron transport system: A re-examination of the effects of copper chelates on the function of cytochrome P-450.

J. Biol.Chem. 254(23):11839-11846, Dec. 10, 1979.

Wessler, S.

The Thrombotic Process in Atherogenesis: Atherothrombology.

Adv. Exp. Med. Biol. 104:409-417, 1978.

Westerling, R.

Hur farliga aer cigaretterna? (Swed.)

Sven. Farm. Tidskr. 83(5):177-178, Apr. 9, 1979.

Westwood, F. R.

Appendix VI: The tetrazolium-reduction test.

Br. J. Cancer 37(6):949-953, June 1978.

Westwood, F. R., et al.

Cellular progression of neoplasia in the subcutis of mice after implantation of 3,4-benzpyrene.

Br. J. Cancer 39(6):761-772, June 1979.

Wexler, H. and Rosenberg, S. A.

Pulmonary metastases from autochthonous 3-methylcholanthrene-induced murine tumours.

JNCI 63(6):1393-1395, Dec. 1979.

Whitaker, C. J., et al.

Oral and pharyngeal cancer in the North-west and West Yorkshire regions of England, and occupation.

Br. J. Ind. Med. 36(4):292-298, Nov. 1979.

White, D. C.

Recent hospital fires in Scotland - An analysis.

Hosp. Health Serv. Rev. 75(1):20-23, Jan. 1979.

White, R., et al.

Effects of cigarette smoke on elastase secretion by murine macrophages.

J. Lab. Clin. Med. 94(3):489-499, Sept. 1979.

Whitlock, Jr., J. P.

The conformation of the chromatin core particle is ionic strength-dependent.

J. Biol. Chem. 254(13):5684-5689, July 10, 1979.

Whitlock, Jr., J. P. and Gelboin, H. V.

Aryl hydrocarbon (benzo(a)pyrene) hydroxylase induction in cells in culture.

Pharmacol. Ther. 4(3):587-599, 1979.

Whitmire, C. E. and Lopez, A.

Comparison of the effects of beeswax: Trioctanoin and trioctanion vehicles on 3-methylcholanthrene, benzo[a]pyrene, and 7,12-dimethylbenz[a]anthracene subcutaneous carcinogenesis in three strains of mice and one hybrid.

JNCI 61(4):1107-1111, Oct. 1978.

Whitmire, C. E.

Effects of subcutaneous administration of 3-methylcholanthrene and 7,12-dimethylbenz[a]anthracene on spontaneous reticulum cell neoplasms in SJL/J mice.

JNCI 62(3):561-564, Mar. 1979.

Whitmire, C. E.

Effects of subcutaneous administration of chemical carcinogens on leukemia in C58 mice.

JNCI 62(3):555-559, Mar. 1979.

Whittemore, A. S.

Quantitive theories of oncogenesis.

Adv. Cancer Res. 27:55-88, 1978.

Whong, W.-Z. and Ong, T.-M.

Mediated mutagenesis of dimethylnitrosamine in Neurospora crassa by various metabolic activation systems.

Cancer Res. 39(5):1525-1528, May 1979.

Wibaut, F. P. and Voskuul, P.

De pil... tot hoelang? (Dut.)

Ned. Tijdschr. Geneeskd. 122(49):1926-1932, Dec. 9, 1978.

Widow, W., et al.

Roentgenographic chest screening in the detection and survival of patients with lung cancer.

Ann. Thorac. Surg. 26(5):406-412, Nov. 1978.

Wiebkin, P., et al.

Effect of various metabolic inhibitors on biphenyl metabolism in isolated rat hepatocytes.

Biochem. Pharmacol. 28(22):3315-3321, Nov. 15, 1979.

Wiener, F., et al.

Chromosome changes (trisomy 15) in murine T-cell leukemia induced by 7,12-dimethylbenz(a)anthracene (DMBA).

Int. J Cancer 22(4):447-453, Oct. 15, 1978.

Wiklund, O. and Gustafson, A.

Lecithin: Cholesterol acyl transger (LACT) and fatty acid composition of lecithin and cholesterol esters in young male myocardial infarction survivors.

Atherosclerosis 33(1):1-8, May 1979.

Wilcox, R. G., et al.

Verification of smoking history in patients after infarction using urinary nicotine and cotinine measurements.

Br. Med. J. 2(6197):1026-1028, Oct. 27, 1979.

Wiley, J. A. and Camacho, T. C.

Life-style and future health: Evidence from the alameda county study.

Prev. Med. 9(1):1-21, Jan. 1980.

Wilhelmsen, L.

Proceedings of the Meeting of the International Society of Hypertension: Salt and hypertension.

Clin. Sci. 57(Suppl. 5):455s-458s, Dec. 1979.

Wilkinson, S. P., et al.

Changes in plasma renin activity in cirrhosis: A reappraisal based on studies in 67 patients and "low-renin" cirrhosis.

Hypertension 1(2):125-129, Mar.-Apr. 1979.

Williams, C. L., et al.

Validation of students' self-reported cigarette smoking status with plasma cotinine levels.

Am. J. Public Health 69(12):1272-1274, Dec. 1979.

Williams, D. G.

Different cigarette-smoker classification factors and subjective state in acute abstinence.

Psychopharmacology (Berlin) 64(2):231-235, Aug. 8, 1979.

Williams, G. M. and Laspia, M. F.

The detection of various nitrosamines in the hepatocyte primary culture/DNA repair test.

Cancer Lett. 6(4-5):199-206, Apr. 1979.

Williams, R.

De sanitate urbanorum.

Br. Med. J. 2(6205):1617-1622, Dec. 22-29, 1979.

Willis, K. A., et al.

MacAndrew scale scores of smoking and nonsmoking alcoholics.

J. Stud. Alcohol 40(9):906-907, Sept. 1979.

Wilson, J. R., et al.

Vectorcardiographic detection of early hemodynamic abnormalities in chronic obstructive pulmonary disease.

Chest 76(2):160-165, Aug. 1979.

Wilson, J. T., et al.

Drug excretion in human breast milk: Principles, pharmacokinetics and projected consequences.

Clin. Pharmacokinet. 5(1):1-66, Jan.-Feb. 1980.

Wilson, P. D., et al.

Alkaline phosphatase as a marker of transformation in adult mouse bladder epithelium after in vitro exposure to 7,12-dimethylbenz(a)anthracene.

Cell Biol. Int. Rep. 2(4):365-374, July 1978.

Windsor, R. A., et al.

Health promotion and maintenance for patients with chronic obstructive pulmonary disease: A review.

J. Chronic Dis. 33(1):5-12, 1980.

Winne, D.

Influence of blood flow on intestinal absorption of drugs and nutrients.

Pharmacol. Ther. 6(2):333-393, 1979.

Winston, J. M. and Roberts, R. J.

Influence of increasing age on lethality induced by carbon monoxide or hypoxic hypoxia.

Biol. Neonate 34(3-4):199-202, 1978.

Wipf, R. and Stinghe, R.

Enquete sur la prevalence de l'obstruction des petites voies aeriennes dans une populaton d'age scolaire. (Fr.)

Rev. Fr. Mal. Respir. 6(5):483-492, Sept.-Oct. 1978.

Wirth, C. R.

Metastatic Bone Cancer.

Curr. Probl. Cancer 3(11):1-36, May 1979.

Wislocki, P. G., et al.

Tumorigenicity of benzo[a]pyrene 4,5-, 7,8-, 9,10- and 11,12-oxides in newborn mice.

Cancer Lett. 5(4):191-197, Oct. 1978.

Wislocki, P. G., et al.

Tumorigenicity of the diastereomeric benz(a)anthracene 3, 4-diol-1,2-epoxides and the (plus)-and (-)-enantiometers of benz(a)anthracene 3,4-dihydrodiol in newborn mice.

JNCI 63(1):201-204, July 1979.

Witte, J. J.

The hazards of cigarette smoking during pregnancy.

J. Maine Med. Assoc. 69(11):314-316; 320, Nov. 1978.

Wixom, R. L., et al.

Excretion of creatine and creatinine in feces of man.

Proc. Soc. Exp. Biol. Med. 161(4):452-457, Sept. 1979.

Woehler, W., et al.

Inborn Errors of Metabolism in Man. Part II: Connective Tissue and Purine Metabolism, and Endocrinology. Benzpyrene metabolism in human diploid fibroblasts.

Monogr. Hum. Genet. 10:165-170, 1978.

Wojtyniak, B. and Gorynski, P.

Czestosc wystepowania i dynamika nadwagi w grupie doroslych mieszkancow Krakowa. Czesc II. Nadwaga wg wyksztalcenia, srodowiska pochodzenia i nalogu palenia. (Pol.)

Przegl. Lek. 35(8):683-688, 1978.

Wolf, P. A., et al.

Neurological Epidemiology: Principles and Clinical Applications. Prospective investigations: The Framingham Study and the epidemiology of stroke.

Adv. Neurol. 19:107-120, 1978.

Wolf, C. R., et al.

The rabbit pulmonary monooxygenase system: Characteristics and activities of two forms of pulmonary cytochrome P-450.

Chem. Biol. Interact. 21(1):29-43, Apr. 1978.

Wolf, C. R., et al.

The rabbit pulmonary monooxygenase system: Catalytic differences between two purified forms of cytochrome P-450 in the metabolism of benzo(a)pyrene.

J. Biol. Chem. 254(9):3658-3663, May 10, 1979.

Wolf, G. T., et al.

Papers of the Society of Head and Neck Surgeons. Serum glycoproteins in head and neck squamous carcinoma: Correlations with tumor extent, clinical tumor stage, and T-cell levels during chemotherapy.

Am. J. Surg. 138(4):489-500, Oct. 1979.

Wong, L. K., et al.

Oxidative metabolites of 7,12-dimethylbenz(a)anthracene: Further investigation of the K-region epoxide.

Drug Metab. Dispos. 8(1):28-33, Jan./Feb. 1980.

Wood, A. J. J., et al.

Effect of aging and cigarette smoking on antipyrine and indocyanine green elimination.

Clin. Pharmacol. Ther. 26(1):16-20, July 1979.

Wood, A. W., et al.

Metabolic activation of 3-methylcholanthrene and is metabolities to products mutagenic to bacterial and mammalian cells.

Cancer Res. 38(10):3398-3404, Oct. 1978.

Wood, A. W., et al.

Biological activity of benzo[e]-pyrene. An assessment based on mutagenic activities and metabolic profiles of the polycyclic hydrocarbon and its derivatives.

J. Biol. Chem. 254(11):4408-4415. June 10, 1979.

Wood, A. W., et al.

Mutagenicity and tumorigenicity of phenanthrene and chrysene epoxides and diol epoxides.

Cancer Res. 39(10):4069-4077, Oct. 1979.

Wood, C.

The association of psycho-social factors and gynaecological symptoms.

Aust. Fam. Physician 7(4):471-478, Apr. 1978.

Wood, C., et al.

Subjective recording of fetal movement.

Br. J. Obstet. Gynaecol. 86(11): 836-842, Nov. 1979.

Wood, J. D. and Mayer, C. J.

Serotonergic activation of tonic-type enteric neurons in guinea pig small bowel.

J. Neurophysiol. 42(2):582-593, Mar. 1979.

Woodhill, J. M., et al.

Drugs, Lipid Metabolism, and Atherosclerosis: Low fat, low cholesterol diet in secondary prevention of coronary heart disease.

Adv. Exp. Med. Biol. 109:317-330, 1978.

Woodward, J. G. and Daynes, R. A.

Cell-mediated immune response to syngeneic UV induced tumors: I. The presence of tumor associated macrophages and their possible role in the in vitro generation of cytotoxic lymphocytes.

Cell. Immunol. 41(2):304-319, Dec. 1978.

Woolcock, A. J.

Proceedings of the Aspen Lung Conference: Conference summary.

Chest 77(2 Suppl.):326-330, Feb. 1980.

Woolcock, A., et al.

Proceedings of the Aspen Lung Conference: The influence of bronchitis and asthma in infancy and childhood on lung function in schoolchildren.

Chest 77(2 Suppl.):251, Feb. 1980.

Worden, J. K., et al.

Respiratory disease in Vermont: A population survey for planning a public education program.

Prev. Med. 9(1):120-134, Jan. 1980.

Wright, D. J. and Pandya, A.

Smoking and gastric juice volume in outpatients.

Can. Anaesth. Soc. J. 26(4):328-329, July 1979.

Wright, M.

Panel discussion: Role of the knowledge of high risk groups in occupational health policies and practices.

Environ. Health Perspect. 29:143-153, Apr. 1979.

Wylie, C. M. and Bear, M. R.

Should we discourage cigarette smoking in elderly patients?

Geriatrics 33(9):95-104, Sept. 1978.

Wylie, C. M. and Slee, V. N.

Community healthy surveillance through hospital discharges.

Univ. Mich. Med. Cent. J.44(2):60-64, Apr.-June 1978.

Wynder, E. L.

Proceedings of the American Cancer Society and National Cancer Institute National Conference on Nutrition in Cancer: Dietary habits and cancer epidemiology.

Cancer 43(5, Suppl.):1955-1961, May 1979.

Wynder, E. L.

Workshop on Carbon Monoxide and Cardiovascular Disease: Introduction.

Prev. Med. 8(3):261-263, May 1979.

Wynder, E. L. and Stellman, S. D.

Impact of long-term filter cigarete usage on lung and larynx cancer risk: A case-control study.

JNCI 62(3):471-477, Mar. 1979.

Wynder, E. L. and Hoffmann, D.

Tobacco and health: A societal challenge.

N. Engl. J. Med. 300(16):894-903, Apr. 19, 1979.

Wynder, E. L. and Hoffmann, D.

Smoking and health: Pathogenic and preventive considerations.

Bull. Schweiz. Akad. Med. Wiss. 35(1-3):83-98, Mar. 1979.

Wyndham, C. and Safe, S.

A comparison of the in vitro metabolism of biphenyl and 4-chlorobiphenyl by rat liver microsomes.

Can. J. Biochem. 56(10):993-997, Oct. 1978.

Wyndham, C. H.

The role of physical activity in the prevention of ischaemic heart disease: A review.

S. Afr. Med. J. 56(1):7-13, July 7,1979.

Yaffe, S. J.

Drugs and pregnancy.

Clin. Toxicol. 13(4):523-533, 1978.

Yagasaki, O., et al.

Effect of loperamide on acetylcholine and prostaglandin release from isolated guinea pig ileum.

Jpn. J. Pharmacol. 28(6):873-882, Dec. 1978.

Yalow, R. S., et al.

Plasma and tumor ACTH in carcinoma of the lung.

Cancer 44(5):1739-1792, Nov. 1979.

Yamada, H.

Experimental and clinical study on closing volume: Part 2. Clinical study on closing vulume. (Jpn.)

Bull. Chest Dis. Res. Inst. Kyoto Univ. 11(1-2):15-28, Mar. 1978.

Yamada, S., et al.

An alteration in sensitivity to cholinergic agents on guinea-pig ilea and atria after repeated administration of an organophosphate and an antagonism by a carbamate.

Arch. Int. Pharmacodyn. Ther. 241(1): 32-44, Sept. 1979.

Yamaguchi, K., et al.

Ultramicro analysis of benzo[a]pyrene in food.

Chem. Pharm. Bull. (Tokyo) 26(11):3600-3602, Nov. 1978.

Yamamura, M., et al.

Inhibition of 7,12-dimethylbenz[a]-anthracene-induced mammary tumorigenesis in rats by a synthetic protease inhibitor, N,N-dimethylamino-[p-(p'-guanidinobenzoyloxy)]benzilcarbonyl-oxyglycolate.

Gann 69(6):749-752, Dec. 1978.

Yamasaki, H., et al.

Benzo(a)pyrene 7,8-dihydrodiol-9,10-oxide modification of DNA: Relation to chromatin structure and reconstitution.

Chem. Biol. Interact. 23(2):201-213, Nov. 1978.

Yamaura, I., et al.

Effects of benzo(a)pyrene adducts on DNA synthesis in vitro.

Chem. Biol. Interact. 23(3):399-407, Dec. 1978.

Yamagita, T.

The International Challenge of Drug Abuse: Drug dependence studies in laboratory animals.

Natl. Inst. Drug Abuse Res. Monogr. Ser. 19:179-190, 1978.

Yanai, R. and Nagasawa, H.

Prolactin binding in pregnancy-dependent mammary tumors in GR/A mice.

Endocrinol. Jpn. 25(5):511-514, Oct. 1978.

Yamaura, S., et al.

Pharmacological studies on the cough-like reflex induced by chemical stimulation. (Jpn.)

Folia Pharmacol. Jpn. 74(3):345-352, Apr. 1978.

Yang, C. S., et al.

Analysis of the aryl hydrocarbon hydroxylase assay.

Biochem. Pharmacol. 27(19):2321-2326, 1978.

Yang, J. A., et al.

Inhibition of DNA synthesis in cultured lymphocytes and tumor cells by extracts of betel nut, tobacco, and miang leaf, plant substances associated with cancer of the ororespiratory epithelium.

Cancer Res. 39(12):4802-4809, Dec. 1979.

Yang, S. K., et al.

Proceedings of the International Symposium on Microsomes and Drug Oxidations. Mechanism of microsomal activation of benzo[a] pyrene to diol-epoxides: The separation and characterization of intermediates and products.

Biochem. Pharmacol. Suppl.:403-410, 1977.

Yang, S. K., et al.

Enzymatic formation of an 8,9-diol from 8-methylbenz [a]anthracene.

Biochem. Biophys. Res. Commun. 90(4): 1136-1141, Oct. 29, 1979.

Yanysheva, N. Ya., et al.

The Blastomogenic effect of benzo(a) pyrene in its multiple entry into respiratory organs. (Russ.)

Gig. Sanit. No. 7:8-11, July 1978.

Yarnell, J. W. G. and St. Leger, A. S.

Respiratory illness, maternal smoking habit and lung function in children.

Br. J. Dis. Chest 73(3):230-236, July 1979.

Yeager, Jr., H., et al.

Aspen Lung Conference: Immunology of the Lung. Alveolar macrophage-lymphocyte interaction: Alterations in smokers and in sarcoidosis.

Chest 75(2, Suppl.):289, Feb. 1979.

Yernault, J.-C., et al.

Sex and age differences in intrathoracic airways mechanics in normal man.

J. Appl. Physiol. 46(3):556-564, Mar. 1979.

Yokota, T., et al.

Propionibacterium acnes-mediated humoral immune responses to tumor-specific antigens on rat liver cells transformed in vitro by chemical carcinogens.

JNCI 61(6):1525-1529, Dec. 1978.

Yokoyama, K.

Effect of perfluorochemical (PFC) emulsion on acute carbon monoxide poisoning in rats.

Jpn. J. Surg. 8(4):342-352, Dec. 1978.

Yoshida, D. and Matsumoto, T.

Changes in mutagenicity of protein pyrolyzates by reaction with nitrite.

Mutat. Res. 58(1):35-40, Sept. 1978.

Yoshida, H.

Studies of partial hepatectomy on canine cirrhotic liver induced by diethylnitrosamine. (Jpn.)

J. Nara Med. Assoc. 29(6):723-739, Dec. 31, 1978.

Yoshida, K., et al.

Nicotine induced release of noradrenaline from hypothalamic synaptosomes.

Brain Res. 182(2):361-368, Jan. 27, 1980.

Yoshimori, M., et al.

Malignant tumor of the pancreas. (Jpn.)

Jpn. J. Gastroenterol. 75(7):1080-1089, July 1978.

Yoshinaga, K., et al.

Effects of nicotine on early pregnancy in the rat.

Biol. Reprod. 20(2):294-303, Mar. 1979.

Yotti, L. P., et al.

Comparative study of X-ray and UV induced cytotoxicity, DNA repair, and mutagenesis in Down's syndrome and normal fibroblasts.

Pediatr. Res. 14(2):88-92, Feb. 1980.

Young, G. P., et al.

Treatment of duodenal ulcer with carboxolone sodium: A double-masked endoscopic trial.

Med. J. Aust. 1(1):2-5, Jan. 13, 1979.

Younoszai, M. K.

Effect of maternal smoking on hemoglobin and hematocrit of the newborn. (Letter to the Editor.)

Am. J. Clin. Nutr. 32(10):1983, Oct. 1979.

Yu, G. S. M., et al.

Renal oncocytoma: Report of five cases and review of literature.

Cancer 45(5):1010-1018, Mar. 1, 1980.

Yuhas, J. M., et al.

Multicellular tumor spheroid formation by breast cancer cells isolated from different sites.

Cancer Res. 38(9):2486-2491, Aug. 1978.

Zajdela, F. and Latarjet, R.

Inhibition of skin carcinogenesis in vivo by caffeine and other agents.

Natl. Cancer Inst. Mongr. 50:133-140, Dec. 1978.

Zalokar, J. B.

Pulmonary dysfunction, smoking, and coronary heart-disease. (Letter to the Editor.)

Lancet 1(8130):1348-1349, June 23, 1979.

Zamel, N., et al.

Decrease in lung recoil pressure after cessation of smoking.

Am. Rev. Respir. Dis. 119(2):205-211, Feb. 1979.

Zbar, B., et al.

Eradication by immunization with mycobacterial vaccines and tumor cells of microscopic metastases remaining after surgery.

Cancer Res. 39(5):1597-1603, May 1979.

Zdichynec, B.

Biodoza a histaminova patergometrie u chronickych kuraku. (Czech)

Fysiatr. Reumatol. Vestn. 56(4):198-201, Aug. 1978.

Zdichynec, B.

Neurovegetativni reaktiva, zmeny biodozy a histaminove patergometrie u dlouhodobych kurakue cigaret. (Czech)

Cesk. Dermatol. 53(4):262-266, Aug. 1978.

Zdichynec, B.

Risk factors and survival prognosis in men younger than 40 years and men older than 60 years with myocardial infarction: (Retrospective clinico-epidemiological study).

Cor Vasa 20(4):271-276, 1978.

Zdzienicka, M., et al.

Mutagenic activity of furfural in Salmonella typhimurium TA100.

Mutat. Res. 58(2-3):205-209, Nov. 1978.

Zehle, A. and Kovarik, U.

Spaetergebnisse nach aortogemoralem Gefaessersatz. (Ger.)

Med. Klin. 73(35):1192-1201, Sept. 1, 1978.

Zehm, S. J.

Symposium on Malignant Disease of the Oral Cavity and Related Structures: Dental diseases and oral malignant disease.

Otolaryngol Clin. North Am. 12(1): 21-27, Feb. 1979.

Zenser, T. V., et al.

Cooxygenation by prostaglandin cyclo-oxygenase from rabbit inner medulla.

Kidney Int. 16(6):688-694, Dec. 1979.

Zenz, C.

Workshop on Carbon Monoxide and Cardiovascular Disease: The epidemiology of carbon monoxide in cardiovascular disease in industrial environments: A review.

Prev. Med. 8(3):279-288, May 1979.

Zielhuis, R. L. and Van der Kreek, F. W.

Calculation of a safety factor in setting health based permissible levels for occupational exposure.

Int. Arch. Occup. Environ. Health 42(3-4):203-215, Jan. 15, 1979.

Zisman, F., et al.

Symposium of the International Research Group on Colour Vision Deficiencies. Colour Vision Deficiencies IV: Spectral sensitivities of acquired color defects analyzed in terms of color opponent theory.

Mod. Probl. Ophthalmol. 19:254-257, 1978.

Zitting, A., et al.

Radiographic and physiological findings in patients with asbestosis.

Scand. J. Work Environ. Health 4(4): 275-283, Dec. 1978.

Zittoun, R., et al.

Hyperleucocytose due au tabagisme. (Fr.)

Nouv. Presse Med. 7(39):3554, Nov. 11, 1978.

Zubrod, C. G.

Selective toxicity of anticancer drugs: Presidential address.

Cancer Res. 38(12):4377-4384, Dec. 1978.

zur Hausen, H., et al.

Tumor initiators and promoters in the induction of Epstein-Barr virus.

Proc. Natl. Acad. Sci. USA 76(2):782-785, Feb. 1979.

Zuskin, E., et al.

Airway responsiveness in workers processing polyester resins.

JOM 21(12):825-827, Dec. 1979.

Zuspan, F. P. and Davis, N.

The effect of smoking and oral contraceptives on the urinary excretion of epinephrine and norepinephrine.

Am. J. Obstet. Gynecol. 135(8):1012-1015, Dec. 15, 1979.

Zwang, G. and Dermange, H.

Troubles d'origine iatrogenique ou toxique de la physiologie sexuelle. (Fr.)

Concours Med. 100(47-48):7857-7870, Dec. 23-30, 1978.

Zwicker, G. M., et al.

Clinical and pathological effects of cigarette smoke exposure in beagle dogs.

Arch. Pathol. Lab. Med. 102(12):623-628, Dec. 1978.

Zytkovicz, T. H., et al.

Competitive binding and metabolism of several carcinogenic polycyclic aromatic hydrocarbons by AKR mouse embryo cells in culture.

Cancer Res. 38(8):2307-2313, Aug. 1978.